HEALTH UNIT COORDINATOR:

21st Century Professional

Donna J. Kuhns, CHUC

Health Unit Coordinator Instructor
Aurora Health Care
Milwaukee, Wisconsin

Patricia Noonan Rice, BA, CHUC

Association Management and Staff Development Provider
Rockford, Illinois

Linda L. Winslow, BS, CHUC

Staff Development Coordinator
Marquette General Health System
Marquette, Michigan

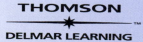

THOMSON ™

DELMAR LEARNING

Australia Canada Mexico Singapore Spain United Kingdom United States

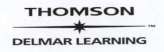

THOMSON

DELMAR LEARNING

Health Unit Coordinator: 21st Century Professional
By Donna J. Kuhns, Patricia Noonan Rice, and Linda L. Winslow

Vice President, Health Care Business Unit:
William Brottmiller

Editorial Director:
Cathy L. Esperti

Acquisitions Editor:
Marah Bellegarde

Developmental Editor:
Debra Flis

Editorial Assistant:
Jadin Babin-Kavanaugh

Marketing Director:
Jennifer McAvey

Marketing Channel Manager
Tamara Caruso

Marketing Coordinator:
Michele Gleason

Production Editor:
Anne Sherman

Technology Project Manager:
Victoria Moore

Library of Congress Cataloging-in-Publication Number
Kuhns, Donna J.
  Health unit coordinator: 21st century professional / Donna J. Kuhns, Patricia Noonan Rice, Linda L. Winslow.
    p. ; cm.
  Includes bibliographical references and index.
  ISBN 1-4018-2705-5 (alk. paper)
  1. Hospital ward clerks—Outlines, syllabi, etc. [DNLM: 1. Hospital Units—organization & administration. 2. Personnel, Hospital. WX 159 K957h 2005] I. Rice, Patricia (Patricia Noonan) II. Winslow, Linda L. III. Title.
  RA972.55.K845 2005
  362.11'068—dc22
                            2004024694

Notice to the Reader

Publisher does not warrant or guarantee any of the products described herein or perform any independent analysis in connection with any of the product information contained herein. Publisher does not assume, and expressly disclaims, any obligation to obtain and include information other than that provided to it by the manufacturer.

The reader is expressly warned to consider and adopt all safety precautions that might be indicated by the activities described herein and to avoid all potential hazards. By following the instructions contained herein, the reader willingly assumes all risks in connection with such instructions.

The publisher makes no representations or warranties of any kind, including but not limited to, the warranties of fitness for particular purpose or merchantability, nor are any such representations implied with respect to the material set forth herein, and the publisher takes no responsibility with respect to such material. The publisher shall not be liable for any special, consequential, or exemplary damages resulting, in whole or part, from the reader's use of, or reliance upon, this material.

CONTENTS

SECTION 2: *Coordination of the Unit/ Department*   63

PREFACE

A shortage of health care workers is the identified need for the upcoming decade. The need is great and will continue as the baby boomer generation retire and increase their use of the health care system. The health unit coordinator position was originally developed out of necessity during the nursing shortage of World War II. Administrative and nonclinical tasks were delegated from the nurse to the health unit coordinator. The U.S. Department of Labor Bureau of Labor Statistics states, "RN positions will grow faster than average for all occupations through 2010. Thousands of job openings will also result from the need to replace experienced nurses who leave the occupation as the median age of the RN populations continues to rise." The nursing shortage is expected to continue; therefore, the need for the health unit coordinator position will continue to exist. The inexperienced RN relies even more heavily on the health unit coordinator to perform the delegated tasks. The rapid changes in the health care field provide an avenue for the health unit coordinator to fill an important niche in the health care profession.

Because the Department of Labor classifies the health unit coordinator position with general office clerks, the exact number of employed health unit coordinators is unknown. Looking at the number of hospital beds gives some indication of how many health unit coordinators may be employed in inpatient settings. The American Hospital Association states there are 983,628 registered staffed hospital beds across the United States. It is not uncommon for hospitals to employ health unit coordinators at a ratio of 1 health unit coordinator to 20 beds or patients for two to three shifts. This calculation puts the number of health unit coordinators at approximately 100,000 within the hospital setting. A recent Health Care Advisory Board analysis of the number of inpatient beds needed to care for our aging population indicates that we will face a shortage of beds in the future. The analysis indicates that we will need an additional 176,000 beds by 2005. These additional beds will increase the number of health unit coordinators needed in the workforce.

We believe that health unit coordinating will be a profession that is attractive to the new wave of health care workers. We believe that health unit coordinating should be introduced in the high school and community college curriculums as a health care profession. Students graduating with skills in health unit coordinating will be prepared to work in a variety of health care settings.

APPROACH

Health Unit Coordinator: 21st Century Professional was written as a core textbook for a community college academic course or an in-house health care facility-based training program. It is also appropriate for an adult education or high school course. The book is organized so that each chapter can be studied as a stand-alone topic or used with a combination of chapters. This design addresses the flexibility issues faced by health unit coordinator educators and learners. The book is also ideal as a reference for the practicing health unit coordinator, and as a study guide for the national certification exam.

The book conforms to the Health Unit Coordinator national certification exam content outline that is based on the national job analysis performed by the Certification Board's testing agency. The authors bring in-depth knowledge of the health unit coordinator profession through their experience as practitioners, supervisors, and educators. Throughout the book, the professional association standards and information are used to support health unit coordinating as a health care profession.

The importance of the team approach in the working environment is emphasized throughout the book. A special feature called "Through the Eyes of a Health Care Professional" reinforces the team approach to providing health care through real-world presentations.

ORGANIZATION

The book is organized into eight sections. Section 1 discusses the health unit coordinator's responsibilities as a health care team member. Chapter 1 explains that from the beginning of the profession health unit coordinators were an asset to the nurse and physician staff in dealing with the many nonclinical tasks associated with patient care. Section 1 emphasizes the professionalism of health unit coordinators and the important role they have as a member of the health care team in the various health care facilities.

Section 2 focuses on essential knowledge the health unit coordinator needs in order to work together with all departments within a health care facility. The many personnel on the nursing unit and at the workstation and the health unit coordinator's responsibilites are presented, such as ordering patient and office supplies. Chapter 10 is devoted to a safe and healthy environment for both the nursing staff and the patients, and includes JCAHO and CDC references.

Section 3 discusses the management of health care information. Chapter 11 addresses confidentiality, including government rules and regulations for ways to keep all patient information confidential, including the computerized patient care record and includes HIPPA references. Chapter 12 focuses on patient rights and responsibilities and how those rights and responsibilities are communicated to the patient. Chapter 13 discusses patient record chart forms a health unit coordinator will work with on a daily basis and how to maintain a complete and current record. Chapter 14 discusses the patient record, beginning with the admission process and proceeding all the way through the health care stay until discharge.

Section 4 focuses on communication skills that the health unit coordinator will use every day. Communication with physicians, nurses, and all health care facility staff, as well as communication with patients and the public are addressed. Chapter 17 discusses orientation and training personnel as a responsiblitiy of today's health unit coordinators and addresses the training process from the perspective of the trainee and trainee. The many new communication devices seen in the health care setting today are also included in this section.

Critical thinking is the focus of Section 5. Key areas addressed are problem identification, priorization, decision making, and multitasking. Chapter 19 is devoted to diversity because cultural and generational diversity are so prominent in our society today. Ethics in the health care setting is also addressed.

Section 6, prior to order transcription, is an introduction to medical terminology. It can be covered in a short orientation setting and can be a stepping stone for programs that require a full medical terminology course. Common prefixes, suffixes, and word roots are included as well as short pictorial views of the body's structure and its components. Chapter 22 presents abbreviations and is designated as a separate chapter for instructors who teach this content as a separate segment in the curriculum.

Section 7 may be considered the most important part of the text. It is located toward the back of the book because without the knowledge of what the orders are or knowledge of the departments that carry out the orders, the transcription task would be quite difficult. This section goes through the transcription process from reading the initial order to notifiying departments of the orders. An in-depth look at the process for diagnostic, therapeutic, and support departments is included. Separate chapters on medication order transcription as well as pre- and post-operative order transcription are included.

Section 8, on professional development, rounds out the book with detailed information about career opportunities, résumes, interviews, and follow-up. Certification and recertification as well as career ladders are addressed because of the importance for health unit coordinators to stay current with the many changes and health care advances made in this fast-changing environment.

ADDITIONAL TOOLS

INSTRUCTOR'S MANUAL TO ACCOMPANY *HEALTH UNIT COORDINATOR: 21ST CENTURY PROFESSIONAL*

The *Instructor's Manual* includes several features to assist you in instructing health unit coordinators, including lesson plans, teaching tips and strategies, quizzes, and answers to the review questions in the book. ISBN 1-4018-2706-3

COMPUTERIZED TESTBANK TO ACCOMPANY *HEALTH UNIT COORDINATOR: 21ST CENTURY PROFESSIONAL*

The Computerized Testbank includes over 700 questions with answers organized according to the 32 chapters in the textbook. Rationales for correct answers reinforce learning. This CD-ROM testbank assists you in creating personalized unit tests. Features include:

◆ An interview mode or "wizard" to guide you through the steps to create a test in less than five minutes

◆ The capability to edit questions or to add an unlimited number of questions

◆ Online (Internet-based) testing capability

◆ Online (computer-based) testing capability

◆ A sophisticated word processor

◆ Numerous test layout and printing options

ISBN 1-4018-2708-X

TRANSCRIPTION PRACTICE CD-ROM

The transcription practice CD-ROM includes order sets for 25 conditions that allow learners clinical practice transcribing doctor's orders. Order sets may be printed, transcribed, and then checked for accuracy against the answer keys included on the CD-ROM. See "How to Use the Health Unit Coordinator Transcription Practice CD-ROM" on pages xv and xvi for details.

ACKNOWLEDGMENTS

The completion of this book would not have been possible without the support of our families, our colleagues, and our editor, Debra Flis. A special thank you to Robert Kuhns, who shared his many years of experience with us by being our first-line editor, supporter, and mentor.

We also acknowledge the support and assistance from our fellow colleagues, health unit coordinators, and health care staff who provided encouragement and expert advice throughout this project.

To all of you who answered a technical question, made a suggestion, provided a sounding board, recommended a resource, searched for a form or photograph, or shared access to your facility, we thank you. Your contribution was significant and helped shape the final project.

Specifically, we thank Wendy Csik for her hospitality and energetic assistance during the photo shoot at All Saints Health Care.

We also thank health unit coordinators in general who have provided us with motivation and support throughout this project. Their dedication to quality patient care and their belief in their profession were the catalysts behind the project.

REVIEWERS

The authors and Thomson Delmar Learning acknowledge the instructors who reviewed the manuscript and provided valuable feedback.

Sandy Ayres, BBA, CHUC
Health Unit Coordinator Specialist
Eau Claire, Wisconsin

Debra L. Ebert, RN, MSN, MEd
Waukesha County Technical College
Pewaukee, Wisconsin

Diane K. Fox, RN
Health Unit Coordinator Instructor
Brewster Technical Center
Tampa, Florida

Lori Katz, CHUC, MEd
Health Unit Coordinator Instructor
Hennepin Technical College
Brooklyn Park, Minnesota

Cecil Pope, AA, CHUC
Nursing Informatics Coordinator
Scott & White Memorial Hospital
Temple, Texas

Shirley Walker Powell, BA, CHUC
Education Specialist II, Corporate Education
TriHealth
Cincinnati, Ohio

ABOUT THE AUTHORS

The authors have over 60 years experience teaching and training health unit coordinators in a variety of health care settings.

Donna J. Kuhns, CHUC, has been employed by Aurora Health Care in Milwaukee, Wisconsin for over 27 years, where she has worked as a health unit coordinator and health unit coordinator instructor. Currently, she is the Health Unit Coordinator Instructor for the metro region. She is called upon by surrounding regions for health unit coordinator orientation advice and is sought out by other departments for health unit coordinator expertise. Donna has served as both a Regional Representative and an Education Board Director of NAHUC.

Patricia Noonan Rice, BA, CHUC, of Rockford, Illinois, has worked as both a health unit coordinator and a health unit coordinator instructor. Her teaching experience includes hospital-based and community college health unit coordinator programs, staff development programs, and workshops and seminars. Currently, she owns a business that provides association management and education support. She is a past Education Board Director of NAHUC.

Linda Winslow, BS, CHUC, has been employed at Marquette General Health System, Marquette, Michigan, for over 34 years. She has worked as a nurse aide, health unit coordinator, and health unit coordinator educator. Currently, she is the Staff Development Coordinator in Education Services responsible for coordinating health unit coordinator education. Additional responsibilities include coordinating conferences, consumer library services, and computer education. Linda serves as the Education Board Director of the National Association of Health Unit Coordinators (NAHUC).

How to Use the Health Unit Coordinator Transcription Practice CD-ROM

SYSTEM REQUIREMENTS

Operating System: Microsoft Windows 98 SE, Windows 2000 or Windows XP
Processor: Pentium PC 500 MHz or higher
RAM: 64 MB of RAM (128 MB recommended)
Adobe Acrobat Reader

INSTALLATION INSTRUCTIONS

1. Insert CD into your computer's CD drive. Health Unit Coordinator Transcription Practice should start automatically. If it does not, go to step 2.

2. From My Computer, double-click the icon for your CD drive.

3. Double-click the *HUC.exe* file to start the program.

GETTING STARTED

A key skill of the Health Unit Coordinator's role is transcribing doctors' orders. The Transcription Practice CD-ROM lets you practice this skill with order sets for twenty-five conditions. For your convenience, order sets may be printed, transcribed in a separate notebook, and then checked for accuracy against the answer keys included on the CD-ROM.

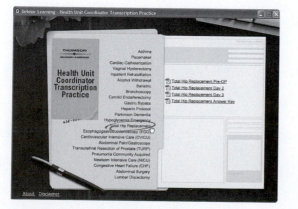

MAIN SCREEN

The main screen lists conditions covered on the cd-rom. Click on a condition to view a list of all the related order sets.

ORDER SET

From the list of order sets available for each condition, click on the first order set. **Read the handwritten set of orders. On a blank sheet of paper, write the translation of the order, which department carries out the order, and what forms if any would be needed to complete the set of orders.** When you have completed transcribing the first order set, return to the opening screen and work through the remaining order sets.

ANSWER KEY

When you have finished transcribing all order sets related to a condition, click on the answer key. Check your answers against the answer keys provided for each order set.

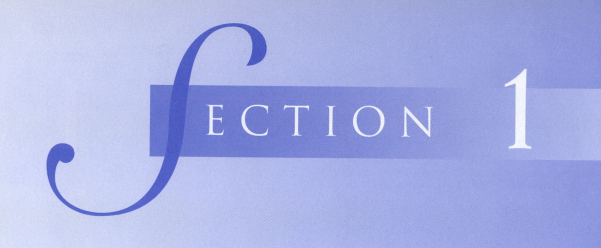

SECTION 1

Health Unit Coordinating

History of Medicine and Health Unit Coordination

Learning Objectives

Upon completion of this chapter and review questions, the learner should be able to:

1. Identify major events in the history of medicine that helped shape health care today.

2. Define the term *coordination*.

3. Differentiate between Social Security and Medicare.

4. Explain why the Education Board of the National Association of Health Unit Coordinators was formed.

5. List five groups of people with whom health unit coordinators communicate during a workday.

6. List at least four other titles used instead of health unit coordinator.

7. Name the first physician to practice sports medicine.

Key Terms

coordination The arrangement or harmonious functioning of parts for the most effective results.

floor clerk An early title for health unit coordinator.

floor secretary An early title for health unit coordinator.

Medicaid A U.S. program administered by each individual state to provide medical assistance for people with low incomes and resources.

Medicare A U.S. federal health insurance program designed to provide all older adults with medical coverage at an affordable cost.

National Association of Health Unit Coordinators (NAHUC) The only professional association for health unit coordinators.

paper requisition A paper form used for ordering tests from hospital departments.

Social Security A U.S. government program that provides financial support for people faced with disabilities, illness, old age, or unemployment.

station clerks An early title for health unit coordinator.

station coordinator An early title for health unit coordinator.

unit clerk An early title for health unit coordinator.

unit communicator Another title for health unit coordinator.

unit coordinator Another title for health unit coordinator.

unit secretary An early title for health unit coordinator.

ward clerk An early title for health unit coordinator.

ward secretary An early title for health unit coordinator.

Abbreviations

DRG Diagnosis Related Groups

HUC Health Unit Coordinator

ICD International Classification of Disease

NAHUC National Association of Health Unit Coordinators

PERSONAL HEALTH

To be active and happy and to enjoy life is the desire of every person. It is difficult to enjoy life if you are not healthy. A simple example is the common cold. Think about the party that you plan on attending Friday night. You talk about the party with your friends all week, the excitement is building, and finally Friday is here. You wake up early, because you're very cold—no wait, you feel quite warm. You have a temperature of 100°F. Your arm and leg muscles ache, your nose is running, and your stomach is upset. You find yourself spending the day and night in bed. So much for the party.

That cold hampered your plans for just one night. Imagine the limitations on people so ill that they need to spend days or weeks in a hospital. When you are ill, especially ill enough to require hospitalization, you count on the best care, including the latest technology and best professionals. In this chapter, you will review some of the historical discoveries that made medicine what it is today and how you, as the professional health unit coordinator, assist in providing the best possible care during a hospital or long-term facility stay.

PHYSICIANS

The practice of medicine goes back as far as 3000 B.C., when an Egyptian, Sekhet'eanach, is recorded as having "healed the king's nostrils." Imhotep and other Egyptian doctors recommended plants and herbs, as well as surgery and magic charms for healing treatments. Some of the early medical treatments have been proven to have healing properties; for example, honey has antibacterial properties and was used to heal wounds. Other "medicine" was believed to have religious, magical, or mystical characters. One common form of medical treatment or cure, which dates back more than 5,000 years and is still practiced, is acupuncture. Although this type of treatment is practiced for patients with arthritis, migraine headaches, ulcers, and asthma, scientists still do not understand how it works.

Hippocrates (460 B.C.–399 B.C.) became known as the Father of Medicine. He was regarded as the greatest physician of his time. He rejected the views that illnesses were caused by superstitions, evil spirits, or disfavor from the gods. He was the first physician to believe that feelings, thoughts, and ideas come from the brain and not the heart. He was also the first physician to correctly describe the symptoms of pneumonia. He believed in the natural process of healing and in good health practices, which included rest, a good diet, fresh air, and cleanliness. Hippocrates's medical practice and teachings were based on facts from observations and the study of the human body. He believed that the body must be treated as a whole and not as just a series of parts. Hippocrates practiced medicine throughout Greece and Asia Minor. He founded a school on the island of Cos, Greece, and began teaching his ideas.

In A.D. 144–145, Aelius Nicon, a Roman architect and builder, stated that, in a dream, a god told him to allow his son Galen to study medicine. So he did. Galen studied and practiced medicine for years. During his studies, Galen proved to the world that the vessels called arteries contain blood, not air, as had been the earlier belief. Years later, Galen was appointed the physician assigned to gladiators. During this time, Galen gained valuable and practical experience in trauma and sports medicine, and also continued his studies in theoretical medicine and philosophy.

FLORENCE NIGHTINGALE AND NURSES

In the early 1800s, nursing was a charitable act, not an act of work, which a cultured lady of that day entered. In 1846, Florence Nightingale began to read and teach herself about hospitals and sanitation. She continued her studies in nursing and became known as an expert, traveling from her native England through Europe. In 1853, Nightingale decided to serve God by serving the "sick poor." In 1854, during the Crimean War, Florence Nightingale was asked by the Secretary of War to nurse British soldiers. Nightingale saw this as an opportunity to show the value of female nursing in military hospitals and assembled 38 nurses to go to the Barrick Hospital in Turkey. Because of this work, Nightingale was viewed as a heroine by the troops and the public back home. In 1860, she published a small booklet titled *Notes on Nursing*, which became very popular. Millions of copies of this book were sold all over the world. In 1860, the Nightingale Training School for Nurses opened at St. Thomas Infirmary, Southwark, London. The school was a success, and Nightingale is credited for having invented modern nursing as we know it today. Physicians and nurses in the past, as well as now, provided health care with the patient's dignity and well-being as the main objectives. The image of physicians and nurses throughout history has been one of healing, caring, and respect.

People relate to the roles of physicians and nurses because of their long history and current practice of clinical, or hands-on, patient care. The health unit coordinator has little if any actual patient contact or clinical patient care. This may be one reason most people are unfamiliar with health unit coordinators. Another reason people are unfamiliar with a health unit coordinator is that the title, as well as the role, has changed through the years. In the past, and even today in some health care facilities, health unit coordinators are known as unit secretaries.

This chapter will explain how medical advances and other technology advances have changed the role of health unit coordinators and why health unit coordinators are considerably more than a secretary for physicians and nurses. The roles and responsibilities of physicians and nurses in any health care setting today are fast paced and ever changing. The health unit coordinator provides consequential assistance by coordinating and carrying out needed tasks for physicians and nurses.

MEDICAL ADVANCES

Discoveries and inventions throughout the ages have led to the modern practice of medicine. Some of the most significant ones are discussed here.

ANCIENT DISCOVERIES

Medical discoveries date far back into the past and helped shape medicine as we know it today. There are far too many discoveries to cover in this chapter, so we list only some of the more influential and interesting ones in Table 1-1. Many of these discoveries played a role in changing medicine from an art or a philosophy into a science.

TABLE 1-1 Ancient Medicine	
CHINA *(These concepts are still practiced today.)*	The Yin and Yang theory, that two forces flow through everything in nature, including the human body Acupuncture to treat or cure arthritis, migraine headaches, ulcers, and asthma
EGYPT	Mummy-wrapping, which preserved bodies for a long period of time, so the Egyptians learned much about the body, and turned Egyptians into experts in bandaging wounds
ISRAEL	A system of health laws to prevent the spread of germs and disease, such as banning pork because pork was thought to contain tapeworms and trichina worms and separating ill people from healthy people, thereby preventing epidemics
INDIA	Some of the first surgical procedures, including a cesarean section and plastic surgery First observation that bubonic plague occurred when rats were nearby and that mosquitoes spread malaria
GREECE	Some of the first hospitals, aqueducts to bring fresh drinking water to Rome, and an extensive sewage system to remove waste from the streets of Rome

MIDDLE AGES A.D. 400–A.D. 1400

The Middle Ages of Europe, often known as the Dark Ages, lasted from the middle of the fifth century to the period known as the Renaissance, or the middle of the fifteenth century. As you read through the following list, you will see why this long period is referred to as the Dark Ages.

The Romans' aqueducts and sewage systems were forgotten.

Cities were overcrowded.

Garbage was tossed into the streets, and dirty water accumulated in pools throughout the streets.

Bubonic plagued killed approximately 100 million people.

Medical care was mainly available only to the wealthy.

Doctors were discouraged from dissecting the human body or cadavers.

Not all was gloomy about the Middle Ages. Some key advances were made as well in Europe and Asia (see Table 1-2).

TABLE 1-2 Middle Ages Major Advancements	
ITALY	First European medical school, requiring its students to pass certain courses and meet certain standards before they could become doctors
ASIA	Muslims translated ancient Greek medical texts, preserving much of the earlier medical knowledge

RENAISSANCE

As society moved out of the Middle Ages and into the Renaissance, discoveries other than medical technology began to affect the medical world. The printing press is a prime example. In 1440, the first printing press was constructed. The printing press enabled people to share medical findings in a much shorter period of time than in the past. In 1590, the microscope was invented, and the discovery of bacteria followed shortly thereafter.

LATE EIGHTEENTH TO THE TWENTIETH CENTURY

The discovery that germs and bacteria caused diseases was a major breakthrough in the late 1700s and early 1800s. Edward Jenner developed a vaccine for smallpox, which had reached epidemic proportions. Diseases such as anthrax, leprosy, tuberculosis, tetanus, and pneumonia were all identified in the 1800s. Scientists realized that, once they had isolated the germs and bacteria that caused these diseases, they could vaccinate against them. Louis Pasteur created vaccinations against anthrax and rabies during this period.

Medical Instruments

Medical instruments created in the nineteenth century made diagnosing a patient quicker and more accurate. The stethoscope, invented in 1816, let the physician listen to sounds inside the body, such as the heart and lungs. The fever thermometer, developed in 1850, helped the physician measure a patient's temperature. The ophthalmoscope was also designed in 1850 to help the physician look at the structure of the eye. In 1895, X-rays were invented to see through the human body.

In the twentieth century, the discoveries of the past were enhanced and expanded at a rapid pace. Major advances in treatment for the mentally ill were made. Thirteen vitamins and their benefits were discovered. Many types of radiology techniques, such as computerized tomography and magnetic resonance imaging, were developed. Radiation therapy and open-heart surgeries are all possible because of medical discoveries of the twentieth century and the past.

Medical Specialties

There are so many advances being made so quickly in medicine that many physicians select a specific type of medicine to practice. Table 1-3 describes some types of physicians.

TABLE 1-3	Types of Physicians
ALLERGISTS	Specialize in allergies
ANESTHESIOLOGISTS	Administer anesthesia during surgery or other major procedures
CARDIOLOGISTS	Specialize in the study and treatment of the heart
EPIDEMIOLOGISTS	Deal with the causes, distribution, and control of diseases
GERONTOLOGISTS	Specialize in aging and diseases associated with aging
INTERNISTS	Experts on treating problems of the internal organs
ONCOLOGISTS	Specialize in cancer
PODIATRISTS	Treat foot diseases
RADIOLOGISTS	Specialize in performing and reading x-rays and other radioactive exams

HISTORY OF HOSPITALS

Hospitals go back as far back as the Roman Empire. The word *hospital* comes from the Latin word *hospitalis*, meaning house of guests. The purpose of very early hospitals was to care for orphans, the aged, the blind, and the sick. These were followed by hospitals that provided first aid to injured soldiers. Finally, hospitals started taking care of the general public. The first hospital established in the New World was in Mexico City during 1506. The health care in hospitals at that time did not require much coordination because they offered limited tests and treatments. Early hospitals had physicians and nurses and a few other personnel to work in departments such as the kitchen and housekeeping. World War II brought huge numbers of casualties to the hospitals, making the coordination of work difficult for the physicians and nurses who staffed the hospitals. It was then that floor secretaries were hired to complete some of the paperwork, perform receptionist-type duties, order supplies, and run errands—all tasks that were previously done by nurses. In the 1950s, unit coordinators began transcribing physician orders in addition to their other duties. *Transcribing* in this sense is communicating to the various hospital departments which of their services were needed in the care of the patient. The health unit coordinator would transcribe physician orders by calling the departments or ordering the medical tests or treatments on **paper requisitions**, as shown in Figure 1-1. There were numerous requisition forms, usually a different requisition form for every hospital department.

More hospitals were built and others expanded as the population grew. Hospitals also had to stay current with new developments and technology. Existing hospitals needed to accommodate such advances, so additions were built. Hospital departments such as

DIAGNOSIS:

ST. LUKE'S MEDICAL CENTER • MILWAUKEE, WISCONSIN

BLOOD BANK A

WHITE - CHART   PINK - BLOOD BANK   BLUE - NURSE   CARD - DATA

05-222000 REV. 3/88   S VHA +PLUS ™

DATE NEEDED	HOUR NEEDED	☐ PRE OP ☐ PREVIOUS TRANSFUSIONS
URGENCY:	☐ STAT ☐ GIVE ☐ HOLD	☐ SURGERY
TYPE	TYPE AND Rh	
XMCH	CROSSMATCH	# UNITS
STS	SURGICAL TYPE AND SCREEN	
ABSC	ANTIBODY SCREEN	9754
DCT	DIRECT COOMBS TEST	9756
ICT	INDIRECT COOMBS TEST	
FUHT	FUTURE HEART	9767
TFOL	TRANSFUSION REACTION FOLLOW-UP	9765
TITR	ANTIBODY TITER	
9090	THERAPEUTIC PHLEBOTOMY	
	OTHER	
	OTHER	

PLATELET ANTIBODY STUDIES
PLATELET ANTIBODY STUDIES DRUG RELATED
(INDICATE DRUGS BELOW)
HLA B27 TYPING
HLA TYPING — COMPLETE
INDICATE REASON:
PLATELET/WBC RECIPIENT
DIALYSIS PATIENT
ORGAN DONOR
OTHER

REMARKS:

TECHNOLOGIST   DATE
BLOOD BANK A

ROOM NO.   DATE
PATIENT
HOSP. NO.   AGE
DOCTOR   UNIT

INDICATIONS FOR TRANSFUSION:

☐ BLOOD LOSS (EST. AMT.) _____ ML
☐ HYPOVOLEMIA (SHOCK)
☐ COAGULATION DEFECT _____
☐ ANEMIA: HGB _____ HCT _____
☐ EXTRACORPORAL CIRCULATION
☐ OTHER _____

DR. SIGNATURE

Figure 1-1 • *An old test requisition (Courtesy of Aurora Health Care, Milwaukee, WI)*

cardiac services, emergency room, laboratory, medical records, and pharmacy were added. At some hospitals, large departments such as radiology divided into specialty areas such as ultrasound and computerized tomography (CT). Physical medicine added departmental sections such as occupational therapy and rehabilitation. The health unit coordinator communicates with all of these hospital departments throughout the course of the day.

Specialty hospitals and health care facilities also began to emerge with the advances in medicine. Children's hospitals, veteran's hospitals, hospitals for the mentally ill, and nursing homes were established to provide places that could handle and treat specific types of patients.

Hospitals began to focus on retaining records of the patient's stay. They recognized the necessity of keeping track of the care and treatment given to patients during their hospitalization. These records included the tests that were requested as well as the test results. Patient vital signs, such as temperature, pulse, respiration, and blood pressure, were recorded on the patient's chart, often by unit secretaries or health unit clerks.

AGING POPULATION

Life expectancy in the 1700s was 30 years old. As you can imagine, medical advances and technology improvements have increased that number dramatically. In the United States, life expectancy had almost doubled in the twentieth century. Statistics show that people born in 1900 had an average life expectancy of 47. The life expectancy for those born in 1950 is approximately 73. Those born in the year 2000 have a life expectancy of close to 90 years. The reasons for the increase vary.

Life expectancy in poorer countries is appreciably lower. Malnutrition, economic underdevelopment, and the lack of medical resources, including medications, are just some of the factors for the lower life expectancy in many poor countries today.

GOVERNMENT ASSISTANCE

Government concern for the economic well-being and health of the people dates back to ancient times. For example, during the times of the ancient Greeks, economic security took the form of urns filled with olive oil. Olive oil was very nutritious and could be stored for long periods of time in the urns. Stockpiling olive oil was the Greeks' form of economic security.

Health unit coordinators need not know all the historical background of government assistance. However, some working knowledge of how a government's assistance affects its people and health care organizations is beneficial to the health unit coordinator. Two of the programs in the United States we will discuss are **Social Security** and **Medicare**.

Social Security was designed for people who face economic challenges brought on by disabilities, illness, old age, and unemployment. The Social Security Act was passed in 1935, after the Great Depression. It was originally designed to pay retired workers age 65 or older an income after retirement; payments were based on payroll tax contributions. One of the first tasks that needed to be completed before payment could be made was to register employers and workers who qualified for the insurance benefits. When they were identified, they were assigned a number—hence, the beginning of Social Security numbers. There have been numerous amendments to the Social Security Act, some of which included expanding benefits to spouses and minor children in case of the premature death of the worker. However, it was realized in the 1950s, that, with people living longer, the greatest single cost of economic security was the high cost of medical care.

After years of debate, in 1965 Congress passed a bill adopting Medicare. Medicare is a health insurance program designed to provide all older adults with medical coverage at an affordable cost. It provides for hospitals to be paid a reasonable compensation for treating Medicare patients. The federal government administers Medicare. There is also the **Medicaid** program, which provides medical assistance for people with low incomes and resources. The states administer Medicaid according to their individual standards. To standardize the payment system, the **Diagnosis Related Groups (DRG)** system was adopted. The Diagnosis Related Groups system is based on the **International Classification of Disease (ICD)**. ICDs are also known as ICD-9-CM codes, which are standardized numbers assigned to specific diagnoses and operations. Most medical tests need an ICD-approved reason for the hospital to be reimbursed for the test. The health unit coordinator is responsible for including appropriate ICD-approved reasons when requesting services from the various diagnostic departments.

COORDINATOR OF HEALTH CARE

The term **coordination** means the arrangement, or harmonious functioning of parts for the most effective results. The health unit coordinator (HUC) coordinates or arranges the patient's medical chart from the beginning of the hospital admission stay. The HUC arranges and places in a chart holder admission forms and other forms that the doctors and nurses will use to document the care and progress of a patient. The health unit coordinator also needs to ensure that the patient's chart is current by filing any necessary reports during the hospital or long-term health care stay. The health unit coordinator transcribes the orders or arranges medical tests, treatments, and even meals during a patient's stay in a health care facility.

Communication between doctors and nurses, and between physicians and various departments, involves time and coordination. The health unit coordinator facilitates communication for the doctors, nurses, patients, family members, and friends as needed. Health unit coordinators must have good customer service skills and strong organizational skills.

COMMUNICATION TECHNOLOGY AFFECTING HEALTH UNIT COORDINATORS

An important role of the health unit coordinator is communication. Greeting visitors, answering phones, and paging nursing staff via a unit intercom are all part of the HUC role as a communicator. The difference in the nursing units of the 1960s and today are illustrated in Figures 1-2 and 1-3.

Communication advances as well as advances in diagnostic procedures and treatment of patients make keeping records of a patient's stay in a health care facility crucially important. As the technology at the nursing stations or units has changed, so have the titles of health unit coordinators. Some of the titles used between the 1940s and the 1960s were **floor clerks**, **floor secretaries**, **unit secretaries**, **ward clerks**, **ward secretaries**, **station clerks**, **station coordinators**, **ward clerks ll**, and **unit clerks**.

Medical tests and treatments ordered by the patient's physician are now most often requested by the health unit coordinator, who enters the test or procedure into the nursing unit's computer; the performing department then receives the electronic request. Paging nurses and physicians involves finding the correct pager numbers or contacting physicians' offices or answering services. Communication to physician offices and other health care facilities may require faxing of some information. All these changes resulted in more changes in the nursing unit and more changes in the health unit coordinator's title. Titles used from 1960 to the current time include floor secretaries, unit clerks, unit secretaries, ward clerks, ward secretaries, **unit coordinators**, **unit coordinators ll**, **unit communicators**, and **health unit coordinators (HUCs)**.

EDUCATION FOR HEALTH UNIT COORDINATORS

Until the 1960s, floor secretaries learned their role and responsibilities through on-the-job training. Then, in August 1966, Ruth Stryker published an article in *Nursing Outlook*. Minnesota's vocational education system, after findings from a hospital study, showed that the floor secretary did a great deal of managing in the form of coordination of patient and unit activities, such as scheduling patient exams and ensuring that the nursing unit had clerical as well as patient supplies on hand. With this realization, Minnesota started a hospital station secretary program in vocational schools. San Antonio, Texas offered the first college credit for the program in 1968, and New Hampshire Vocational Technical College in Manchester offered the first associate's degree program for unit coordinating beginning in 1987. Today, many cities throughout the United States offer a diploma or certificate program at their community colleges and vocational-technical colleges.

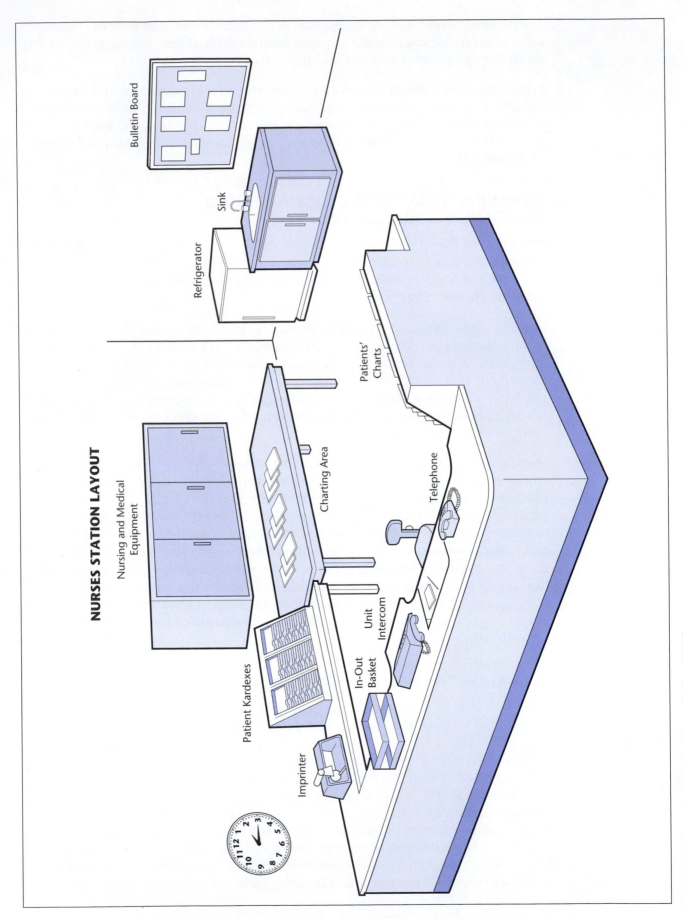

NURSES STATION LAYOUT

Bulletin Board

Sink

Refrigerator

Nursing and Medical
Equipment

Charting Area

Patients'
Charts

Telephone

Patient Kardexes

Unit
Intercom

In-Out
Basket

Imprinter

Figure 1-2 • *A workstation of the 1960s*

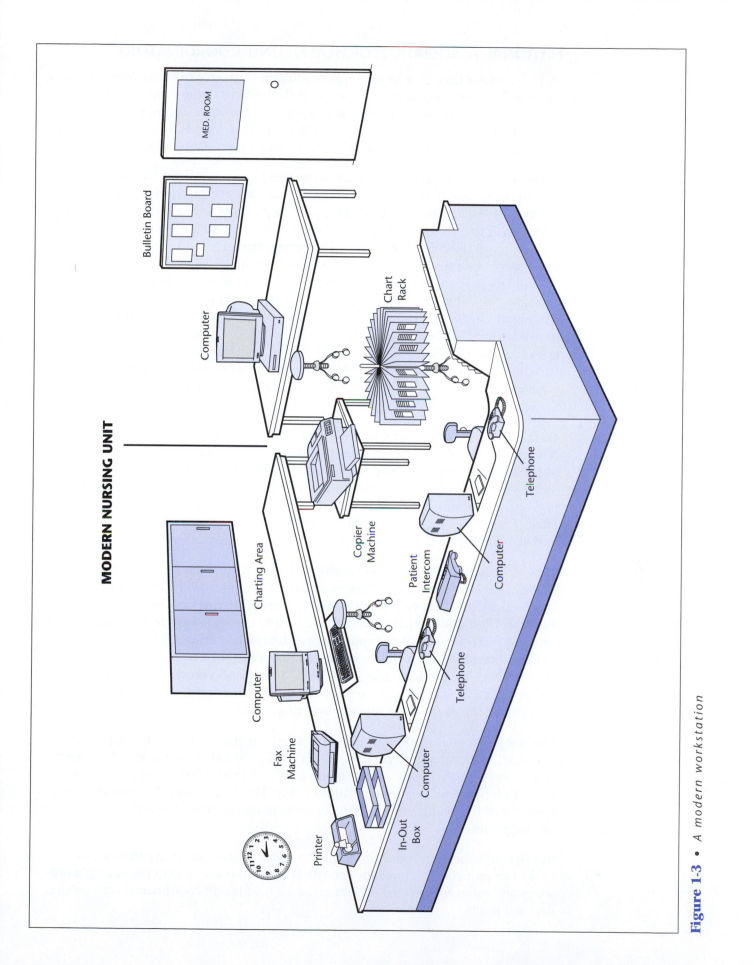

Figure 1-3 • *A modern workstation*

NATIONAL ASSOCIATION OF HEALTH UNIT COORDINATORS

In 1977, Myrna LaFleur, a health unit coordinator instructor from Phoenix and founding president of the National Association of Health Unit Coordinators (NAHUC), conducted a national survey to identify the health unit coordinating programs that existed throughout the country. The survey revealed that there were at least 52 programs in adult education centers, community colleges, and vocational-technical schools.

In the late 1970s, Wisconsin established the first known organization for ward clerks, and, in the spring of 1980, Arizona formed a state association for health unit coordinators. In 1980, LaFleur was asked to speak to a group of unit coordinators and unit managers at the Upper Midwest Hospital Conference in Minneapolis, Minnesota. LaFleur found the conference quite invigorating. She returned home and looked up the survey responses from 1977, when she had inquired if anyone was interested in the formation of a national association for unit coordinators. LaFleur contacted the persons who had indicated an interest and invited them to meet in Phoenix, Arizona. On August 23, 1980, the founding members of NAHUC held the first meeting. They were Kay Cox (California); Helga Hegge (Minnesota); Carolyn Hinken (New Mexico); Estella Johnson, Connie Johnston, Kathy Jordan, and Winnie Starr (Arizona); Velma Kerschner (Texas); and Jane Pedersen (Wisconsin). During the weekend, they worked out a constitution and selected the title National Association of Health Unit Clerk/Coordinators.

The association formally dropped the term *clerk* from the title in 1990. The **National Association of Health Unit Coordinators (NAHUC)** is an association made up of practicing health unit coordinators, health unit coordinator educators, and supervisors. Its mission is to promote health unit coordinating as a profession through education and certification complying with the NAHUC Standards of Practice, Standards of Education, and Code of Ethics. These Standards and the Code of Ethics are explained in detail in Chapter 2 of this textbook.

There are numerous benefits from becoming a member of the association. You will receive *The Coordinator*, a quarterly newsletter with topics of interest and reports from around the United States. For certified health unit coordinators, *The Coordinator* offers a contact hour questionnaire that may be used as credits toward recertification. Benchmarking and leadership development opportunities are available. Members receive notifications of regional workshops and a discount to such workshops. Members also receive a NAHUC pin to wear and a NAHUC information brochure, which includes the Standards of Practice and the Code of Ethics. Networking with other coordinators throughout the country is a valuable benefit as well.

The NAHUC logo is made with five outer segments (Figure 1-4). These segments represent doctors, nursing staff, patients, visitors, and hospital departments. These five segments are the main entities that a health unit coordinator coordinates throughout a patient's hospital or long-term health care stay. The circle connecting the segments is symbolic of the health unit coordinator's role in coordinating the activities among the five segments.

In 1984, an education board was formed to assist in standardizing formal education for health unit coordinators. The education board also assists with organizing workshops and other educational opportunities for health unit coordinators on local and national levels.

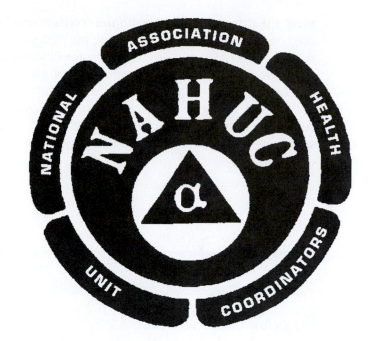

Figure 1-4 • *National Association of Health Unit Coordinators logo (Courtesy of the National Association of Health Unit Coordinators)*

The first NAHUC annual convention was held in San Antonio, Texas, in June 1982. At this convention, the Code of Ethics and Standards of Practice for unit coordinating were adopted. The Code of Ethics and Standards of Practice apply to all health unit coordinators, whether or not they are a member the National Association of Health Unit Coordinators.

The annual conference is a wonderful time for networking with other health unit coordinators from throughout the United States. It also is an opportunity to learn more about the role of the health unit coordinator. There are usually up to 15 educational sessions offered within a 3-day period.

A subsidiary Certification Board was established, and the first National Certification Examination was given in May 1983. There are hundreds of certified health unit coordinators today. Certified members may demonstrate broad knowledge or dedication in a specialized field of work. Specialization is discussed in Chapter 2.

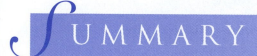

SUMMARY

Although patients and the public may not know of health unit coordinators, the duties of the health unit coordinator are very important. The tasks of the floor secretary started out to be quite minimal and only similar to those of a receptionist in nature. Even so, floor secretaries were recognized as a valuable member of the nursing team. As medical discoveries advanced and the floor secretary's role and responsibilities grew, the title changed to health unit coordinator. However, no matter what title is used, the responsibility for arranging the patients' charts, for keeping the charts current, and for efficiently placing orders for diagnostic tests and treatments is an important aspect of health care. A health unit coordinator must be able to handle more than one task at a time—all while maintaining the professionalism of the role. As well as the healing, caring, and respectful nature of physicians and nurses, transcribing and communicating the physicians' orders will always be best accomplished by professional people who are willing to remember that what they do will affect the patient outcome.

REVIEW QUESTIONS

1. Define the term *coordination*.

2. List at least four other titles used instead of health unit coordinator.

3. Explain why the Education Board of the National Association of Health Unit Coordinators was formed.

4. Define DRG.

5. Define ICD.

6. List five groups of people with whom health unit coordinators communicate during a workday.

7. Describe the difference between Social Security and Medicare.

Match the type of physician in the left column to the specialty in the right column.

8. Allergist

9. Anesthesiologist

10. Cardiologist

11. Epidemiologist

12. Gerontologist

13. Internist

14. Oncologist

a. A physician who specializes in aging and diseases associated with aging

b. A physician who specializes in treating internal organ problems

c. A physician who specializes in the study and treatment of the heart

d. A physician who specializes in the study and treatment of allergies

e. A physician who treats foot diseases

f. A physician who specializes in the study and treatment of cancer

g. A physician who administers anesthesia during surgery or other major procedures

15. Podiatrist

    h. A physician who deals with the causes, distribution, and control of diseases

16. Radiologist

    i. A physician who specializes in performing and reading x-rays and other radioactive exams

THROUGH THE EYES

OF A HEALTH CARE PROFESSIONAL

Health unit coordinators who have been in the role for 20 or more years have vivid memories of the many changes throughout the years. When asked, they quickly mention the change from a single-line phone to a multiple-line phone, the change from the use of the paper requisitions to the computer, and the high use of pagers and cell phones, which they did without for years. Do they see these changes as good? How do the changes affect the health unit coordinator? Most health unit coordinators feel that the use of pagers was definitely a positive change; people can be reached more quickly, and the noise level of the nursing unit has decreased. Because of computers, exams can be ordered and completed, and the results recorded much more quickly than was once possible; thus the length of a patient's stay is shorter. However, even with all the technology, there is no decrease in the workload. As Joanne Wice, certified health unit coordinator, St. Lukes Medical Center, Milwaukee, WI, puts it, "Our profession has evolved into a special niche requiring greater medical and practical knowledge. As technology takes us into the future, there will be increasing respect for our profession."

REFERENCES

http://www.NAHUC.org Accessed January 15, 2003.

http://ssa.gov/history/early.html Accessed January 20, 2003

http://www.beacon11c.com/hcref/cclookup/icddescription.htm Accessed January 24, 2003.

http://www.countryjoe.com/nightgale/nutting.htm Accessed January 10, 2003.

http://www.nursingworld.org/pressrel/nnw/nnwpled.htm Accessed January 10, 2003.

Brindell Fradin, D. (1989). *Medicine: Yesterday, today, and tomorrow.* Chicago, IL: Children Press.

LaFleur-Brooks, M. (1998). *Health unit coordinating* (4th ed.). Philadelphia: Saunders.

Kerschner, V. (1992). *Health unit coordinating principles and practices.* Clifton Park, NY: Thomson Delmar Learning.

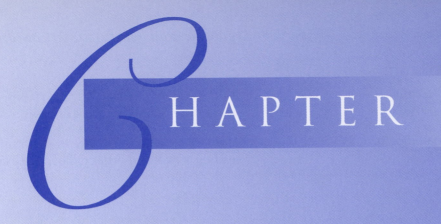

CHAPTER 2

Profession of Health Unit Coordinating

Learning Objectives

Upon completion of this chapter and review questions, the learner should be able to:

1. Define *job description*.

2. Compare the terms *clinical* and *nonclinical*.

3. List the responsibilities of health unit coordinating.

4. Compare selected job descriptions of health unit coordinating.

5. Identify the criteria for a profession.

6. Discuss how health unit coordinating does or does not meet the criteria for a profession.

7. Discuss the purpose for being recognized as a profession.

Key Terms

autonomy The state of functioning independently, without outside influence, or being self-reliant.

career levels, or **career ladders** Grade levels of increasing complexity and responsibility within a job description.

certification Compliance with a set of standards defined by nongovernmental organizations.

clinical care Direct, hands-on care.

competency The skills and/or abilities of an individual to perform the requirements of the job description.

job description A written document describing the duties, responsibilities, skills, qualifications, and reporting relationships of a particular job.

medical staff The licensed physicians who have privileges to admit and attend to patients in the health care facility.

nonclinical Indirect patient care or duties; care or duties performed without having direct physical or hands-on contact with the patient.

terminal competency The end goal of training; what a student has learned at the end of the training course.

THE HEALTH UNIT COORDINATING PROFESSION

The meaning of the word *coordinating* that is applicable to the health unit coordinating profession is to harmonize in a common action; to work together harmoniously. Therefore, it follows that a health unit coordinator is one who facilitates the activities of people in a health unit to work together smoothly and harmoniously in a common action, which is the delivery of health care to patients.

As a professional health unit coordinator, one will be expected to conform to the standards and ethics of the health care profession. One will be expected to practice the principles of the health unit coordinator's profession and to apply the appropriate skills and methodologies required to fully and competently meet the responsibilities of the job.

The job of a professional health unit coordinator is interesting, fulfilling, and wide in scope. The health unit coordinator acts as the communications liaison among all of the various departments in the health care facility, including nurses, physicians, other professional staff, ancillary staff, patients, and visitors. Health unit coordinators transcribe physicians' orders, maintain patient and unit records, and order supplies and services. In short, they are a vital force in facilitating the team effort required in a health care unit. This chapter explores the coordinator's responsibilities and how those responsibilities fulfill the criteria for a profession.

JOB DESCRIPTION

A **job description** is a written document that describes the duties, responsibilities, skills, qualifications, and reporting relationships of a particular job. Susan Heathfield, a noted human resource specialist, states that "job descriptions should be based on objective information obtained through job analysis, an understanding of the competencies and skills required to accomplish needed tasks, and the needs of the organization to produce work." In other words, a job description should state what to do and what to know to do it. Job descriptions should clearly identify and spell out the responsibilities of a specific job. Job descriptions may also include information about working conditions, tools, equipment used, knowledge and skills needed, and relationships with other positions. Competency assessment is a tool used within the job description to provide an expanded view of the position. Competency lists augment the job description by listing the skills needed to be competent at the job.

It is beneficial for most employers to have a job description for every position. A job description is a communication tool that is important for an organization's success. Poorly written job descriptions create workplace confusion, hurt communication, and make people feel uncertain about what is expected from them. Well-written job descriptions clearly define job responsibilities. People cannot be held accountable for responsibilities they do not know about or do not understand. A well-written job description will help both the employer and the employee understand the job expectations.

HEALTH UNIT COORDINATOR JOB DESCRIPTIONS

Health unit coordinator job descriptions will vary, often depending on the size, or other attributes, of the specific health care facility. A health unit coordinator working in a large health care facility may have specialized duties because of the many specialized services offered by the facility. For example, a health unit coordinator in a large neonatal intensive care unit may work mainly on processing the admission, transfer, and discharge paperwork. There may be another health unit coordinator assigned to the same unit who is responsible only for the transcription of physicians' orders.

A health unit coordinator in a small or rural health care facility may perform a greater variety of tasks. Because of the smaller number of employees, a health unit coordinator in a rural hospital may work under a wider or broader job description. A wider job description would include a larger number of duties. For example, a health unit coordinator might also pick up and deliver supplies in addition to ordering them, or perform medical records duties that, in a larger facility, would be performed by administrative personnel.

One thing is certain; most health unit coordinator job descriptions will have a sentence that says, "Perform other duties as assigned." Such a sentence allows for flexibility and change within the job. Variety and change are what make the health unit coordinating profession exciting. One day is never the same as the one before.

HEALTH UNIT COORDINATOR COMPETENCIES

Job descriptions in recent years have been expanded to include an additional component called competencies. **Competencies** are the skills, knowledge, abilities, and behaviors required to perform a job. The competencies are what are reviewed during an evaluation. Employees must be competent to function in the position for which they are hired. Competency assessment is an ongoing process that is subject to continual change, just as the health care world continues to change. Each facility must create its own definition of competency assessment and define how it is to be used in the evaluation process.

NONCLINICAL HEALTH CARE TEAM MEMBER

The health unit coordinator is a nonclinical health care team member. Health unit coordinators perform **nonclinical** duties. Nonclinical duties are those activities that do not involve direct patient care. It is care given without having direct physical or hands-on contact with patients (Figure 2-1). The term **clinical care** is used within health care to describe direct patient care (Figure 2-2). *Clinical* describes hands-on patient care.

For example, the health unit coordinator provides indirect patient care by transcribing physicians' orders, maintaining patient and unit records, answering visitor questions, ordering tests and treatments, and making sure supplies are available. Although all of these activities are necessary to ensure that the patient receives the best care available, they are all indirect, nonclinical services. Competent performance of these indirect duties facilitates patient care. The health unit coordinator enhances patient care by efficiently and accurately transcribing physician's orders and by relieving the nurses of clerical duties. Although health unit coordinators may never physically touch the patients, the duties they perform contribute significantly to the patients' care.

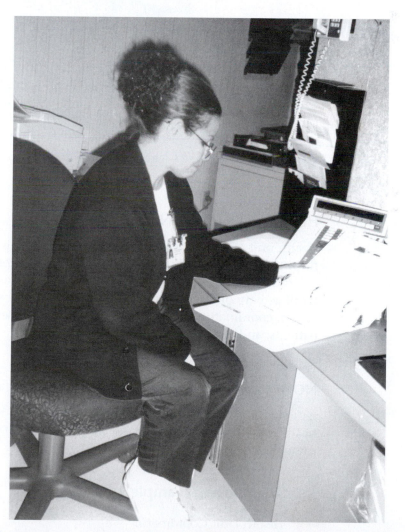

Figure 2-1 • *Health unit coordinators provide nonclinical care for the patient. (Courtesy of All Saints Healthcare, Racine, WI)*

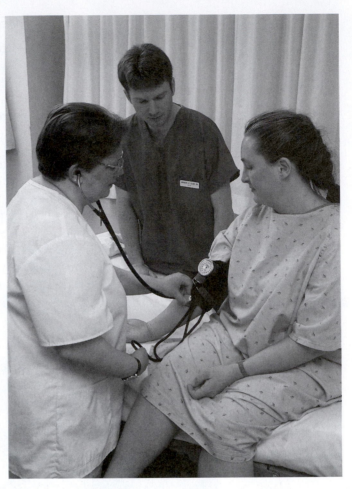

Figure 2-2 • *A health team member providing clinical care to the patient*

HEALTH CARE SETTINGS

Health unit coordinators work in a variety of settings, including hospitals, clinics, nursing homes, rehabilitation centers, surgical centers, and physicians' offices (Figures 2-3 and 2-4). Within the settings, the health unit coordinator can be found at the center of activity of the workstations. The health unit coordinator is in the middle of the action, coordinating requests from physicians, nurses, health care staff, support staff, patients, and visitors.

NONCLINICAL DUTIES

As stated, the health unit coordinator performs the nonclinical duties in a variety of health care settings. A selection of three health unit coordinator job descriptions lists some of the nonclinical duties.

Job Description: Example 1

Health Unit Coordinator

Reports to: Unit Services Manager   Department: Patient Services

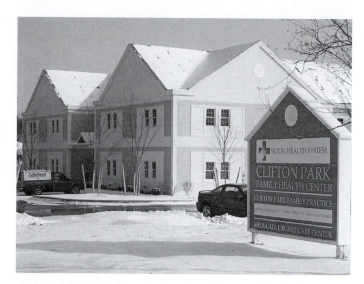

Figure 2-3 • *Health care provided within a family practice clinic setting*

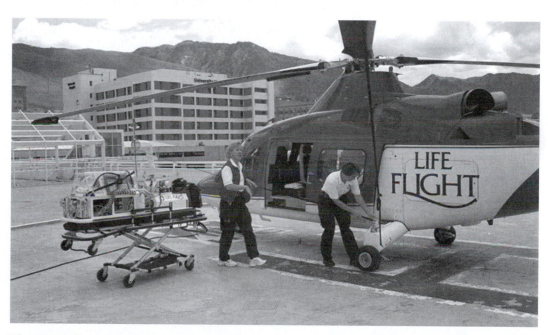

Figure 2-4 • *Health care provided within a hospital setting that offers trauma services*

Job Function

Performs the nonclinical support activities involved in patient care, including transcribing physicians' orders, maintaining records, ordering supplies, and serving as communication liaison for the unit.

Duties and Responsibilities

1. Utilize knowledge of diagnostic tests, pharmacology, nursing procedures, therapies, and medical terminology to transcribe physician's orders.

2. Utilize knowledge of human relations to coordinate requests from patients, visitors, and staff.

3. Handle telephone communications, including answering the workstation phones, forwarding calls, using the paging system, and taking messages.

4. Perform the clerical transactions involved in admissions, discharges, and transfers.

5. Maintain patient records in the manner appropriate for a legal document.

6. Manage unit supplies, including inventory records, disbursements, reordering as required.

7. Perform other duties as required.

Competencies, Knowledge, and Skills

1. Sufficiently skilled in human relations to tactfully handle patients and visitors who may be under intense stress.

2. Knowledge of diagnostic tests, pharmacology, nursing procedures, therapies, and medical terminology.

3. Ability to accurately transcribe physicians' orders.

4. Working knowledge of data entry and word-processing programs.

Desirable Qualifications

1. Ability to work with a minimum of supervision.

2. Successful completion of a health unit coordinator training program.

3. National health unit coordinator certification.

Job Description: Example 2

Health Unit Coordinator

Reports to: RN Nursing Unit Manager   Department: Nursing

Job Function

Responsible for the coordination and management of the nursing unit and activities associated with the unit's patients.

Duties and Responsibilities

1. Transcribe (communicate and coordinate) the therapeutic and diagnostic orders of the **medical staff**.

2. Independently establish priorities for multiple tasks.

3. Utilize effective written and verbal communication skills and problem-solving skills when working with physicians, hospital staff, patients and families, students, vendors, and so on.

4. Operate various communications and office equipment.

5. Maintain patient charts and unit records and, using discretion, protect confidentiality.

6. Manage unit supplies.

7. Calculate and enter patient charges.

Competencies, Knowledge, and Skills

1. Transcribe orders per physician priority and established procedures utilizing computer skills.

2. Ability to work with a minimum of supervision.

3. Utilize excellent customer service skills at all times.

Desirable Qualifications

1. High school graduate and completion of health unit coordinator training program.

2. Two years of experience as a health unit coordinator.

3. Familiarity with medical terminology.

4. Working knowledge of office equipment and computers.

Job Description: Example 3

Health Unit Coordinator

Reports to: Assistant Clinical Director   Department: Nursing

Job Function

The health unit coordinator is the professional responsible for managing nonclinical activities of patient care areas in health care facilities. Performs nonclinical support functions in a confidential manner.

Duties and Responsibilities

1. Transcribe orders and schedule diagnostic and therapeutic services for patients as requested by written physician orders.

2. Arrange/coordinate all nursing unit communication and activities.

3. Assemble and maintain the patient record as a medical legal document according to facility policy and procedures.

4. Organize and communicate with other departments in an effort to provide quality patient care. Act as liaison with other departments and agencies providing patient services.

5. Use communication devices such as telecommunication systems, computer terminals, and fax machines.

6. Maintain an orderly, equipped, and supplied nursing unit.

Competencies, Knowledge, and Skills

1. Demonstrates knowledge and skills in use of communication systems.

2. Demonstrates ability to be flexible, be organized, and function in stressful situations.

3. Ability to meet the customer's expectations using appropriate resources within the system.

Desirable Qualifications

1. Satisfactory completion of a health unit coordinator program.

2. National health unit coordinator certification.

3. Two years of experience as a health unit coordinator.

4. Excellent human relations skills.

SIMILARITIES OF JOB DESCRIPTION SUMMARIES

The three job descriptions are different, as one would find if collecting job descriptions from different health care facilities. Each health care facility writes its job descriptions to meet its unique needs. Even though there are differences, there are some common nonclinical duties in each of the job descriptions. Most health unit coordinator job descriptions will include nonclinical coordination duties such as:

◆ Transcribing orders

◆ Scheduling tests and treatments

◆ Maintaining supplies and equipment

◆ Communicating via phones, computers, faxes, pagers

◆ Providing customer/guest service

The above are examples of nonclinical duties. It is not necessary to fully understand the duties at this time. These duties will be discussed in detail in later chapters.

CAREER LADDERS

The job summaries discussed so far have been described as one level. However, it is a growing trend for job descriptions to be written in levels or ladders. Health care facilities may write the health unit coordinator description in levels or ladders. **Career levels** or **career ladders** are job descriptions written on two or more levels. The levels or ladders allow for growth and advancement within the same job position. Career levels and ladders are often used by health care facilities as recruitment and retention tools. Health care facilities that have career levels recognize that it is important to give employees a chance to grow and advance. Growth opportunities can help retain existing employees and recruit new employees. Career ladders will be discussed again in Chapter 32.

CRITERIA FOR A PROFESSION

What makes a job a profession? Who decides when a job becomes a profession? The NAHUC Web site lists the criteria of a profession according to Wilson and Neuhauser (1982) from their book *Health Services in the United States*. According to Wilson and Neuhauser, "For a group to become a profession, they must meet the following criteria:

1. Have a national association.

2. Have a formal education.

3. Have certification.

4. Have a code of ethics.

5. Have an identified body of systematic knowledge and technical skill.

6. Have members that function with a degree of autonomy and authority under the assumption that they alone have the expertise to make decisions in their area of competence."

A critical examination of the health unit coordinator's job will determine if it meets those criteria to qualify as a profession.

NATIONAL ASSOCIATION

The first criterion is to have a national association. A national association gives professionals the opportunity to:

◆ Network nationally with other people in the same profession

◆ Unite under a common mission

◆ Have a voice or vote in issues that affect their profession

Health unit coordinators have a national professional association. It is the National Association of Health Unit Coordinators, Inc. (NAHUC). The history of the association was discussed in Chapter 1. According to their mission statement, the National Association of Health Unit Coordinators is dedicated to promoting health unit coordinating as a profession through education and certification, complying with the NAHUC Standards of Practice, Standards of Education, and Code of Ethics.

FORMAL EDUCATION

Formal education is standardized or organized instruction or schooling. It is a broad term used to describe instruction other than on-the-job training. On-the-job training, or OJT, is the term used to describe training or orientation that is given by an employer to an employee.

Health unit coordinators have formal education. There are a variety of types of training programs across the nation. Training may be offered at community colleges, vocational and technical schools, and health care facilities (Figure 2-5). The professional

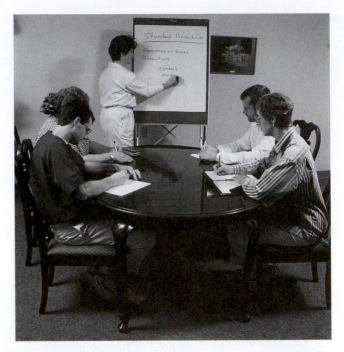

Figure 2-5 • *Health unit coordinators receive formal education in a classroom setting.*

association, NAHUC, states that there have been formal education programs for health unit coordinators since the 1960s. NAHUC has also developed essentials and guidelines for formal health unit coordinator education programs. The terminal competencies are listed in the Essentials and Guidelines for Health Unit Coordinator Education Programs (Figure 2-6). A **terminal competency** is what a student has learned by the end of the training. NAHUC lists their recommendations for what a student in a formal health unit coordinator program will be able to do upon graduation.

CERTIFICATION

The On-line Medical Dictionary defines **certification** as "compliance with a set of standards defined by non-governmental organizations." Individuals apply for certification on a voluntary basis, and receipt of certification verifies achievement of a professional status, for example, certification for a medical specialty.

Health unit coordinators have a certification process. The professional association, NAHUC, offers a certification exam program (Figure 2-7). The National Health Unit Coordinator Certification Examination is designed to measure knowledge and skills in areas of health unit coordinator job performance. Review for the examination is recommended. The examination is geared neither to geographic nor to specialty areas. The examination is prepared, administered, and graded by a testing agency. The testing agency selects the questions for the exam from a bank of questions that have been written by health unit coordinator practitioners and educators.

Certification denotes a process by which the National Association of Health Unit Coordinators grants recognition for basic knowledge (or competency) to an individual who has met certain predetermined qualifications specified by NAHUC. Certification is a voluntary process and is granted for 3 years. Maintaining certification is accomplished

ESSENTIAL III F

Terminal competencies shall include, but not be limited to, the following:

The graduate will be able to:

1. Demonstrate responsibilities and accountability to the nursing personnel, medical staff, hospital departments, patients and visitors.

2. Operate the nursing unit communication systems: telephones, pagers, imprinter devices, and computers.

3. Record telephoned doctors' orders; diagnostic test values, vital signs, and census data.

4. Order daily diets and laboratory tests.

5. File reports on charts.

6. Transcribe doctors' orders utilizing basic knowledge of anatomy, physiology, disease processes, medical terminology, and accepted medical abbreviations without requiring the cosignature of a nurse.

7. Perform nonclinical tasks for patient admission, transfer, discharge, and preoperative and postoperative procedures.

8. Manage the nonclinical functions of the nursing unit.

9. Maintain the nursing unit supplies.

10. Prepare patient consent forms.

11. Maintain the patient chart.

12. Coordinate scheduling of patients' tests and diagnostic procedures.

13. Transcribe medication orders, utilizing concepts of drug categories, automatic stop dates, automatic cancellations, time scheduling, and routes of administration.

14. Practice within the medical and ethical framework of health unit coordinating.

15. Schedule diagnostic procedures that require patient preparation.

16. Communicate effectively with patients, visitors, and members of the health care team.

Figure 2-6 • *Terminal competencies from the National Association of Health Unit Coordinators Essentials and Guidelines for Health Unit Coordinator Education Programs.*
(Courtesy of the National Association of Health Unit Coordinators)

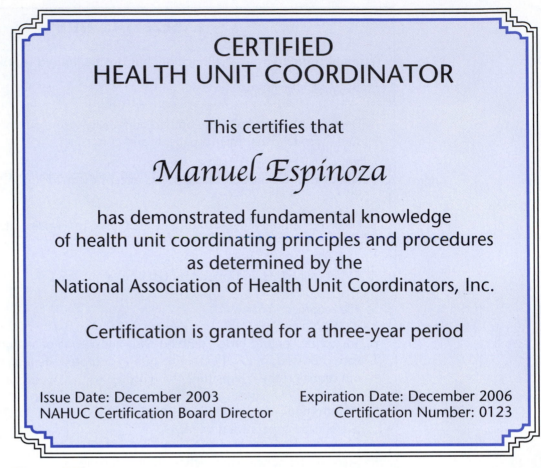

CERTIFIED
HEALTH UNIT COORDINATOR

This certifies that

Manuel Espinoza

has demonstrated fundamental knowledge
of health unit coordinating principles and procedures
as determined by the
National Association of Health Unit Coordinators, Inc.

Certification is granted for a three-year period

Issue Date: December 2003   Expiration Date: December 2006
NAHUC Certification Board Director   Certification Number: 0123

Figure 2-7 • *Health unit coordinators may become certified.*

by recertifying. Certification enhances the personal and professional growth of the health unit coordinator and offers the certificant the right to use the title Certified Health Unit Coordinator (CHUC). Certification says to the employer, other health professionals, and consumers that one is actively participating in professional growth and development. Recertification is the process to demonstrate continued competency to practice. There are two ways to recertify:

◆ Acquiring 36 NAHUC contact hours every 3 years. NAHUC provides continuing educational opportunities for CHUCs to meet this requirement.

◆ Retaking and passing the certification examination before the certification expiration date.

CODE OF ETHICS AND STANDARDS OF PRACTICE

A code of ethics is a set of statements that address broad ethical or moral principles or beliefs. A professional code of ethics lists the ethical and moral responsibilities of a professional; it is a guide for professional conduct. Health unit coordinators have a code of ethics that was developed by NAHUC (Figure 2-8).

NAHUC has also developed Standards of Practice for health unit coordinators. The Code of Ethics and the Standards of Practice promote high standards and a framework of accepted behaviors for health unit coordinators.

CODE OF ETHICS

This code of ethics is to serve as a guide by which Health Unit Coordinators may evaluate their professional conduct as it relates to patients, colleagues, and other members of the health care profession. This code of ethics shall be subject to monitoring, interpretation, and periodical revision by the association's Board of Directors.

Therefore, in the practice of our profession, we the members of the National Association of Health Unit Coordinators, Inc. accept the following principles:

Principle One:

Members shall conduct themselves in such a manner as to gain the respect and confidence of the patients, health care personnel, and community, as well as respecting the human dignity of each individual.

Principle Two:

Members shall protect the patients' rights, including the right to privacy.

Principle Three:

Members shall strive to achieve and maintain a high level of competency.

Principle Four:

Members shall strive to improve their knowledge and skills by participating in educational and professional activities and sharing the benefits of their attainments with their colleagues.

Principle Five:

Unethical and illegal professional activities shall be reported to the appropriate authorities.

Figure 2-8 • *The National Association of Health Unit Coordinators Code of Ethics (Courtesy of the National Association of Health Unit Coordinators)*

The Standards of Practice can be used as guidelines for job performance and evaluation. The NAHUC Standards of Practice are as follows:

A Standard of Practice is a statement of guidelines serving as a model of performance by which practitioners shall conduct their actions.

These Standards are set forth to obtain the best possible service from practitioners for the purpose of providing the organization and competency needed to coordinate the health unit in exemplary fashion enabling the best possible care for the patient.

The National Association of Health Unit Coordinators, Inc. (NAHUC) has formulated standards of practice to encompass all health units. There will be ongoing evaluation and revision in order to keep pace with the advancement of technology and the changing of the health unit's objectives and function.

Purpose

The purpose of the NAHUC Standards is to specify guidelines for health unit coordinators to follow. These standards have as their objectives:

> Define the realm of the health unit coordinators in the health care system.

> Specify the primary responsibility of the health unit coordinator in the nonclinical area of health care.

Basic Assumptions

> Health unit coordinators provide the nondirect, nonclinical patient care for health services.

> Standards for these services are established by health unit coordinators, supervisors and educators, and health care agencies.

> Health unit coordinators accept responsibility for their competency through individual growth, continuing education, and certification.

> Health unit coordinators are responsive to the changing needs and growth of health care.

Criteria for Statements of Standards

A standard is used as a model for the action of practitioners. Criteria used in establishing the NAHUC Standards for health unit coordinators are:

> A standard is established by an authority, in this instance, the National Association of Health Unit Coordinators, Inc.

> A standard is founded on appropriate knowledge.

> A standard is broad in scope, relevant, attainable, and definitive.

> A standard is subject to continued evaluation and revision.

Standards of Practice for Health Unit Coordinators

Standard 1—Education

Health Unit Coordinator personnel shall be prepared through appropriate education and training programs for their responsibility in the provision of nondirect patient care and nonclinical services.

Guidelines

Education shall be set forth by adopted NAHUC Educational Standards.

Standard 2—Policy and Procedure

Written standards of health unit coordinators' practice and related policies and procedures shall define and describe the scope and conduct of non-clinical service provided by the health unit coordinator. These standards, policies, and procedures shall be reviewed annually and revised as necessary. These revisions will be dated to indicate the last review, signed by the responsible authority, and implemented.

Guidelines

Policies shall include criteria based on job description.

Personnel policies shall be included.

Policies will include the philosophy and objectives of the health care organization.

Operational and nonclinical policies and procedures will be included.

Standard 3—Standards of Performance

Written evaluation of health unit coordinators shall be criteria based and related to the standards of performance as defined by the health care organization.

Guidelines

Standards of performance shall define functions, responsibilities, qualifications, and accountability, reflecting autonomy of practice.

Review shall be on at least an annual basis with evaluation to reflect the current job requirements.

Standards of performance shall be available to health unit coordinators.

Standard 4—Communication

The health unit coordinator shall appropriately and effectively communicate with nursing and medical staff, all ancillary departments, visitors, guests, and patients.

Guidelines

There shall be a written organizational plan that defines authority, accountability, and communication.

The organization shall assure that health unit coordinator service functions are fulfilled.

Health unit coordinators shall hold meetings no less than six times per year to define problems and propose solutions. A record shall be maintained documenting the content of these meetings for the purpose of monitoring and evaluating their direction.

Standard 5—Professionalism and Ethics

The health unit coordinator shall take all possible measures to assure the optimal quality of nondirect, nonclinical patient care. The optimal professional and ethical conduct and practices of NAHUC members shall be maintained at all times.

Guidelines

Health unit coordinators shall participate in staff development.

Services shall be provided according to approved policies.

All required meetings shall be attended.

All current competencies shall be maintained.

Standard 6—Leadership

The health unit coordinator shall be organized to meet and maintain established standards of nonclinical services.

Guidelines

Services should be directed by a qualified individual with appropriate education, experience, and knowledge of health unit coordinator services.

Leadership and guidance shall be provided to the health unit coordinator.

Responsibility and authority shall assure:

Hospital policy and procedures are followed.

Hospital goals and objectives are met.

Reasonable steps are taken to assure optimal quality of patient care is provided.

It is desirable that the health unit coordinator leader has an Associate Degree in health service management.[1]

---

[1]The Standards of Practice were reprinted with permission from the National Association of Health Unit Coordinators.

AN IDENTIFIED BODY OF SYSTEMATIC KNOWLEDGE AND TECHNICAL SKILLS

The criterion for having an identified body of systemic knowledge and technical skills can be broken down. It could be restated as a known core of organized information and procedural abilities. In other words, it is recognized that the job duties require one to know a specific set of information and to be able to demonstrate a specific set of skills. Health unit coordinators have an identified body of systematic knowledge and technical skills. What health unit coordinators need to do and what they need to know to do it have been identified. This information is published in the *Final Report of the 1996 Job Analysis*, published by the testing agency Assessment Systems, Inc. The job analysis was performed to determine the health unit coordinator tasks and the knowledge necessary to adequately complete the tasks. Health unit coordinator tasks based on national survey results were compiled. A list of tasks and the knowledge required to perform the tasks were developed. NAHUC also developed the Health Unit Coordinator Entry Level Competencies, based on the results of the job analysis. These documents prove that health unit coordinators have an identified body of systemic knowledge and technical skills.

AUTONOMY

One of the criteria of a profession is that members function with a degree of autonomy and authority under the assumption that they alone have the expertise to make decisions in their area of competence. **Autonomy** is defined as the state of functioning independently, without outside influence, or as being self-reliant. Health unit coordinators are independent and self-reliant. A health unit coordinator:

◆ Works effectively under pressure to process stat (immediate) orders and requests and meet deadlines

◆ Maintains composure and functions effectively during emergency situations

◆ Coordinates a variety of unit activities simultaneously

◆ Independently prioritizes, organizes, and performs work: transcribing, coordinating nonclinical activities, ordering supplies, and so on

◆ Double-checks own work

◆ Detects and correct errors

The health unit coordinator makes decisions. A health unit coordinator:

◆ Determines which preparations, consents, equipment, and forms are required when transcribing physician orders

◆ Investigates and resolves nursing unit/ancillary department concerns

◆ Has frequent telephone and personal contact with physicians, students, patients, visitors, nursing staff, and ancillary departments to coordinate daily activities, address concerns, retrieve and provide information, offer assistance and support, request services, and so on

◆ Possesses unique skills (when a health unit coordinator is absent, a registered nurse must substitute)

◆ Is the information systems expert at the workstation and provides computer training and troubleshooting for the staff

HEALTH UNIT COORDINATING IS A PROFESSION

On the basis of Wilson and Neuhauser's criteria, health unit coordinating is a profession. In Chapter 1, we learned about the history of health unit coordinating. In this chapter, we have demonstrated that, through its history, health unit coordinating has met the criteria for a profession. As an occupational group meets and exceeds the above-mentioned criteria, they become increasingly professional. Health unit coordinating still faces challenges in becoming recognized as a profession. Health unit coordinating is viewed as a female profession with a strong clerical focus. Health unit coordinating must move beyond that perception by educating the public on the roles and responsibilities of health unit coordinators. This education is best accomplished by providing information to the community through media, schools, speaking opportunities, health fairs, community involvement, and job fairs. Moving past that perception is difficult even for health unit coordinators, because often the health unit coordinator is the only person with that title on the unit for that given shift. Health unit coordinators are often the only nonclinical employee within a clinical department, not part of the clinical patient care staff but still a member of the patient care team and the nursing department.

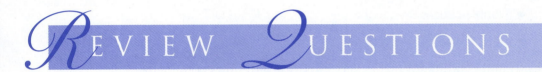

SUMMARY

The health unit coordinator performs nonclinical duties in a variety of settings. The health unit coordinator job description should describe the duties, responsibilities, required qualifications, and reporting relationships of the position. The role of a health unit coordinator is an important one. Even though the health unit coordinator may never come into direct physical contact with the patients, he or she can affect the quality of patient care. Because the health unit coordinator transcribes and processes physicians' orders before the nurse cosigns them, the health unit coordinator has a great responsibility for the patients' welfare. Health unit coordinating meets the criteria for a profession: it has a national association and a code of ethics; requires formal education, certification, and specific knowledge and skills; and has autonomous, self-reliant members.

REVIEW QUESTIONS

1. Define *nonclinical*.

2. Define *job description*.

3. List five nonclinical duties commonly performed by a health unit coordinator.

4. List the six criteria of a profession.

5. What is the purpose of the national association for health unit coordinators?

6. Define *certification*.

7. What documents show that health unit coordinators have an identified body of knowledge and skills?

8. Define *autonomy*.

9. List two nonclinical duties a health unit coordinator performs autonomously.

10. In your own words, explain why you think health unit coordinating is or is not a profession.

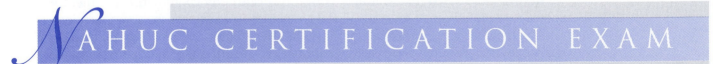

NAHUC CERTIFICATION EXAM

CONTENT AREAS

IV. B. 1   Review job-related publications (e.g., NAHUC Standards of Practice, journals)

IV. B. 3   Pursue and maintain certification

THROUGH THE EYES

OF A HEALTH CARE PROFESSIONAL.

A health unit coordinator who worked on a busy oncology unit at a large teaching hospital compared her job to that of an air traffic control specialist. This comparison interested me, so I looked for a job description of an air traffic control specialist.

The Federal Aviation Administration (FAA) defines an air traffic control specialist as one who provides for the safe and orderly flow of air traffic. It is their function to:

Direct air traffic so it flows smoothly, efficiently, and, above all, safely

Give pilots taxiing and takeoff instructions, air traffic clearances, and advice based on their own observations and information from other sources

Transfer control of aircraft to the ARTCC controller when the aircraft leaves their airspace and receive control of aircraft coming into their airspace from controllers at adjacent facilities

Be familiar with the aircraft identification and positions of the aircraft under their control, aircraft types, and speeds, and the location of navigational aids and landmarks in the area

After reading both the health unit coordinator and the air traffic control specialist job descriptions, I could easily compare the responsibilities. The health unit coordinator on that busy oncology unit also:

Provided safe and orderly traffic flow for the smooth running of the department. She had to be aware of the comings and goings of the patients and the staff. She had to know what supplies and equipment were needed to make sure there were no delays in patient care.

Gave instructions and advice. She had to communicate the physicians' orders to the appropriate staff. She had to obtain test results for the staff. She had to instruct visitors about regulations.

Transferred control of the patients' care. When transcribing orders, she scheduled appointments and referrals to staff to provide various aspects of the patients' care.

Was familiar with surroundings and landmarks. She used her knowledge of her facility to accurately transcribe the physicians' orders. She had to know about medications, treatments, and tests that were ordered for the patient. She had to know how to operate communication devices (see Table 2-1).

(continues)

(continued)

TABLE 2-1 Comparison of Job Descriptions

Air Traffic Controller	Health Unit Coordinator
Direct air traffic so it flows smoothly, efficiently, and safely.	Provide safe and orderly traffic flow for the smooth running of the department. Must be aware of the comings and goings of the patients and the staff. Must know what supplies and equipment are needed to avoid delays in patient care.
Give pilots taxiing and takeoff instructions, air traffic clearances, and advice based on own observations and information from other sources	Give instructions and advice. Communicate the physicians' orders to the appropriate staff. Obtain test results for the staff. Instruct visitors about regulations.
Transfer control of aircraft to the ARTCC controller when the aircraft leaves the airspace and receive control of aircraft coming into the airspace from controllers at adjacent facilities.	Transfer control of the patient's care. When transcribing orders, schedule appointments and referrals to staff to provide various aspects of the patients' care.
Be familiar with the aircraft identification and positions of the aircraft under their control, aircraft types, and speeds, and the location of navigational aids and landmarks in the area.	Be familiar with surroundings and landmarks. Use knowledge of the facility to accurately transcribe physicians' orders. Be familiar with medications, treatments, and tests. Know how to operate communication devices.

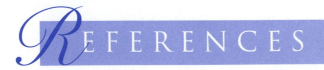

REFERENCES

Accreditation Board, a Committee of the NAHUC Board of Directors. (1995). *Essentials and guidelines for health unit coordinator education programs.* Rockford, IL: Author.

Heathfield, S. Why effective job descriptions make good business sense. *http://www.human resources.about.com/library/weekly/aa080402a.htm* Accessed January, 2004.

History of NAHUC. *http://www.nahuc.org/nahuc_hi.htm* Accessed January, 2004.

http://www.faa.gov/careers/employment/atc.htm Accessed December, 2003.

National Association of Health Unit Coordinators, Inc. (2002). *Information handbook.* Rockford, IL: Author.

The On-line Medical Dictionary. *http://www.cancerweb.ncl.ac.uk/cgi-bin/omd?certification* Accessed December, 2003.

Wilson, F. A., & Neuhauser, D. (1982). *Health services in the United States.* Cambridge, MA: Ballinger.

Health Care Team

Learning Objectives

Upon completion of this chapter and review questions, the learner should be able to:

1. Define health care team.

2. List at least five clinical professions that could be part of a health care team.

3. List at least two nonclinical professions that could be part of a health care team.

4. Explain the benefits of diverse health care teams.

Key Terms

clinical provider   One who provides direct patient care, care given with direct hands-on contact with the patient.

health care team   A team of health care providers who provide clinical and non-clinical care to the patient.

inpatient   A patient who usually spends more than 24 hours in the health care facility and meets the criteria set forth by the health care facility to be an inpatient.

nonclinical provider   A provider who provides only indirect care for the patient. Nonclinical providers do not provide care at the bedside or by touching the patient.

nursing care team   A team of clinical and nonclinical nursing staff who provide care to the patient.

outpatient   A patient who usually requires health care for less than 24 hours and meets the criteria set forth by the health care facility to be an outpatient.

Abbreviations

BSN Bachelor of Science in Nursing

CNA Certified Nurse Aide

DO Doctor of Osteopathic Medicine

JCAHO Joint Commission on Accreditation of Health Care Organizations

LPN Licensed Practical Nurse

MD Doctor of Medicine

NP Nurse Practitioner

PA Physician's Assistant

RN Registered Nurse

RT Respiratory Therapist

HEALTH CARE SETTINGS

Health care is provided to patients in a variety of settings. The care can be provided in an outpatient or inpatient setting. An inpatient setting is defined as a setting where care is provided continually. These settings are open for patient care 24 hours a day, 7 days a week, 365 days a year. In order to be an inpatient in this setting, the patient must require a certain level of care. An **inpatient** is a patient who usually spends more than 24 hours in the health care facility and meets the criteria set forth by the health care facility to be an inpatient. Examples of inpatient settings are hospitals, health systems, long-term care facilities, and nursing homes.

An **outpatient** is a patient who usually requires health care for less than 24 hours and meets the criteria set forth by the health care facility to be an outpatient. An outpatient can be provided care in a setting that is not available for 24-hour care. Examples of outpatient care settings are doctors' offices, clinics, and health centers. These settings are often closed during some hours of the 24-hour day.

Both outpatient and inpatient settings can vary according to the guidelines set forth by the health care facility and the state regulations. The health care providers in both inpatient and outpatient settings can be either clinical or nonclinical. **Clinical providers** are patient health care providers who provide direct patient care. Clinical providers are also called hands-on care providers. They provide direct care to the patient. This care is often provided at the bedside. **Nonclinical providers** provide only indirect care for the patient. Nonclinical providers do not provide care at the bedside or by touching the patient.

HEALTH CARE ACCREDITING ORGANIZATION

Patient health care providers must undergo training in order to attain the necessary qualifications to provide care for patients. For clinical providers, the required qualifications are defined by state regulations. State examining boards, after determining that the required qualifications have been fully met, license an individual to provide patient care at certain levels. For example, a physician will be licensed to provide care at a different level than a nurse.

Health care facilities are subject to a variety of state and national regulations, depending on the level of patient care they provide. A variety of municipal, state, and national agencies and groups validate that the specific health care facilities are meeting the regulations. They evaluate a facility by physically visiting the health care facility and by conducting a survey of the facility to validate that it is in fact providing care at the level it is licensed to provide. The surveyors will meet with the management staff, interview the unit and department staff, interview the patients, and conduct chart and document reviews. They provide this service so that the public can be confident that the health care system is providing care at the level required. The results from these surveys are public. If the surveyors identify areas that do not meet the standards, they will require the facility to correct the identified area.

The predominant accrediting and surveying agency for health care facilities in the United States is the Joint Commission on Accreditation of Health Care Organizations (JCAHO). JCAHO is an independent nonprofit group that deals with quality of patient care issues and the safety of the environment in which care is provided. JCAHO's mission statement is "To continuously improve the safety and quality of care provided to the public through the provision of health care accreditation and related services that support performance improvement in health care organizations" (JCAHO, 2003).

JCAHO surveys health care organizations throughout the United States and the world. In the United States alone, JCAHO surveys, evaluates, and accredits over 17,000 health care organizations. The survey team is made up of physicians, nurses, respiratory therapists, laboratory technologists, pharmacists, and health care administrative personnel. The accreditation process must be renewed every 3 years for health care organizations and every 2 years for laboratories. Health care organizations choose to have the JCAHO accreditation because it benefits their organization. Some of the benefits of being accredited by JCAHO are:

- ◆ Leads to improved patient care

- ◆ Demonstrates the organization's commitment to safety and quality

- ◆ Supports and enhances safety and quality improvement efforts

- ◆ May substitute for federal certification surveys for Medicare and Medicaid

- ◆ Helps secure managed care contracts

- ◆ Enhances the health care organization's image to the public

- ◆ Fulfills licensure requirements in many states

◆ Is recognized by insurers and other third-party payers

◆ Strengthens community confidence in the health care organization

This accreditation is universally recognized in the health care community. As a member of the health care team, you will be involved in surveys and accreditation processes.

HEALTH CARE TEAM

A **heath care team** is a group of health care workers who are members of different disciplines, each providing a different service to the patient (Mosby, 2002). A health care team can have clinical and nonclinical members. Clinical health care providers are the team members who provide hands-on care to the patient. Clinical providers typically provide care at the patient's bedside, but they can also provide the care at locations away from the bedside. Patients may receive care in the respiratory care department, where they would be taught breathing techniques to reduce shortness of breath. A physical therapy department team member might provide patient care by reteaching a patient who has had a stroke how to walk. Using equipment in the physical therapy department, the patient can practice the skills learned in a safe environment. These health care team members, although not delivering bedside care, are called direct care providers because they provide direct care to the patient.

Nonclinical providers are team members who indirectly provide care to the patient, that is, without touching the patient directly. Nonclinical providers are also called indirect care providers. Indirect care providers facilitate the direct care required by patients. These indirect providers perform behind-the-scenes services, often never connecting a patient face to a patient name. A physical therapist aide in the physical therapy department is an example. He or she is responsible for preparing and setting up the equipment and supplies the physical therapist will need to provide the direct patient care.

The makeup of the health care team is directed by the needs of the patient. The health care team's role is to provide care for the patient. The members of a health care team can vary during the patient's health system encounter. The team may increase as needs are identified and decrease as issues are resolved or completed.

Team members may be part of the admission process and not be involved in the patient care again until discharge. Dietitians, for example, may see patients during the admission process to provide the dietary plan for the health system stay. They then will not see the patient again until just before the patients' discharge, when they will provide the patient with recommendations for dietary intake at home.

Members of the health care teams are as varied as the patients and their health care conditions. Health care professionals from many disciplines can be members of patient health care teams. For example, a multidisciplinary team could include social workers, dietitians, pharmacists, and therapists. They provide education, treatment, evaluation, and a varied perspective of the patients and their needs. Because health care facilities continually strive to provide the highest quality of care possible, the varied perspectives of all the health care team members are of utmost importance and value. A patient health care team can improve responsiveness, reduce or eliminate errors, and elevate the level of care provided to the patient.

Often, a patient care plan will be the tool used to communicate with the health care team members. This document is in the patient chart. Each health care team member should review the care plan before seeing the patient. Patient care plans are either handwritten or are electronic documentation of what needs to be provided to each patient by the health care team members. The plan is reviewed by all health care providers during each shift and is rewritten by the providers as the patient condition warrants. For example, a patient care plan may state:

Reinforce the importance of activity by

◆ Encouraging the patient to get up to use the bathroom

◆ Encouraging the patient to sit in a chair to eat meals

◆ Walking with the patient in the hallway twice on each shift, day and evening

Each team member will continue to follow the plan and reinforce the information or skill identified as needing to be reinforced or introduced for that day. This is the concept of building on information already in place. Patients are more likely to recall the information if it is repeated often.

Health care teams reduce errors by frequently double-checking the plan of care for each patient. Frequent review of the patient care plan increases the team members' knowledge of the events that are taking place and that should be taking place with the individual patient. It is easier to prevent errors if many eyes are watching and many ears are listening. Health care teams also reassure patients because patients generally perceive that, with several people looking out for them, they are receiving a high level of care.

HEALTH CARE TEAM MEMBERS

The health care team is composed of both clinical and nonclinical providers. Ideally, a health care team will consist of a physician, members from the nursing staff, including a health unit coordinator; and members from the support staff. The role of each team member is to provide the appropriate level of care to the patient. Each patient receives individual care to meet his or her needs. Patient care plans are written by the health care team and followed by all health care team members.

PHYSICIAN

The physician's role in the health care team is to assess the patient and to direct the patient care process. The physician has completed a course of education and passed examination and testing requirements to meet the license requirements of the state in which she or he will practice. Physicians practice under the state licensing privileges and clinic, hospital, or health system physician bylaws.

A physician may be either a doctor of medicine (MD) or a doctor of osteopathic medicine (DO). A doctor of medicine diagnoses, treats, and educates patients on medical diseases and disorders. A doctor of osteopathic medicine treats, diagnoses, and educates patients on medical diseases and disorders, with emphasis on the connection between body, mind, and emotions.

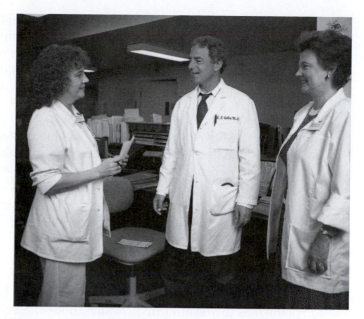

Figure 3-1 • *The physician directs the health care team.*

Physicians who choose to specialize require further education and additional certification. Specialists are referred to as a doctor of the medical specialty. A doctor of cardiology is called a cardiologist; a doctor of neonatology is a neonatologist; and a doctor of radiology is a radiologist.

One of the newest specialists to be seen in hospitals is a hospitalist. A hospitalist is a doctor who specializes in treating patients who are in the hospital. This specialty was created to improve patient care in the hospital. The hospitalist is not intended to replace the patient's primary physician but rather to provide quality care for the patient while he or she is a hospital patient. The hospitalist is based in the hospital, where he or she can watch patients closely, respond to the patients' needs quickly, and save money for the hospital and the patients.

The primary physician directs the patient care process by ordering the services the patient requires. The health care team members discuss the physician orders with the physician when questions arise (Figure 3-1). After the assessment, the physician will write orders to request treatments, tests, procedures, medications, and other services required. The health unit coordinator is responsible for transcribing these orders.

PHYSICIAN'S ASSISTANT AND NURSE PRACTITIONER

The physician may employ a physician's assistant (PA). The PA is an employee of the physician or of the health system and practices within the scope of the license and job description. The PA often writes patient orders and directs patient care under the supervision of a physician. The health system defines the scope of the PA's practice, or what the PA is able to do in the health care facility.

A PA is a graduate of a physician's assistant program and then passes a certification test given by the state in which he or she will practice. Other states may accept the certification or license or require that the PA take another certification test to practice as a PA in their state. Hospitals also grant practicing privileges and limitations based on their own physicians' bylaws.

A physician may employ a nurse practitioner (NP) to support the physician's practice. The NP may provide patient assessment, write physician orders, take calls, and provide other services as defined by the scope of practice and licensing of the state in which the NP is practicing. Usually, the NP practices under the supervision of a physician. The health care facility will also define the scope of practice for a NP in the facility.

Physician's assistants and nurse practitioners have enabled physicians to expand their practices by having a health care professional provide care to patients within their scope of practice. With the addition of these health care professionals to the health care team, patients and other team members have access to another level of health care professional to provide quality patient care. PAs and NPs are often on the patient care unit for longer periods of time than the physician and are able to assist the nursing staff by answering questions and addressing concerns.

NURSING STAFF

The nursing staff plays an important role in the health care team. Nursing staff can be defined as the health care providers, both clinical and nonclinical, who are part of the nursing service department. Members of the nursing staff, often called the **nursing care team**, include both clinical and nonclinical staff; case managers, registered nurses (RNs), licensed practical nurses (LPNs), nursing assistants (aides), and health unit coordinators. These are the members of the health care team who spend the greatest amount of time with the patient and family, and they work closely with each other. It is important that each member of the nursing staff know the roles and responsibilities of the other members of the nursing staff. The nursing staff provides direct and indirect care for the patient. They provide personal care, dispensing of medications, treatments, emotional support, and education, and they arrange for tests and procedures so that all things happen in a timely fashion. The nursing staff coordinates and carries out the orders of the physicians and their representatives (PAs and NPs) (Figure 3-2).

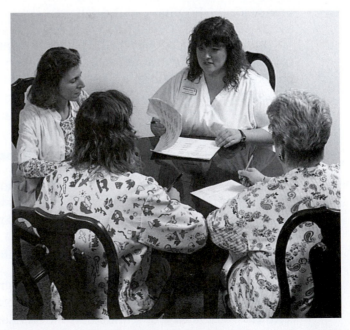

Figure 3-2 • *The nursing staff shares information about patient care in a private area.*

Nurse Case Manager

Nurse case managers are the health care team members who direct the patient care ordered by the physician in the health care setting. The case manager uses the team approach to provide the services and care the patient needs in the most effective and efficient way. The intent is to provide high-quality patient care using all the available resources wisely. The nurse case manager is a registered nurse (RN). The following is an example of the roles and responsibilities of the position of nurse case manager.

Nurse Case Manager Position Summary: The nurse case manager manages the care of the patient or specific patient grouping to provide quality care within the financial constraints of the health care system. The nurse case manager is a Registered Nurse.

Responsibilities/Competencies

1. Provides direct patient care.
2. Assesses patient and home/family circumstances.
3. Recommends resources, equipment, and support services.
4. Coordinates recommended services.
5. Coordinates nursing care team.
6. Demonstrates knowledge of medications, diagnoses, tests, procedures.
7. Provides education to patient, family, caregivers, significant others.
8. Researches current trends and recommends system changes.
9. Serves on assigned committees.
10. Participates in other projects and duties as assigned.

Registered Nurse

Registered nurses (RNs) are members of the health care team. They are registered in the state in which they practice. To be a registered nurse, an individual must have completed a defined education program and fulfilled the licensing requirements of the state in which he or she is registered. The education program must meet requirements set forth by the state in which the course is provided. RNs may receive a diploma, an associate's degree, or a bachelor's degree, depending on the education program they attend. Diploma programs associated with or provided through a health care facility were popular through the 1970s. There are few hospital-based programs still available in this country. Associate degree programs for registered nurses are offered by many community colleges. These programs have become popular because they usually take only 2 years to complete. They often are attractive to licensed practical nurses (LPNs), who have already completed an LPN program. Bachelor of science in nursing (BSN) programs are offered throughout the country at universities and colleges. These programs usually take 4 years to complete.

Registered nurses practice within their scope of practice as defined by their license, their job description, and the facility in which they work. The shortage of employees in this profession has affected health care facilities across the country. The following job description provides an example of the roles and responsibilities of the registered nurse.

Registered Nurse Position Summary: Performs the functions of a registered nurse in the care of all assigned patients and works with assigned team members.

Responsibilities/Competencies

1. Demonstrates planning, treatment, direct care, and education of assigned patients.

2. Creates a plan of care and implements the plan for each patient assigned.

3. Coordinates care for assigned patients.

4. Directs and supervises the work of ancillary staff.

5. Maintains unit, department, and patient confidentiality.

6. Dispenses medication to patients according to health system policies and procedures.

7. Demonstrates collaboration and decision making with health care team members.

8. Assists and directs other staff in the care of patients.

9. Demonstrates continuing professional growth.

Licensed Practical Nurses

Licensed practical nurses (LPNs) are members of the health care team in many health care facilities (Figure 3-3). They have attended an approved program and passed a state test to be licensed as an LPN. These approved programs are often offered at community colleges and may be from 1 to 2 years in length. The scope of practice and the facility in which they are employed define their role on the health care team. Often, the LPN is the team member who most closely assists patients with their needs. The following job description describes the role of the LPN.

Licensed Practical Nurse Position Summary: Performs the functions required of a licensed practical nurse in the care of patients, in collaboration with a registered nurse.

Responsibilities/Competencies

1. Provides care to assigned patients:
   a. Monitors patients
   b. Records information on appropriate forms
   c. Reports information to appropriate person

2. Provides for patient
   a. Physical care
   b. Emotional care
   c. Psychological care
   d. Social care

3. Reviews and follows patient plan of care and participates in patient care conferences.

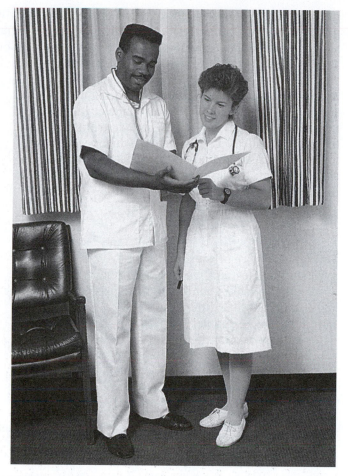

Figure 3-3 • *Licensed practical nurses provide care to patients and are members of the health care team.*

4. Administers medications

5. Performs procedures and treatments within the scope of practice.

6. Ensures patient safety, patient comfort, and patient privacy.

7. Maintains confidentiality for patient, unit or department, and health care facility.

8. Uses correct body mechanics.

9. Demonstrates correct setup and use of equipment and trouble-shoots equipment problems.

10. Provides education to patient and families.

11. Performs other duties as assigned.

Nursing Assistant (Aide)

Nursing assistants (or nurse aides) are members of the health care team who have limited formal education. This education or training may be provided at the work site or through technical programs provided by high schools, technical schools, community colleges, or privately operated programs. Education provided at the work site is called on-the-job training. This form of education usually involves a classroom introduction to the role of the nursing assistant with hands-on training sessions to follow. Each state and facility determine what skills the nursing assistant is able to perform in the health care facility. Nursing assistants who pass a certification test are titled certified nurse aide (CNAs). Some health care facilities require that their nursing assistants be certified. Nursing assistants who work in a long-term care facility must have completed a state-approved training program that is a minimum of 75 hours and must pass an examination to be certified or registered. The role of the nursing assistant is defined by the job description of the health care facility. These direct care providers are supervised and directed by the licensed nursing staff (Figure 3-4). Other job titles that are used for these care providers include care aides, nurse aides, nurse assistants, and certified nurse assistants. The following is an example of the roles and responsibilities of a nursing assistant.

Nursing Assistant Position Summary: The nursing assistant will assist in nursing care under the direction of the registered nurse.

Role/Responsibilities

1. Assists team members in the care of patients.

2. Orients patient and family to unit or department.

3. Interacts with patients of all ages.

4. Reports observations to the registered nurse or team leader.

5. Maintains patient records, and charts.

6. Maintains patient confidentiality.

7. Maintains unit or department confidentiality.

8. Performs other duties as requested.

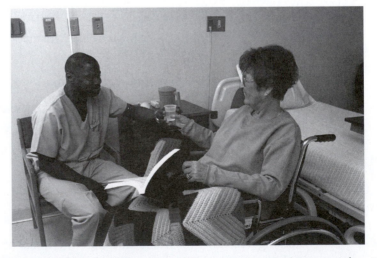

Figure 3-4 • *A nursing assistant provides care to patients under the supervision of the licensed nurse.*

Health Unit Coordinator

The health unit coordinator is the member of the health care team who provides clerical patient care. One description of the position's responsibilities is to transcribe orders and schedule diagnostic and therapeutic services for patients as requested by written physician orders. The health unit coordinator orchestrates all nursing unit communication and activities and interacts with all the nursing staff, communicating information to and receiving information from them to facilitate the quality of patient care (Figure 3-5). The health unit coordinator also communicates with physicians to resolve questions (Figure 3-6).

A health unit coordinator may have obtained the required education through post-secondary opportunities or an on-the-job training program. The health unit coordinator may be certified. Other job titles for this member of the health care team are ward clerk, unit clerk, ward secretary, and unit secretary.

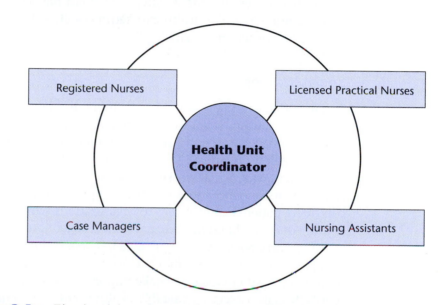

Figure 3-5 • *The health unit coordinator communicates with all the nursing staff members of the health care team.*

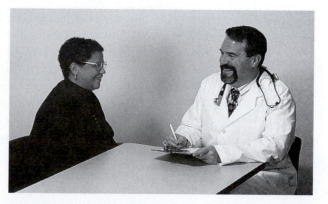

Figure 3-6 • *The health unit coordinator communicates with physicians to resolve questions.*

SUPPORT SERVICES

The staffs of support services are health care professionals who provide clinical and nonclinical services to the patient. Support services may include social workers, therapists, dietitians, pharmacists, and respiratory therapists. These support services are provided to patients who have an identified need. The need may be identified by current health care team members, the family of the patient, or the patient. The service is requested by the physician, and the referral (the physician's request) is communicated to the support service by the health unit coordinator. Communication of the referral may be by phone, computer entry, paper, or all three. The referral information is communicated to the nursing care team by following the procedure used in the health care facility. Patient care plans typically have a specific place to document this information.

Support services provided by members on the health care team are usually services that are visible in the patient areas. These services assist or complement patient care in the health care environment. After the patient has been discharged, support services may continue in a non-health-care setting, such as the patient's home, an extended-care facility, or senior housing.

Social Worker

Social workers assist the patient and family in preparing to have the patient leave the health care setting. Social workers are knowledgeable about the support services available in the community and are familiar with the insurance regulations, state and federal regulations, and all laws governing health care issues in the community in which they work. Social workers are aware of the support groups and support systems that patients may need to use as they prepare to return to their home. Social workers can direct patients and families to organizations within communities that offer needed health equipment and items at a free or reduced rate, meal service, and financial assistance options. Social workers are able to explain the laws and rules regarding extended-care placement. They are often the people who are able to communicate clearly with families and patients as they make important decisions about after-discharge arrangements. Social workers are valuable health care team members for patients and families because of their knowledge of resources and the location of those resources.

Therapists

Physical therapists, occupational therapists, and communication therapists provide therapy to patients when the physician requests these services. The therapy services can be provided in the inpatient and outpatient settings. The services are often started while the patient is in the hospital and continued after discharge. The therapists become members of the health care team, providing a support service to assist the patient in returning to the normal activities of daily living. The therapists set up programs to reach the goals the health care team has set. The health care team tracks the progress of the patient to meet those goals, and the program is adjusted as needed.

Dietitian

Nutritional status affects our healing and growth, and dietary intake affects nutritional status. Dietitians evaluate the patients' nutritional status and make recommendations for nutritional intake. They are important health care team members, observing the patients' intake, reviewing the patients' health history, and being knowledgeable about the patients' diagnoses and how it affects nutritional status. Using all of this information, as well as information from the other health care team members, the dietitian is able to create a nutritional plan for the patient that will meet the goals of the health care team.

Pharmacist

Pharmacists are members of the health care team who monitor the patients' medication. For many years, pharmacists had little to no patient interaction. Now pharmacists can be seen in the patient rooms, monitoring medications, providing information to the patients and families, and meeting with members of the health care team. The pharmacist is an important health care team member, educating the health care team on medications, making recommendations as to medication use, and carefully monitoring the patients' medication regimen for potential drug reactions or interactions.

Respiratory Therapist

Respiratory therapists (RTs) are health care team members who provide care for patients who need assistance with breathing. They provide oxygen therapy and respiratory treatments and perform respiratory testing (Figure 3-7). This support service can be provided as an inpatient service and may need to be continued after discharge. RTs also provide education, teaching patients and families important information about the lungs and the breathing function.

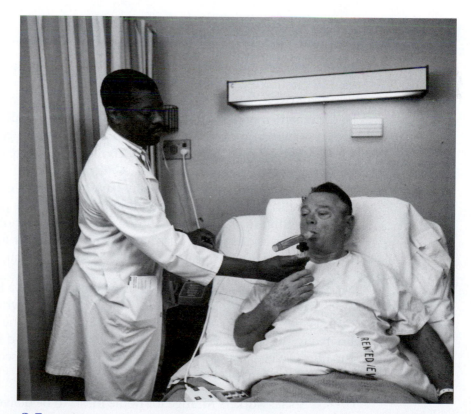

Figure 3-7 • *The respiratory therapist provides care for patients who need assistance with breathing.*

CREATION OF A HEALTH CARE TEAM

Each unit and each patient will have different health care team members. The team is created by the needs of the patient. The health care team members work to resolve those needs by providing the best possible care for the patient. Here is an example of the creation of a health care team.

Mr. Token is admitted to the Medical Nursing Unit. He is a 53-year-old male with a diagnosis of diabetes and renal failure. He is unable to walk alone. He has lost 25 pounds in the last 2 weeks. The nursing care team staff admits Mr. Token to his room and processes his admission. During the admission interview, the registered nurse notes that Mr. Token's knowledge of diabetes is minimal. The nurse makes a note to consult the diabetes educator (adding a member to the health care team). The diabetes educator visits the patient and asks about his food intake at home. The diabetes educator calls the dietitian (adding a member to the health care team). The health unit coordinator, after noting on Mr. Token's admission form that he does not have an insurance carrier listed, calls the social worker (adding a member to the health care team) to offer options for financial assistance. The physician who comes to see Mr. Token notes his difficulty with walking and orders a physical therapy consultation (adding a member to the health care team).

As one can see, Mr. Token now has a multidisciplinary health care team in place: a diabetes educator, a dietitian, a social worker, and a physical therapist, as well as the nursing staff and his physician. All team members are taking an active role in his health care.

HEALTH CARE TEAM COMMUNICATION

All members of the health care team need to communicate with each other to provide quality care for the patient. Health care team members may communicate with each other in person or by reviewing the documented information. This information may be documented on the patient chart in specific areas as defined by the health care facility's charting process. One health care provider may communicate with another in an informal setting. To ensure patient confidentiality, the team members should hold these conversations in areas where the information can be kept private. All units and departments in the health care facility have areas where conversations can be held privately. Health care teams may meet formally to discuss a patient and the plan of care. These meetings may be called staffings, patient plans, or discharge planning meetings if the focus is on discharge. These formal meetings allow for the health care team to discuss the patient and create a plan of care, or a care plan. Here is an example.

Mr. Smith is going to be discharged on Monday. He has a broken right leg and lives alone. He is 65 years old and has no family in the area where he lives. The health care team is meeting to discuss Mr. Smith's discharge plan. The health care team members invited to the staffing are the social worker, the registered nurse, the physical therapist, the nurse aide, and the health unit coordinator. After discussion, the team decides on the following care plan for Mr. Smith.

Social worker: Arrange for home meals to be delivered

Registered nurse: Explain the discharge plan to Mr. Smith

Physical therapist: Teach crutch walking before discharge

Health unit coordinator: Arrange for doctor visits and transportation to appointments

Nurse aide: Reinforce crutch walking skills and review discharge plan

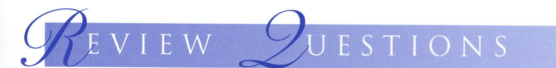

SUMMARY

Health care teams play an important role in the delivery of health care to patients. Teams can reduce the length of stay for patients, thereby reducing the cost of health care. Members of the teams share information and create patient care plans that provide the best possible care for patients. Often, all team members participate in "staffings," or meetings in which information and observations are discussed with goals then being formulated and plans being written. The frequency of these meetings depends on the patient's condition. Members of the team can be both clinical and nonclinical health care providers. Families and patients may also be active in these meetings.

REVIEW QUESTIONS

1. Explain the difference between clinical and nonclinical providers.

2. List five advantages of being accredited by JCAHO.

3. List four professions that may have members on a health care team.

4. List two advantages for patients that health care teams provide.

5. Explain why health care providers would choose to be members of health care teams.

THROUGH THE EYES

OF A HEALTH CARE PROFESSIONAL

As the nonclinical health care provider, the health unit coordinator relies on the clinical care team members to communicate necessary information so that the clerical aspects of patient care can be performed. All team members need each other to provide the best possible care for patients. The health unit coordinator shares with the clinical providers the patient information they need to know to perform their jobs, while protecting patient confidentially at all times. In turn, team members provide the health unit coordinator with patient information. Working as a team member is important to the flow of patient care.

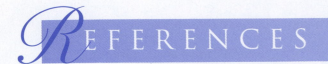

REFERENCES

Joint Commission on Accreditation of Health Care Organizations. *http://www.jcaho.org* Accessed November 2003.

Mosby's medical nursing and allied health dictionary (6th ed.). (2002). St. Louis, MO: Mosby.

Powell, S. (1996). *Nursing case management.* New York: Lippincott.

Simmers, L. (2004). *Diversified health occupations essentials* (6th ed.). Clifton Park, NY: Thomson Delmar Learning.

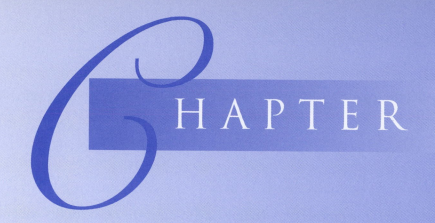

CHAPTER 4

Patient Care Delivery Systems

Learning Objectives

Upon completion of this chapter and review questions, the learner should be able to:

1. Explain three systems used to deliver patient care.

2. Describe the team model.

3. Discuss the importance of the patient care delivery systems.

Key Terms

case management   A management system in which the case manager reviews patient care and changes systems to reflect the best possible treatment with the best possible outcomes.

critical thinker   A member of the patient care delivery team who makes the critical decisions for the patients on the team, usually a registered nurse.

focused care   A patient care delivery system in which the patient is the focus of the care provided.

patient care   The process of providing care to meet the needs of the patient in the health care system.

team care   A system in which different members of a nursing care team provide patient care to the meet the patient's needs.

total patient care A patient care delivery system in which one care provider on each shift provides the entire care for a patient.

WHAT IS PATIENT CARE?

Patient care is the process of providing care to meet the needs of the patient in the health care system. It can be provided either directly or indirectly. It is directly provided when there is direct interaction between the patient and the caregiver. That interaction can be provided by a variety of health care workers. Indirect care is provided to patients through the health care system when the provider does not come into direct contact with the patient but rather provides care through a series of events or actions. An example of indirect patient care would be the patient care that is provided by a health unit coordinator.

HOW IS PATIENT CARE DELIVERED?

Patient care is provided by systems, and health care providers deliver it. The systems are designed to provide the best possible care to patients. Health care organizations use three main systems in providing health care to patients. Each unit or department within an organization uses the same basic system to meet patient care needs. These systems are total patient care, team care, and focused care.

TOTAL PATIENT CARE

Total patient care is a system in which one person provides all the health care needs for a patient on the assigned shift. When that care provider returns from a day off she or he again assumes the care of the same patient, provided of course, the patient is still in the unit or department. Most often in this system, registered nurses provide the total care.

The health unit coordinator interacts with each patient care provider in this delivery system as the need arises. For example, if the laboratory calls to verify whether a patient has been given a prescribed antibiotic dose, the health unit coordinator will contact the person providing care for that patient to obtain the information required by the lab. The health unit coordinator is responsible for the health care clerical needs of all the patients in the assigned unit or department.

TEAM CARE

Team care is a system in which different members of a nursing care team provide patient care to the meet the patient's needs. The team members may be registered, certified, licensed, or skilled. The state in which the health facility is located and the health facility itself determine the required professional level of each team member. Team care systems are designed to meet the needs of the health care system. Team members are assigned responsibilities on the basis of their skill and license levels. Health unit coordinators have defined responsibilities, within the team system, to provide the clerical patient care.

FOCUSED CARE

Focused care is a care delivery system that uses a variety of professional health care members to provide care to patients. The system uses a team approach, with a registered nurse being the team leader, or **critical thinker**. The role of the critical thinker is to solve problems, direct the health care team members, and coordinate the care of the patients who are part of the patient group. Other team members may include licensed practical nurses (LPNs), nurse aides, and registered nurses (RNs). It is these members who provide direct patient care. The health unit coordinator, another member of the team, provides indirect patient care. The health unit coordinator would contact the team leader to provide or request information concerning the patients. It would be the responsibility of the team leader to transmit the patient information that is required by the team members in performing their part in patient care. The focused care system became popular in the 1990s as health care facilities looked for ways to provide quality care and contain health care costs. The health unit coordinator is responsible for the clerical care for all patients that reside in the department or unit.

CASE MANAGEMENT

Case management is a patient management system that uses a case manager (a registered nurse) to review and analyze data regarding patient population types. The case manager then makes system changes, based on data gathered, to provide optimal care for patient types in the health care system. The changes are based not only on information gathered throughout the health care system but also on information gathered from similarly sized health care systems that provide similar services throughout the country. The goal of case management is to provide patients with the services and care that will afford them the shortest possible hospital stay with the best possible results. As health care systems look to provide the best possible care for patients, case managers become a valuable resource in the patient care delivery system. Health unit coordinators assist case managers by gathering data and providing needed information.

GOALS OF PATIENT CARE DELIVERY SYSTEMS

The goals of any patient care delivery system are to provide the best possible care for the patient population served and to provide it in the most cost-effective method. The system that is used in any specific health care facility can be a combination of team nursing and total patient care, as unique to its area as is its patient population. The health unit coordinator plays an important role in the patient care delivery system by providing the nonclinical portion of patient care.

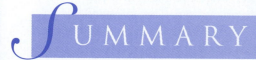

SUMMARY

Patient care delivery systems provide care to patients in health care systems. The systems are developed to meet the needs of both the patients and the health care providers. Health care is provided to patients through health care teams or through individual health care providers. Health care systems are continually evaluated and reviewed by case managers and peers in a never-ending quest to ensure that the best possible care is provided through the best possible system for the wisest use of health care dollars. The health unit coordinator provides nonclinical patient care.

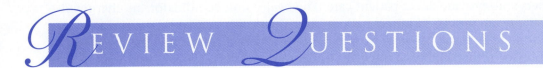

REVIEW QUESTIONS

1. List the members of the focused care team.

2. Describe the total patient care delivery system.

3. Explain the value to the patient of patient care delivered by patient care teams.

4. Name three goals of patient care delivery systems.

5. Explain the value of case management.

6. "All patient care delivery systems are the same." Is that statement true or false?

7. List who can deliver hands-on patient care.

8. What items are considered when deciding how patient care will be delivered at a health care facility?

9. "The health unit coordinator provides clerical patient care." Is that statement true or false?

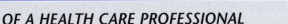

THROUGH THE EYES

OF A HEALTH CARE PROFESSIONAL

When patient care is delivered using the focused care model, the critical thinker and the health unit coordinator rely on each other to share information that is important in delivering care to the patient. The communication allows each member to function in the role assigned. It is important that the health unit coordinator understand how care is provided to the patient, which system is used, and the roles and responsibilities of each member in the delivery system. This knowledge enables the health unit coordinator to contact the correct co-worker regarding the information, thereby saving time. The health unit coordinator has a key role in the delivery system.

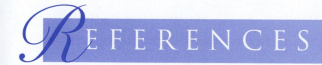

Porter-O'Grady, T. (1995). *The leadership evolution in health care.* Gaithersburg, MD: Aspen.

Powell, S. (1996). *Nursing case management: A guide to success in managed care.* Philadelphia: Lipponcott-Raven.

Sloane, R. M. (1999). *Introduction to health care delivery organizations* (4th ed.). Chicago: Health Administration Press.

Wilkinson, J. (1996). *Nursing process: A critical thinking approach* (2nd ed.). Menlo Park, CA: Addison-Wesley Nursing.

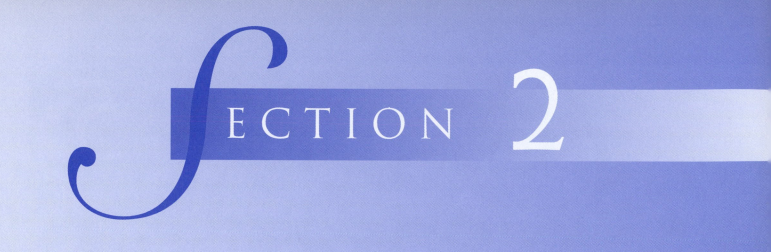

SECTION 2

Coordination of the Unit/Department

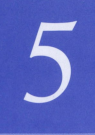
Your Department

Learning Objectives

Upon completion of this chapter and review questions, the learner should be able to:

1. Define key terms.

2. List the supplies and equipment at the health unit coordinator work area.

3. List the reference material at the health unit coordinator work area.

4. List sources of information for the patient activity form.

5. Describe the types of requests made of the health unit coordinator.

Key Terms

acuity The severity of the patient's condition and the level of care needed for the patient.

acute A rapid onset and a short but severe course.

chronic Long-lasting and recurrent.

department A division, a section, or a separate part of a whole; a unit.

drug formulary A listing of medications available in the facility's pharmacy.

dumbwaiter Small mechanical pulley elevator large and sturdy enough to allow for portable equipment and supplies to be sent up vertically through the floors of the facility.

patient classification system   A manual or computerized method used to determine patient acuity levels. The patient classification system addresses criteria such as the tasks and characteristics associated with each patient. It is a method of determining, validating, and monitoring individual patient care requirements over time.

Physician's Desk Reference (PDR)   A medication reference book.

pneumatic tube system   Similar to the pneumatic tube system used at drive-through banks. Items that fit into the plastic tube receptacle can be routed through the facility's pneumatic tube system.

unit   A division, a section, a subgroup with a special function; a department.

unit census   A list of the names of all the patients within the unit and demographic information about each patient.

THE WORK ENVIRONMENT OF THE HEALTH UNIT COORDINATOR

Traditionally, the health unit coordinator worked in the inpatient nursing unit in a hospital. As health care services have evolved, so has the health unit coordinator work environment. It is feasible that a person with health unit coordinating skills could work in any facility that provides health care. Examples of health care facilities include hospitals, clinics, physicians' offices, surgery centers, rehabilitation centers, and nursing homes. In addition to working in an inpatient nursing unit, a health unit coordinator may work in an outpatient department such as outpatient services or dialysis, a physician's office or clinic, or a long-term facility such as substance abuse rehabilitation or an extended-care facility for the elderly. Within the facility, the employer will assign the health unit coordinator to work in a unit or department where patients receive some type of service or treatment.

WORKING IN AN INPATIENT OR OUTPATIENT SETTING

In Chapter 3, inpatient and outpatient health care facilities were defined. A department in which the patient receives care for a period of less than 24 hours is an outpatient department. When a patient receives services from an outpatient department, it is planned for the patient to go home after the service or treatment is completed. An example of an outpatient department would be the laboratory or same-day surgery.

A department in which a patient receives care for more than 24 hours is an inpatient unit. When the patient receives services from an inpatient unit, it is planned for the patient to stay overnight, or longer, at the health care facility. Inpatient health care facilities may be divided into short-term, **acute** care facilities or long-term, **chronic** care facilities. An example of a short-term health care facility would be a hospital, and an example of a long-term health care facility would be a nursing home.

Patients who need health care may use any combination of the inpatient and outpatient departments and both the short-term and long-term health care facilities. For example, a patient may go to a health care facility for outpatient diagnostic exams. During the outpatient exam, it may be determined that the patient needs surgery. The patient would then have the surgery in a short-term health care facility and recover in an inpatient department. Then, if it is determined that the patient needs additional recovery and therapy, the patient could be sent to a long-term inpatient rehabilitation facility.

DEFINITIONS OF DEPARTMENTS

Health care facilities are separated into divisions. The specialized divisions provide unique services or tasks. The divisions or departments within a health care facility are created to best manage the delivery of services to their customers. Departments within the health care facility may be open for set hours such as 7:00 A.M. to 5:00 P.M., or they may be open to provide 24-hour care, 7 days a week, 365 days a year. Among the departments are diagnostic and treatment departments, departments that offer various types of services and support for the patient and patient family members, and, of course, the nursing department. The nursing department is composed of nurse managers, nurse specialists, and nurses as the caregivers, along with nursing assistants, unit aides, and health unit coordinators. The number and type of departments will depend on the size and structure of the health care facility. A small facility may have only a few departments, or the departments may provide more than one type of service. For example, in a smaller facility, there may be one inpatient nursing unit that provides care for patients with medical, surgical, and neurological diagnoses. At larger facilities, there might be a separate nursing unit to provide health care to each separate group of medical patients, surgical patients, and neurological patients. Still larger facilities may have many departments and be very specialized. For example, they may have a separately functioning inpatient nursing unit for various categories of surgical patients, such as a separate nursing unit for orthopedic surgical patients, one for gastrointestinal surgical patients, and one for urological surgical patients.

The terms **unit** and **department** may be used interchangeably to describe the divisions of services within the health care facility. However, the term *unit* is usually used to refer to an area that provides nursing services to inpatients. Nursing units are divided into areas in which patients require similar types of nursing care. The term *unit* has replaced the term *ward*. For example, the term *unit* is used for the intensive care unit, the orthopedics unit, or the pediatrics unit nursing areas. These areas are where patients are receiving continuous nursing care. Usually the term *department* is used to refer to an area that provides services to outpatients or an area that provides one-time or limited-time services. The term *department* is used for the emergency department, the radiology department, and the physical therapy department.

Outpatient Departments

An outpatient department provides services to patients during set or scheduled hours. Generally, outpatients come to the health system for a specific reason at a specific time. It is anticipated that the outpatient will leave the facility after the appointment. Outpatient services can be one-time or ongoing services. Typical health care services offered by departments in outpatient facilities are:

> *Emergency department (ED).* A department that provides immediate medical attention. Many of the services offered by this department are on a one-time basis, but some medical problems require follow-up treatments in other departments of the health care facility (Figure 5-1).

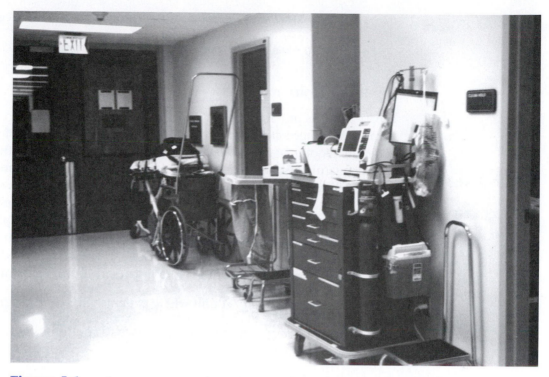

Figure 5-1 • *An emergency department of a hospital (Courtesy of All Saints Health Care, Racine, WI)*

Emergency room (ER). Another name for the emergency department.

Genetics. A department that provides genetic testing or tests that provide information about inherited diseases. This service would probably be done in just one or two visits.

Hemodialysis. A department with dialysis machines that are used to cleanse blood for patients whose kidneys are not able to filter blood. Usually this is an ongoing service, perhaps done every few days.

Outpatient surgery (OPS). A unit where a patient will go before and after an operation that does not require an overnight stay. It is usually a one-time service.

Physical Medicine & Rehabilitation (PM&R). A department or group of departments that provides services to patients needing physical, occupational, vocational, or speech/communication therapy. The service provided by this department is usually ongoing.

Prenatal clinic. A department that provides ongoing services to patients during their pregnancy.

Radiology (x-ray). A department with equipment that makes images of internal organs and bones. This is usually a one-time service.

Same-day surgery (SDS). Another name for outpatient surgery. As its name implies, it is typically a one-time service.

Sleep lab. A department that diagnoses and treats sleep disorders.

Sports medicine. A department that provides health services for athletes.

Trauma services. A department that treats serious or critical bodily injuries.

Inpatient Units

Inpatient units provide services to patients who generally come to the health system because they need care for more than a short, specified period of time. Inpatients generally require 24-hour-a-day nursing care. Inpatient stays at the health care facility may be planned (scheduled in advance), or they may be unplanned. An example of a planned inpatient stay would be the case of a patient who has orthopedic surgery scheduled in advance for a specific date and it is known that the surgery will require the patient to be hospitalized for an overnight period. An example of an unplanned inpatient stay would be the case of a patient who goes to the emergency department with a rapid onset of chest pain and nausea and then is admitted to the cardiac inpatient unit for further monitoring. Other inpatient health care units are:

Cardiology (cardio). A unit where patients with heart diagnoses are admitted.

Endocrinology. A unit where patients with conditions related to internal ailments or hormonal secretions are admitted.

General (Gen). Same as medical unit.

Medical (Med). A unit where patients with medical diagnoses are admitted (Figure 5-2).

Nephrology. A unit where patients with kidney diagnoses are admitted.

Neurology (Neuro). A unit where patients with nervous system diagnoses are admitted.

Oncology (Onc). A unit where patients with cancer are admitted.

Operating room (OR). The department where surgery is performed.

Orthopedic (Ortho). A unit where patients with orthopedic or bone diagnoses are admitted.

Pediatrics (Peds). A unit where children are admitted.

Postanesthesia care unit (PACU). The department where surgical patients recover after receiving a general anesthetic during an operation.

Preoperative unit (Pre-op). The department where a patient is prepared for an operation.

Progressive care unit/step down. A unit with special monitoring equipment. It may be a unit that provides a level of care between intensive and general.

Pulmonology. A unit where patients with lung or respiratory diagnoses are admitted.

Surgical (Surg). A unit where patients with scheduled inpatient surgery are admitted.

Telemetry. A cardiac unit with special heart-monitoring equipment.

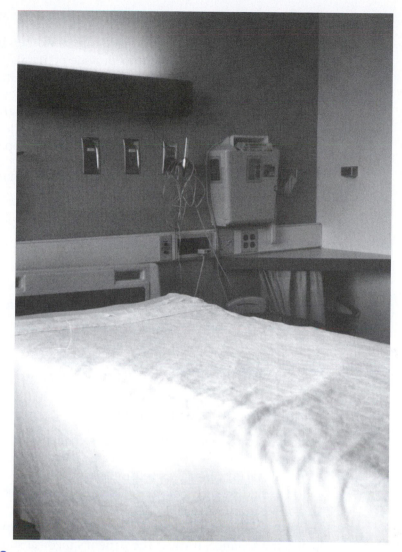

Figure 5-2 • *A medical inpatient bed in a hospital (Courtesy of All Saints Health Care, Racine, WI)*

Intensive Care Units

Intensive care units provide care to patients who need an elevated level of care. In an intensive care unit, the health care staff-to-patient ratio is lower than that of a general inpatient unit. An intensive care nurse may be responsible for only one or two patients, depending on the level of care required. Intensive care units are equipped with specialized monitoring equipment and technology and are often named for the type of patients they serve. Examples of some intensive care units are:

> *Coronary intensive care unit* (CICU)
>
> *Medical intensive care unit* (MICU)
>
> *Neonatal intensive care unit* (NICU)
>
> *Pediatric intensive care unit* (PICU)
>
> *Surgical intensive care unit* (SICU)

Mother/Baby Inpatient Units

Mother/baby inpatient units provide care to women before, during, and after pregnancy. That is, mother/baby units provide prenatal, perinatal, and postnatal care. The departments that provide care to the newborn infant (neonatal units) are also included in the mother/baby units. The trend in most health care facilities is to have the mothers and babies in the same room rather than having separate areas for each. However, a separate nursery unit is staffed to provide care for the babies who are not in the mothers' room. Examples of mother/baby departments are:

High-risk perinatal (HRP). The department that provides services to patients with high-risk pregnancies.

Labor and delivery (L&D). The department where mothers in labor are admitted and babies are delivered.

Nursery. A unit for newborns.

Postpartum (PP). The department where patients are admitted after they have a baby.

Postpartum recovery (PPR). The department where patients who have delivered a baby recover.

Long-Term Units or Facilities

Long-term care facilities provide care to patients who need a longer duration of care than can be provided by an acute care facility. Before a patient is admitted to a long-term care facility, he or she must meet the criteria of the facility. For example, a patient who has had surgery may have had a few days of recovery time in an inpatient unit in a short-term care facility. The patient is probably in stable condition but may be unable to perform activities of daily living such as hygiene, getting dressed, or walking without assistance. Because the patient's medical status is stable, the patient no longer needs the type of care provided by the short-term care facility, but he is not ready to care for himself at home either. This patient would be a candidate for a long-term health care facility. Examples of long-term care departments or facilities are:

Behavioral health. A unit or facility for patients with psychiatric or mental illness diagnosis.

Extended-care facility. A facility that provides long-term inpatient care, such as a nursing home.

Home care. A department that provides care and equipment to patients in their homes.

Hospice. A department or facility that provides inpatient or outpatient care to terminally ill patients.

Rehabilitation. A unit or facility for patients with physical disabilities requiring therapy, such as a stroke or motor vehicle accident patient.

Substance abuse/addiction. A department or facility for patients with addiction diagnoses.

HEALTH UNIT COORDINATOR WORKSTATIONS

A health unit coordinator could be employed in almost any one of the outpatient departments or units listed, or at any one of the inpatient departments or units. It takes little imagination to see that the work environment in a coronary intensive care unit of a large facility would be considerably different from what it would be in a mother/baby unit or in a neurology unit. However, regardless of the environment, the patients and their families expect, and are entitled to, efficient, accurate, and understanding health care. The health unit coordinator plays a vital role in providing this expected level of care by carrying out the responsibilities of coordinating the nonclinical activities of the unit.

WORK AREA

The health unit coordinator shares the workstation with the team of health care members described in Chapter 3. The health unit coordinator most likely will have an assigned work area within the workstation. Some health care facilities have centralized workstations (Figure 5-3), and others have decentralized workstations (Figure 5-4). The difference is that, in the centralized workstation, all the patients' charts are kept at the desk, whereas in the decentralized workstation the patients' charts are kept in an individual cabinet outside each patient's room. However, regardless of whether the workstation is centralized or decentralized, the health unit coordinator's work area should have ready access to the phones, the computer or information system, and the intercom or paging system. The health unit coordinator also utilizes imprinters or labeling machines, printers, and facsimile machines. The health unit coordinator needs to know how to operate and maintain the equipment at the work area.

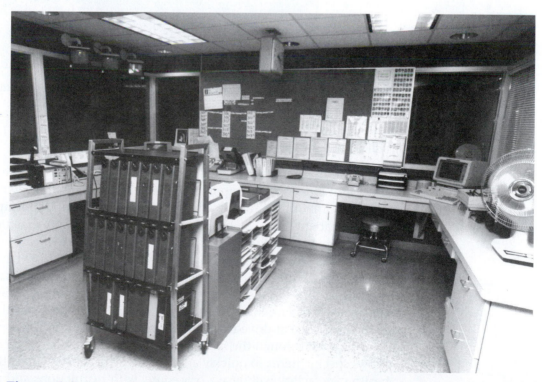

Figure 5-3 • *A centralized workstation* (Courtesy of Aurora Health Care)

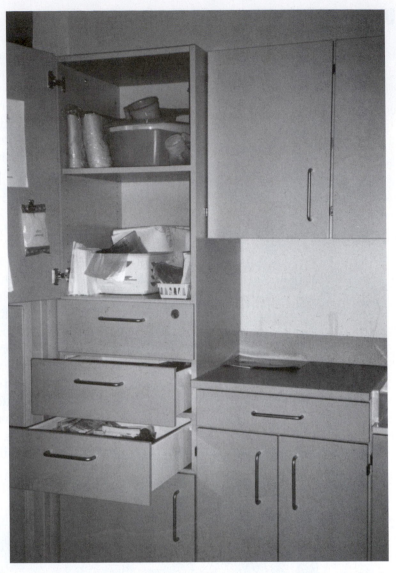

Figure 5-4 • *A decentralized workstation (Courtesy of All Saints Health Care, Racine, WI)*

SUPPLIES AND EQUIPMENT

It is the responsibility of the health unit coordinator to coordinate the ordering, storage, and maintenance of the supplies, forms, and equipment needed to ensure that the unit runs smoothly. Faulty or missing equipment, forms, and supplies can lead to a delay in patient care. The health unit coordinator's responsibilities regarding supplies and equipment are discussed in detail in Chapter 9. The health unit coordinator needs to know where items are stored and how they are ordered. The health unit coordinator also needs to know the delivery and pickup process for supplies and equipment. Many health care facilities use a **pneumatic tube system** interconnected throughout the departments (Figure 5-5). The pneumatic tube system in a health care facility is similar to the ones used at drive-through banks. Items that fit into the plastic tube receptacle can be routed through the facility's pneumatic tube system. The pneumatic tube system allows specific items to quickly arrive at the department where they are needed. The health care facility will have a procedure, with instructions and restrictions, on how to operate the pneumatic tube system.

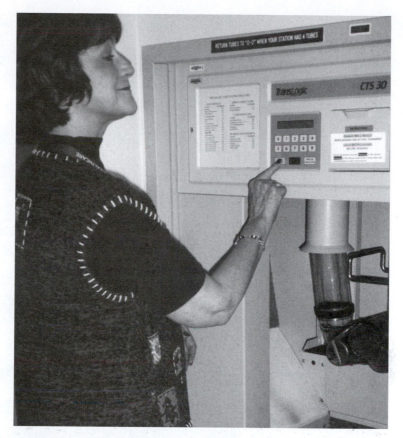

Figure 5-5 • *A pneumatic tube station (Courtesy of All Saints Health Care, Racine, WI)*

Health care facilities may also use dumbwaiters for delivery of supplies. **Dumbwaiters** are small mechanical pulley elevators large and sturdy enough to allow for portable equipment and supplies to be sent up vertically through the floors of the facility (Figure 5-6). The dumbwaiter is a time saver and allows those items transported in the system to arrive quickly. Examples of items that are delivered via the dumbwaiter include linen and equipment needed for patient treatments such as infusion pumps, dressings, and tubing kits. The dumbwaiters are often nicknamed "dummies," so don't be surprised if the health unit coordinator states he is going to the "dummy."

REFERENCE MATERIAL

The health unit coordinator will have a collection of reference material in the work area or access to reference materials on the computer network (Figure 5-7). Reference material may be kept as forms and hard copies in notebook binders or may be kept as files and programs within the computer network. The health unit coordinator needs to know the type and location of reference material available on the unit. Using the reference material will increase the health unit coordinator's knowledge. It is especially important to be able to look up procedures and tests as well as how to correctly spell medical terms. The health unit coordinator may be responsible for the maintenance of some of the reference material on the unit. For example, the health unit coordinator may add, update, and delete the material in the policy and procedure manuals.

The health unit coordinator is a valuable resource person for the health care team. By being familiar with the resource materials, he or she can assist other staff members in

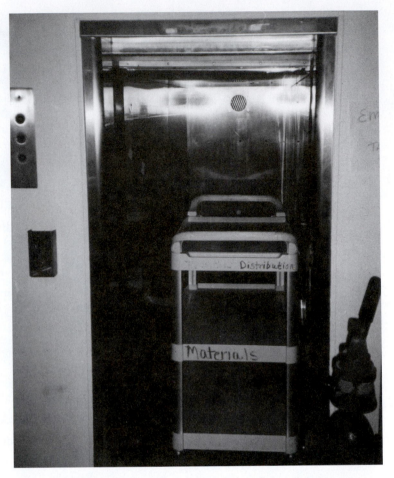

Figure 5-6 • *A dumbwaiter (Courtesy of All Saints Health Care, Racine, WI)*

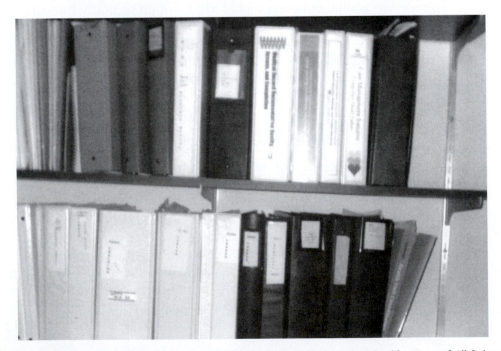

Figure 5-7 • *Reference books used on a patient care unit (Courtesy of All Saints Health Care, Racine, WI)*

the use of these materials. Knowledge of the reference material will assist the coordinator in being a resource person for both staff and visitors. Examples of reference material include:

Medical encyclopedia. A dictionary of medical terms. It may be used to check the spelling and definitions of diagnoses, and surgical and medical procedures.

Physician's Desk Reference (PDR). A medication reference book. It may be used to find a generic or brand name of a medication, assist in the correct spelling of the medication, and answer questions about medication dosages and interactions.

Drug formulary. A listing of medications available in the facility's pharmacy. It may be used to check if a particular medication is used in the facility.

Policy and procedure manuals. Manuals from various departments within the facility that provide the health unit coordinator with a wealth of information. They may be used to find information about visiting regulations, troubleshooting equipment problems, or preparing patients for examinations.

HEALTH UNIT COORDINATOR RESPONSIBILITIES

The health unit coordinator is responsible for maintaining certain facility records and for facilitating the operation of the unit.

DEPARTMENT CENSUS

The health unit coordinator is usually responsible for the department or **unit census**. The unit census lists the names of all the patients within the unit and demographic information about each patient. The census lists the admitting date and physician and the room number of each patient. The health unit coordinator is responsible for manually listing the patients on the census. Usually, the census is generated from the hospital information system.

If a computerized census is used, the health unit coordinator should expect to be responsible for generating and checking the changes once every shift or once every 24 hours. The health unit coordinator can use the census as a reference when the admitting or registration department calls the unit to admit a new patient. An up-to-date census will assist the health unit coordinator in making room assignments or scheduling new patients.

PATIENT ACUITY

The health unit coordinator will also be responsible for entering or tracking information and reports about patient **acuity**. Patient acuity addresses the severity of the patient's condition and the level of care needed for the patient. Health care facilities use **patient classification systems** to determine acuity levels. The patient classification system is a method of determining, validating, and monitoring individual patient care requirements over time. It may be manual or computerized. The patient classification system addresses criteria such as the tasks and characteristics associated with each patient. For example, the Expert Nurse Estimation Patient Classification System (ENEPCS) identifies the uniqueness of each patient using eight categories of care:

Cognitive status

Self-care status

Emotional, psychosocial support needs

Comfort/pain management needs

Family information and support needs

Treatment needs

Interdisciplinary coordination, patient teaching, and documentation needs

Transition planning needs

Patient classification systems such as this greatly assist the health care facility in providing flexible and effective staffing, balancing patient assignments, and preparing budgets. The information provided by a patient classification system can be useful in determining the staffing needs for the upcoming shift. The data entered into patient classification systems by the health unit coordinator consist largely of clinical information determined by clinical staff personnel.

PATIENT ACTIVITY FORM OR BOARD

The health unit coordinator is responsible for knowing where patients are at all times and needs to use some type of tool to track the patients. This tool may be a patient activity form or a patient activity board. Whether using a form or a board, the health unit coordinator must ensure that confidential information is not displayed in sight of visitors. The health unit coordinator may gather information for the patient activity form through a variety of sources, such as:

Change of shift report. The health unit coordinator may listen to the clinical staff's change of shift report to learn about the activities of the patient, or the health unit coordinators may have a nonclinical change of shift report.

Electronic patient tracking system. Some health care facilities use an electronic patient tracking system. With this system, each patient has a unique bar code printed on his or her identification band. The identification band with the bar code is scanned when a patient enters and exits a department. For example, if a patient is going to radiology for tests, the person transporting the patient scans the patient's bar code when the patient arrives in radiology and again when the patient leaves radiology. This scanned information is transmitted by the scanner to the centralized information system. An employee who wants to know the location of a patient can access the scanned information from the computer.

Patient chart/Kardex. The health unit coordinator may access information directly from the patient's chart or Kardex.

Sign in/out form. If someone removes the patient from the department, a form should be signed stating the time of departure, the destination, and the name of the individual who transported the patient (Figure 5-8).

PATIENT TRANSPORTATION LOG

Date

	W/Chart	Cardiac Ser	CT	DX	US	MRI	Pulmonary	PT	OT	Other
Patient name & room # Time– off unit Time returned										
Patient name & room # Time– off unit Time returned										
Patient name & room # Time– off unit Time returned										
Patient name & room # Time– off unit Time returned										
Patient name & room # Time– off unit Time returned										
Patient name & room # Time– off unit Time returned										
Patient name & room # Time– off unit Time returned										
Patient name & room # Time– off unit Time returned										
Patient name & room # Time– off unit Time returned										
Patient name & room # Time– off unit Time returned										

Figure 5-8 • *A sign-in and sign-out form*

COORDINATING REQUESTS

The health unit coordinator is often the central communications person within the health care team and is often the first contact a patient has within a department or unit. Because the health unit coordinator coordinates requests from visitors and staff, communication skills are a key requirement of the health unit coordinator's job.

Family and Visitor Requests

Family and visitors will ask the health unit coordinator about the patient's status. The health unit coordinator must know the facility's policies for release of information about patients. Questions about a patient's condition or treatment should be referred to the clinical team member caring for the patient. Family and visitors will also ask questions about the health care facility. The health unit coordinator needs to be familiar with the policies and procedures about visiting regulations. It is not important for the health unit coordinator to know all the answers to all of the questions. What is important is for the health unit coordinator to know the resources for the answers.

As a health unit coordinator gains experience and knowledge, he or she will be able to determine what questions may be answered and what questions should be referred to another health care team member. For example, if a visitor tells the health unit coordinator that a patient is experiencing pain, the health unit coordinator should know to convey the information to a clinical team member working with the patient. If someone asks the health unit coordinator for directions to another department within the facility, the health unit coordinator should be able to provide the answer directly or else know how to find the answer.

If a clinical team member tells the health unit coordinator that the patient's room is too cold, the health unit coordinator should contact the appropriate party to make a temperature adjustment in the patient's room. However, if a nonclinical team member or a visitor tells the health unit coordinator that the patient's room is too cold, the health unit coordinator should refer this information to the clinical person caring for the patient because the patient may be cold because of his medical condition instead of the room temperature. Until the health unit coordinator gains experience, it is best to err on the side of safety and refer any requests that make him or her uncomfortable or unsure to one of the clinical care providers.

Staff Requests

The health unit coordinator is also the resource for the staff at the health care facility. The health unit coordinator supports the health care team by being their resource person and by answering their requests. Staff requests may include:

- ◆ Location of a patient
- ◆ Location of a chart
- ◆ Contacting a physician or family member
- ◆ Finding the results of a diagnostic test
- ◆ Contacting another department for supplies or equipment
- ◆ Locating the form or process for requesting a day off

The health unit coordinator will also answer requests from the staff of other departments within the health care facility, such as:

◆ Confirming the date and time for a scheduled diagnostic exam

◆ Finding out if a patient has had his meals held for preparation for an exam

◆ Finding phone numbers of the patient's relatives

◆ Assigning a room number for a newly admitted patient

ORGANIZATIONAL SKILLS

The health unit coordinator must use organizational skills to coordinate the work area. Coordinating the work area involves maintaining an adequate supply of forms and supplies to keep the department functioning effectively, operating and troubleshooting the department equipment, and maintaining and updating the patient census and acuity classification system and other department logs. In addition to having good organizational skills, the health unit coordinator must be able to work independently and must have good time management skills.

SUMMARY

Health unit coordinators work in a variety of settings. In this book, the role of the health unit coordinator has been described as the hub or center of activity. This key role is evident when observing the health unit coordinator in the work environment. The health unit coordinator coordinates requests from physicians, nurses, patients, families, visitors, and staff. Whether in an inpatient or an outpatient setting, the work environment will be one of high activity. Although the workstation is a shared area, the health unit coordinator is the most visible resource in the unit. The health unit coordinator maintains control and organization as physicians, nurses, patients, visitors, and staff enter and exit the unit or department.

REVIEW QUESTIONS

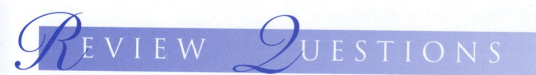

1. Write out the terms for the following abbreviations.
   a. OPS
   b. ONC
   c. OR
   d. Med
   e. Surg

f. Peds

g. ED

h. Ortho

i. Cardio

j. L&D

k. PACU

l. Neuro

Match the request in the left column to the reference in the right column.

2. A health unit coordinator finds the printer is jammed.　　a. PDR

3. A nurse asks for the spelling of an operation.　　b. Medical encyclopedia

4. A health unit coordinator is looking for the generic name for a brand name medication listed in the patient's chart.　　c. Information Systems Policy & Procedure Manual

5. Where might the health unit coordinator obtain information for the patient activity board?

6. "The health unit coordinator is expected to know the answers to all the questions from visitors and staff at the workstation." Is this statement true or false?

NAHUC CERTIFICATION EXAM

CONTENT AREAS

I. A. 4　Prioritize orders and tasks

I. C. 1　Request services from ancillary departments

I. C. 2　Request services from support departments

I. C. 3　Request supplies and equipment

II. D. 1　Maintain a supply of chart forms

II. D. 2　Maintain stock of patient care supplies and equipment

II. D. 3　Maintain stock of clerical and desk supplies

II. D. 6　Maintain unit bulletin board

II. D. 7　Maintain policy and procedures manuals

II. D. 8　Monitor patients' off-unit locations

II. D. 9   Arrange for maintenance and repair of equipment

II. E. 1   Report unit activities to on-coming shift

II. E. 2   Maintain patient census logs

II. E. 3   Record patient acuity

II. E. 4   Record unit/department statistics

II. E. 6   Maintain patient census boards

II. E. 8   Maintain patient assignment board

II. E. 14 Inventory unit equipment

II. F. 7   Respond to patient, physician, visitor, and facility staff requests and complaints

THROUGH THE EYES

OF A HEALTH CARE PROFESSIONAL

I work as a health unit coordinator float. That means that not any one specific department or unit is my "home" unit. Before the beginning of my shift, I report to the nursing office. The scheduler in the nursing office assigns me to a unit or department where there is no unit coordinator available for that particular shift. For example, I may fill in for a health unit coordinator who is sick or on vacation. I enjoy floating from department to department. I have a wide pool of co-workers, and the unit where I am assigned is very grateful their vacancy has been filled. I also get to see a wide range of physician orders. I have learned about the commonly performed tests in many specialty departments. It can be unsettling at times when I never know from one day to the next on which unit I'll be working, but the variety of settings and relationships I have experienced is well worth it to me.

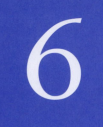
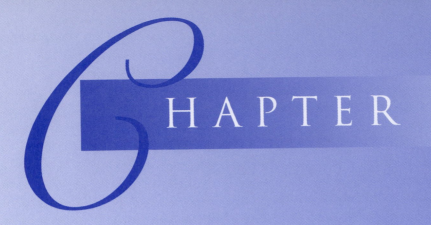

An Introduction to Ancillary Departments

Learning Objectives

Upon completion of this chapter and review questions, the learner should be able to:

1. Define *cardiology*.

2. Define *phlebotomist*.

3. Discuss the various functions of a hospital pharmacist.

4. Discuss three functions of the food management and nutrition services department.

5. Explain in which diagnostic department most endoscopies are performed.

6. Explain the decentralized hospital pharmacy system.

7. Explain pulmonary medicine.

8. List four divisions within the clinical laboratory department.

9. List at least four divisions of the radiology department.

10. Name two distinct areas of the dietary department.

11. Describe three areas in physical medicine.

Key Terms

angiography X-ray study of the inside of the heart and blood vessels. It is done after a dye is injected.

cardiac catheterization A test in which a long tube is passed into the heart through a large blood vessel in an arm or a leg.

cardiology The study of the heart.

clinical laboratory A room or building equipped for scientific experimentation, research, testing, and analysis of body fluids and tissues.

computerized tomography A technique for examining internal structures of the body that shows a detailed cross section of tissue structure. A CT image (called a scan) is a highly accurate picture that shows the relationships of structures to each other.

diagnose To determine the type and cause of a health condition on the basis of a patient's signs and symptoms, laboratory tests, and information about family and occupational background as well as recent injuries or exposure to dangerous substances.

diagnostic departments Areas of a hospital, clinic, or long-term health care facility that examine the patient with specialized equipment to determine the nature or the cause of the disease as well as the extent of the injury or illness.

diagnostic x-ray Electromagnetic radiation of shorter wavelength than visible light. X-rays can go through most substances and are used to investigate the integrity of certain structures.

endoscopic General term regarding visual examination of the body organs or cavities.

gastroenterologist A physician who specializes in gastroenterology.

gastroenterology The study of the stomach, intestines, and related structures such as the esophagus, liver, gallbladder, and pancreas.

gastrology The study of the function and diseases of the stomach.

magnetic resonance imaging A noninvasive diagnostic technique that produces computerized images of internal body tissues and is based on nuclear magnetic resonance of atoms within the body induced by the application of radio waves.

mammography X-ray of the breast and its soft tissues.

nuclear medicine A branch of medicine that uses radioactive chemical elements in the diagnosis and treatment of disease.

occupational therapist A person licensed to work with patients who need help in activities of daily living.

occupational therapy The training of patients with physical injury or illness, mental disease, or learning problems to work and live by themselves despite any health problem that might keep the patient from living a normal life.

pathology The study of the traits, causes, and effects of disease, as seen in the structure and workings of the body.

phlebotomist One who draws blood from a vein.

physical therapist A person who is licensed to assist in testing and treating physically disabled patients.

physical therapy A profession that is responsible for the management of the patient's movement system.

pulmonary medicine Pertains to the lungs and the breathing system.

pulmonologist A physician who specializes in lung diseases.

radiology A branch of medicine that uses radiant energy such as x-rays or ultrasound to prevent, diagnose, and treat disease.

respiratory therapist A person who, under the guidance of a doctor, gives oxygen and helps patients do chest exercises to help patients with breathing difficulties.

respiratory therapy Any treatment that maintains or improves the function of the respiratory tract.

speech therapist A person trained in speech pathology who treats people with disorders affecting normal speech.

speech therapy Therapeutic treatment of speech defects.

therapeutic department A department in which patients receive treatment.

ultrasound The use of high-frequency sound to create images of the internal anatomy.

Abbreviations

ADL Activities of Daily Living

CT Computerized Tomography

MRI Magnetic Resonance Imaging

U/S Ultrasound

HOSPITAL DEPARTMENTS

There are many types of hospitals. There are privately owned hospitals, hospitals for profit, hospitals that are nonprofit, and hospitals that are owned by the state or federal government, such as a veteran's hospital. There are large hospitals and small hospitals (Figure 6-1). No matter the type of hospital, the universal mission is that of providing health care and health care education to their patients and the hospital community.

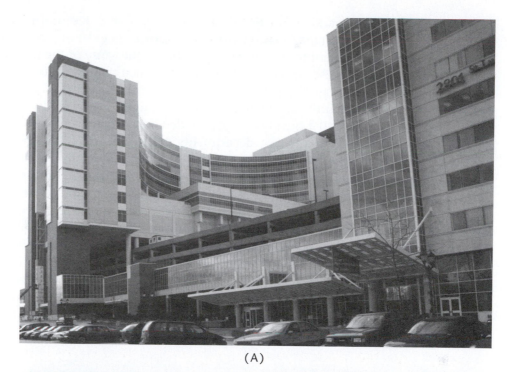

(A)

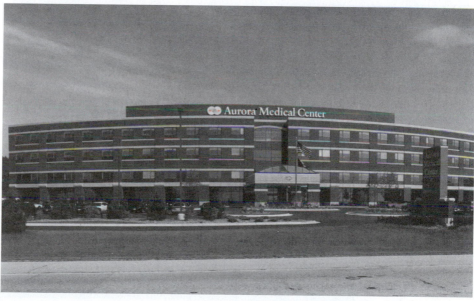

(B)

Figure 6-1 • *(A) A large hospital and (B) a small hospital are just two of many types of hospitals. (Courtesy of Aurora Health Care)*

Providing health care is more than just nursing the sick back to health. Before a patient is treated, the patient's attending physician will write orders describing which tests are needed for the patient's diagnosis. The health unit coordinator will communicate the orders to the correct department. Then personnel trained in a particular specialty and working in a department that has specialized equipment will examine the patient thoroughly.

The term **diagnose** means to determine the type and cause of a health condition on the basis of a patient's signs and symptoms, laboratory tests, and information about family and occupational background as well as recent injuries or exposure to dangerous substances. **Diagnostic departments** examine the patient with specialized equipment to determine the nature or the cause of the disease as well as the extent of the disease, injury, or illness. Other departments, known as **therapeutic departments** are departments in which patients are treated for their illness or injury. The health unit coordinator needs to communicate carefully with these departments to ensure that quality care is provided in an organized and efficient manner. There are numerous ancillary departments within a hospital that provide advanced diagnostic and therapeutic services. Some hospitals have more departments than other hospitals, depending on the size and location of the hospital. In this chapter, we will look at the various diagnostic and therapeutic departments and some of the people who work in those departments. The health unit coordinator will be requesting services from *all* ancillary departments. The health unit coordinator must always order tests and treatments with a focus on the right patient, the right examination or treatment, the right department, and the right date and time. This chapter presents some general information regarding these departments to give the reader a sense of all the services that need coordinating from the workstation. This chapter is an *introduction* to the departments; transcribing information for these departments is addressed in Section 9.

DIAGNOSTIC DEPARTMENTS

The diagnostic departments discussed in this chapter are cardiology; digestive disorders, or GI, lab; clinical laboratory; pulmonary diagnostics; and radiology.

CARDIOLOGY DEPARTMENT

Cardiology is the study of the heart. The cardiology department performs tests related to heart disease. The cardiologist, a physician who specializes in heart disease, will read and analyze cardiac tests, such as an electrocardiogram, and recommend appropriate treatment. Cardiology technicians are trained to use the various diagnostic equipment and perform the tests. The common examinations ordered from the cardiology department are listed in Table 6-1.

TABLE 6-1 Common Cardiology Examinations	
Echocardiogram	An exam using sound frequencies to study the function of the heart
Electrocardiogram (ECG, EKG)	An exam that records electrical impulses of the heart
Holter monitor	A device that monitors heart activity throughout the course of the day. A patient wears electrodes, and the heart activity is recorded on a small tape recorder that the patient wears around the waist or chest. The patient records in a diary physical activity throughout the day.

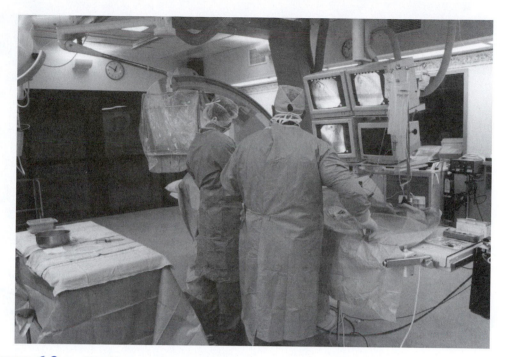

Figure 6-2 • *Cardiac catheterization lab (Courtesy of Aurora Health Care)*

In some hospitals cardiac catheterizations are done in the cardiology department. Larger hospitals may have a separate cardiac catheterization department (Figure 6-2). A **cardiac catheterization** is a diagnostic procedure in which a long tube is passed into the heart through a large blood vessel in an arm or a leg to diagnose heart disease.

DIGESTIVE DISORDERS DEPARTMENT, OR GI LAB

Gastrology is the study of the function and diseases of the stomach. **Gastroenterology** is the study of the stomach, intestines, and related structures such as the esophagus, liver, gallbladder, and pancreas. The GI (gastrointestinal) lab often performs numerous endoscopic studies. **Endoscopic** is a general term regarding the visual examination of the body organs or cavities. The exams are performed using a specific type of endoscope, or a fiberoptic instrument. These endoscopes or fiberoptic instruments can transmit light for better visualization. In addition to visualizing body organs and cavities, endoscopes can be used to administer medications or suction excess fluid as needed. Certain endoscopes can perform excisions, or removal of unwanted material (Figure 6-3).

Most digestive disorders departments are usually open from 8:00 A.M. to 5:00 P.M.

Gastroenterologists are specialists in the diagnosis and treatment of ailments involving the stomach, intestines, and related structures such as the esophagus, liver, gallbladder, and pancreas. They perform most of the examinations in the GI lab. Departmental secretaries and technicians assist them.

Table 6-2 defines common examinations ordered from the GI lab.

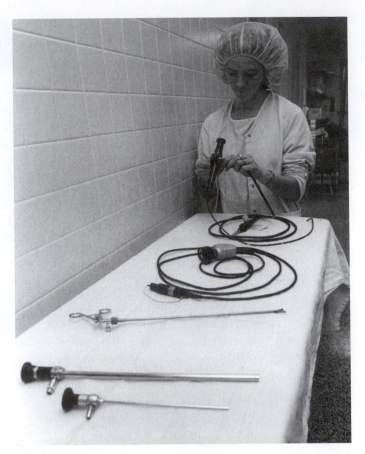

Figure 6-3 • *Endoscope used to perform excisions (Courtesy of Aurora Health Care)*

TABLE 6-2 Common GI Department Examinations	
Bronchoscopy	Visualization of the trachea, bronchi, and bronchial tree using a bronchoscope
Colonoscopy	Visualization of the lining of the large intestine using a colonoscope
Gastroscopy	Visualization of the inside of the stomach by a gastroscope inserted through the esophagus
Proctoscopy	Visualization of the rectum and lower end of the colon using a proctoscope

CLINICAL LABORATORY, OR PATHOLOGY DEPARTMENT

The **clinical laboratory**, or **pathology department**, is an area where tests on blood, urine, sputum, and other body fluids are analyzed for diagnosis of a patient's illness. The advanced laboratory tests and the detailed data from those tests are innumerable. Hospital clinical lab departments are ever growing. Because of such growth, the pathology department is usually divided into various sections or divisions. The size of the hospital usually determines the number of sections of the clinical laboratory.

TABLE 6-3   Laboratory Personnel

Clinical laboratory technologists	Persons who work in any of the various clinical laboratory sections after appropriate training. The clinical assistant may assist in the collecting, preparing, and recording of body fluid specimens. There are different levels of clinical laboratory technicians. Clinical technicians perform multiple procedures on body fluids and tissues. The types of tests one can perform depend on the level of the technician.
Clinical pathology technologists	Persons whose main responsibility is examining and analyzing body fluids, tissues, and cells. They usually have a Bachelor's degree or certificate from a hospital.
Pathologists	Physicians who specialize in disease and work performed in the clinical lab
Pathology assistants	Persons who assist in autopsies, dissections, and processing of tissue
Pathology secretaries	Persons who assist pathologists as a receptionist and by arranging meetings and typing reports
Phlebotomists	Persons who collect, transport, and process blood specimens.

Some of the various sections include blood bank, chemistry, coagulation, cytology, hematology, histology, microbiology, and urinalysis. Large hospitals may have all of these sections separated, whereas small hospitals may group some of these sections together. A department divided up into so many divisions will employ numerous types of personnel in the clinical laboratory. The laboratory personnel for the clinical lab are defined in Table 6-3.

Because most blood specimens are drawn from the patient while in the hospital room, the phlebotomist becomes a familiar person to the health unit coordinator and other staff on the nursing unit.

The laboratory in large health care facilities is open and staffed 24 hours a day, 7 days a week.

PULMONARY MEDICINE

Pulmonary medicine pertains to the lungs and the breathing system. Pulmonary medicine could also be divided into separate divisions such as pulmonary diagnostics, pulmonary rehabilitation, and respiratory therapy. These three areas together encompass both the diagnostic and therapeutic areas of lung disease.

Pulmonary diagnostics is the department that performs tests or examinations on a patient's lungs and breathing system. Pulmonary rehabilitation is the department that assists the patient in living with a lung disease. This assistance may include teaching how to properly use an inhaler or acquiring home equipment such as portable oxygen tanks. The hours of a pulmonary rehabilitation department are usually 8:00 A.M. to 5:00 P.M.

Respiratory therapy is the department that treats patients having lung disease. **Respiratory therapists**, under the guidance of a doctor, give oxygen and help patients do chest exercises to help patients with breathing difficulties. They also collect specimens, evaluate tests, record data regarding the respiratory care, and assemble and check respiratory equipment. Respiratory therapists work with the patient at the bedside, so they become very familiar to the health unit coordinator and the rest of the nursing unit staff. There are many respiratory therapists working throughout the day, but the second shift has fewer respiratory therapists than the first or day shift, and the third or night shift has fewer than the second shift.

A **pulmonologist** is a physician who specializes in lung diseases. Pulmonologists order extensive pulmonary tests to assist in diagnosing the patient and deciding on the plan of care for the patient. Specially trained nurses perform the pulmonary testing in the pulmonary department. Although pulmonologists are always on call, they follow regular office hours.

RADIOLOGY, OR DIAGNOSTIC IMAGING

Radiology is the department that uses radiant energy such as x-rays or ultrasound in the diagnosis or treatment of disease. Today, computers have a major role in this department.

Another name for the radiology department is diagnostic imaging. Depending on the size of the hospital, radiology can consist of many or a few combined departments. Table 6-4 defines the divisions of radiology.

The health unit coordinator needs to differentiate the correct division of radiology when she or he orders a radiology examination. In addition to having a basic knowledge of radiology tests, the health unit coordinator needs to have an understanding of test preparation, such as "nothing to eat after midnight," in order to properly schedule the test. Each hospital will have different preparation instructions (preps). These preps are kept either in a manual or on a Rolodex. Sophisticated computer systems can print out preps as soon as the health unit coordinator orders the test. The health unit coordinator needs to share the prep with the nurse, because there are responsibilities for the nurse to carry out as well as the health unit coordinator to ensure that the patient is ready for the examination.

Radiologists are physicians who use x-rays or other sources of ionizing radiation, sound, or radio frequencies for diagnosis and treatment. Radiology supervisors and managers manage the many facets of the department. Because many radiology examinations can be performed on outpatients, the radiology department has receptionists to greet those patients. Many radiology departments employ their own transcriptionist to type the dictated reports in the department. Radiology retains all x-ray films in the radiology department. Filing clerks file and keep a record of all x-ray films in the department as well as any that are removed from the department. Radiation therapists and radiology technicians perform or will assist in performing the radiology examination. Some radiology departments employ transporters to escort inpatients to the radiology department and then back to their room after the completion of the examination. The health unit coordinator is responsible for knowing where patients are throughout the course of the day, so it is important that the transporters communicate with the health unit coordinator when a patient is escorted off the unit. The health unit coordinator will then keep a written record of when the patient left the unit.

TABLE 6-4   Radiology Divisions

Angiography	X-ray of the inside of the heart and blood vessels. This requires a contrast medium or dye to be injected before the examination.
Computerized tomography (CT)	A technique for examining internal structures of the body that shows a detailed cross section of tissue structure. A CT image (called a scan) is a highly accurate picture that shows relationships of structures to each other (Figure 6-4).
Diagnostic x-ray (Dx x-ray)	Electromagnetic radiation of shorter wavelength than visible light. X-rays can go through most substances and are used to investigate the integrity of certain structures and to destroy diseased tissue (radiation therapy).
Magnetic resonance imaging (MRI)	A noninvasive diagnostic technique that produces computerized images of internal body tissues and is based on nuclear magnetic resonance of atoms within the body induced by the application of radio waves.
Mammography	X-ray of the breast and its soft tissues
Nuclear medicine	A branch of medicine that uses radioactive chemical elements in the diagnosis and treatment of disease
Ultrasound	The use of high-frequency sound to create images of the internal anatomy. Ultrasounds do not use any ionizing radiation.

The hours of radiology departments vary from site to site; typically, radiology is open from 7:00 A.M. to 8:00 P.M. Some facilities have minimal staff in the department 24 hours a day, and some facilities assign staff to be on call to come in and perform procedures as needed. The health unit coordinator needs to know the procedure for contacting radiology personnel during any closed hours.

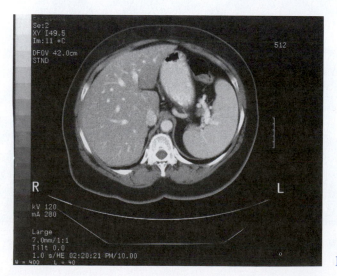

Figure 6-4 • *CT scan*

THERAPEUTIC DEPARTMENTS

The therapeutic departments take an active role in treating the patients' diseases. The main responsibility of most therapeutic departments is the education of the patient. In some cases, the therapeutic departments may work with each other in order to provide the best plan of care for the patient. The therapeutic departments discussed in this chapter are dietary, pharmacy, and physical medicine.

DIETARY DEPARTMENT

Another name for the dietary department is food management and nutrition services. Food management and nutrition services could actually be thought of as two separate departments. The food management department is responsible for ordering and preparing food for patients or residents. Food management is also responsible for preparing food for visitors and for the facility's staff members. This department is staffed with chefs, managers, supervisors, and dietary assistants, who assemble food trays and deliver and collect meal trays. Refer to Figure 6-5 for a picture of a dietary employee at work.

Patients are often required to follow a restricted or special diet, both while in the hospital and when they return home. Nutrition services employ registered dietitians who have extensive knowledge in nutrition and nutritional needs. They assess the patient's needs and assist the patient and, often, family members with hospital menu selections. They also recommend food choices and guidelines for patients in the continuation of their restricted diet at home.

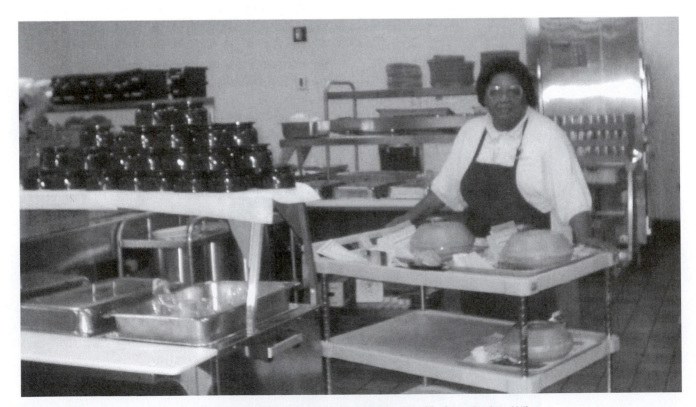

Figure 6-5 • *Dietary personnel at work (Courtesy of All Saints Health Care, Racine, WI)*

PHARMACY

Almost all patients in a hospital or health care facility are offered some type of medication during their stay. Many medications, such as insulin, are given to the patient to maintain good health. Other medications, such as a pain reliever or sleeping medication, may be given for comfort measures.

The pharmacy employs pharmacists who have received at least a bachelor's degree. Pharmacists provide consultation services with physicians, prepare and label medications, calculate proper dosages and double-check for allergies that may interfere with medications ordered by the physician. Pharmacy technicians work under the supervision of pharmacists, assisting with labeling medications, delivering medications to the nursing units, and completing inventory tasks.

In some hospitals, the pharmacy is decentralized. That is, the pharmacists do not work solely in the pharmacy but do certain required tasks in the pharmacy and then complete other tasks on the nursing units. The decentralized pharmacist becomes an invaluable resource on the unit. Pharmacists have an enormous amount of experience reading physician orders and often are able to assist the health unit coordinators in reading illegible orders.

Pharmacists are staffed more heavily during the daytime hours, and there are fewer on the afternoon and night shifts.

PHYSICAL MEDICINE AND REHABILITATION

Physical medicine can be divided into three very different areas: physical therapy, occupational therapy, and speech therapy.

Physical therapy is the department that assesses the muscles and movement of the patient. Different types of treatment are offered. Treatments can range from massage and exercises to application of cold, heat, sound waves, light, water, electricity or ultrasound. **Physical therapists** are licensed individuals who evaluate and treat physically disabled patients. They develop action plans that may include treatments as mentioned above, as well as exercises to improve the physical mobility and strength of the patient. Physical therapy assistants are paraprofessionals who have graduated from an accredited physical therapy assistant course. They assist the physical therapist with the treatments for improving the mobility and strength of the patient. Physical therapy assistants work under the guidance of a physical therapist.

Occupational therapy focuses on the *activities of daily living* (ADLs). It differs from physical therapy in that it teaches the patient to live with the limitations resulting from the illness or injury. **Occupational therapists** are licensed and trained in assessing the patients' physical and mental limitations. After assessing the patient, the occupational therapist develops an exercise and treatment plan. Occupational therapist assistants assist the patient with the prescribed exercises under the supervision of the occupational therapist. Occupational therapy aides may transport patients to and from therapy and assist with routine tasks under the supervision of the occupational therapist.

Speech therapy is the department that concentrates on speech defects. Speech and language pathologists are professionals who evaluate and treat people who have voice, speech, language, swallowing, and hearing disorders. **Speech therapists** are people trained in speech pathology who treat people with disorders affecting normal speech.

The working hours of physical medicine are usually 8 A.M. to 5 P.M., Monday through Friday. Because this department treats outpatients as well as inpatients, some physical medicine departments have Saturday hours as well.

SUMMARY

Hospitals offer a wide variety of diagnostic and treatment opportunities to their patients and community. Correct diagnosis can be made only after the examinations requested by the patient's physician have been completed. The health unit coordinator must arrange for the correct exams from the correct hospital department in order to ensure timely and effective results. To arrange patients' tests in a timely and organized manner, the health unit coordinator must have knowledge of the various departments and their personnel. Health unit coordinators work with *all* the diagnostic and therapeutic departments of the hospital. The health unit coordinator needs to establish working relationships with the personnel from the various departments. The outcome of the patients' hospital stay will be affected by how well the health unit coordinator arranges the many diagnostic and therapeutic services.

REVIEW QUESTIONS

1. Cardiology is the study of _____.

2. Another name for the department of Food Management and Nutrition Services is _____.

3. Gastrology is the study of _____.

4. List four divisions with in the laboratory department.

5. List four divisions of the radiology department.

6. How does a decentralized hospital pharmacy differ from a centralized pharmacy?

7. Name the three areas in physical medicine.

Match the term in the left column to the definition in the right column.

8. Angiography

    a. The study of the stomach, intestines, and related structures such as the esophagus, liver, gallbladder, and pancreas

9. Cardiac catheterization

    b. A test in which a long tube is passed into the heart through a large blood vessel in an arm or a leg.

10. Clinical laboratory

11. Diagnose

12. Diagnostic departments

13. Endoscopic

14. Gastroenterology

15. Occupational therapy

16. Pathology

17. Phlebotomist

18. Physical therapy

19. Radiology

20. Respiratory therapy

21. Speech therapy

c. Areas of a hospital, clinic, or long-term health care facility that examine the patient with specialized equipment to determine the nature or the cause of the disease, as well as the extent of the injury or illness

d. To determine the type and cause of a health condition on the basis of a patient's signs and symptoms, laboratory tests, and information about family and occupational background as well as recent injuries or exposure to dangerous substances

e. General term regarding visual examination of the body organs or cavities

f. A room or building equipped for scientific experimentation, research, testing, and analysis

g. A branch of medicine concerned with radioactive substances, including x-rays, radioactive isotopes and ionizing radiation to prevent, diagnosis, and treat disease

h. The training of patients with physical injury or illness, mental disease, or learning problems to work and live by themselves despite any health problem that might keep the patient from living a normal life

i. The study of the traits, causes, and effects of disease, as seen in the structure and workings of the body

j. One who draws blood from a vein

k. A profession that is responsible for the management of the patient's movement system

l. Therapeutic treatment of speech defects

m. Any treatment that maintains or improves the function of the respiratory tract

n. X-ray study of the inside of the heart and blood vessels, done after a dye has been injected.

NAHUC CERTIFICATION EXAM

CONTENT AREAS

I. C. 1   Request services from ancillary departments

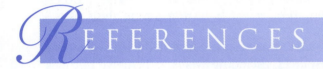

THROUGH THE EYES

OF A HEALTH CARE PROFESSIONAL

There is so much a health unit coordinator is responsible for, having knowledge of the many ancillary departments makes it easier to know where to order the variety of tests and treatments one sees throughout the day. Knowing about the departments will allow one to work through an order that may not be common. Having a thorough knowledge of the departments will help you answer questions from other health unit coordinators when questions do arise.

REFERENCES

American Medical Association. (2002). *Health professions career and education directory 2003–2004.* Chicago: Author.

http://www.hr.edu Accessed March 1, 2003.

Chabner, D. (2001). *The language of medicine* (6th ed.). Philadelphia: Saunders.

Fischbach, F. (2000). *A manual of laboratory & diagnostic tests* (6th ed.). Philadelphia: Lippincott.

The Mosby medical encyclopedia (rev. ed.). (1997). New York: Mosby.

Simmers, L. (1998). *Diversified health occupations essentials* (4th ed.). Clifton Park, NY: Thomson Delmar Learning.

Taber's cyclopedic medical dictionary (19th ed.). (1997). Philadelphia: Davis.

An Introduction to Support Services

Learning Objectives

Upon completion of this chapter and review questions, the learner should be able to:

1. Define support services.

2. Explain the role health unit coordinators have with all support services.

3. List four pieces of information the admitting department must receive from a patient.

4. List three functions of social services.

5. Discuss how the security department provides support to both patients and staff.

6. List when the health unit coordinator should contact a chaplain.

7. Define three areas of responsibility for the business office.

8. Describe three areas of computer services.

9. Discuss the four functions of the hospital information management department.

10. Discuss quality management functions.

Key Terms

business office   Has responsibilities for calculating the patient account and for sending and monitoring the patient's hospital bill.

chaplains   On-call ministers of various faiths who provide spiritual support when needed.

clinical information services   Another name for the medical records department.

computer services department   A department that provides assistance to health care facility personnel regarding computer hardware and software.

direct support services   Services provided face to face with patients to enhance the health care stay, yet not necessarily providing patient care.

environmental services   Another term for housekeeping staff.

hospital information management   Another name for the medical records department.

human resources   The department, also known as employment or personnel, that is responsible for interviewing and offering positions to qualified applicants.

HVAC   A division of the maintenance department focusing on the heating, ventilation, and air conditioning of a health care facility.

indirect support services   Services provided that assist in the care of the patient but do not involve face-to-face contact with the patient.

information services   Another name for computer services.

loss prevention   Another name for the security department.

medical records   The department responsible for storing patient records, coordinating release of information, and tabulating data from records for research purposes.

security department   A department that works to ensure the safety and security of patients, visitors, and health care facility staff.

site support   A division of computer services that assists with software and hardware needs.

support services   Services provided in the health care setting that assist the staff in providing patient care or provide patient assistance.

Abbreviations

CIS   Clinical Information Services

CPR   Cardiopulmonary Resuscitation

HIM   Hospital Information Management

HVAC Heating, Ventilation, and Air Conditioning

ICD International Classification of Disease

IS Information Services

OSHA Occupational Safety and Health Administration

PAS Patient Access Services

SUPPORT SERVICES

In addition to the diagnostic and treatment services provided by health care facilities, many other forms of assistance and support are also available to the patient. These **support services** can be divided into direct and indirect services. **Direct support services** are those that involve face-to-face contact with the patient or the patient's family. The **indirect support services** are provided throughout the health care stay, yet the patient does not see the person performing the services. Health unit coordinators provide mostly indirect services because the majority of their work is completed at the unit workstation. The health unit coordinator contacts departments to request their services. These services range from tasks such as changing a light bulb outside the patient's room to providing home medical equipment.

DIRECT SUPPORT SERVICES

Direct support services include the admitting department, environmental services, security, social services, and pastoral care.

ADMITTING DEPARTMENT

The admitting department, more formally known as patient access services (PAS), has the first contact with patients and patient families at a health care facility. The admitting department is always located by the main entrance of the facility. A tracking board is the center of the admitting department, because admitting is also responsible for bed placement of new patients. The patient access service personnel must be well groomed and courteous at all times. It is important that the admitting department make a very good impression on the patient, for it is true that the first 15 seconds have a lasting impression. PAS personnel take very personal information, such the patient's address and phone number, Social Security number, insurance company and insurance number, the name of the admitting physician, and the reason for being admitted, which is the admitting diagnosis. This information is entered into the hospital's computer system, and various forms that will be needed to start the patient's medical record or chart are printed out. The patient access services personnel must ensure that patient confidentiality is protected; they share with hospital staff only the patient information that pertains to the patient's care. It is very important that this information be entered into the hospital computer carefully and accurately, for once it has been entered it follows the patient throughout the hospitalization. If the wrong insurance information is entered into the registration system, payment of medical bills by the insurance company may be postponed or even denied. If the wrong physician is entered, the patient's test results will go to the wrong physician's office, possibly delaying treatment or increasing the length of the patient's stay. The paperwork that is generated in the admitting department accompanies the patients when they go to the nursing unit. The paperwork is given to the health unit coordinator, who then begins to assemble a chart for use during the patient's stay.

ENVIRONMENTAL SERVICES

Environmental services, or housekeeping, consists of numerous employees. Some environmental services workers are responsible for emptying the trash containers, mopping the floors, and sanitizing the bathrooms of every patient care room on a daily basis. Hanging of clean drapes and room curtains is a routine duty within patient rooms as well. Other environmental service employees may be responsible for maintaining a clean and safe environment around other areas of the health care facility, such as entrances and hallways and business offices. The health unit coordinator needs to contact environmental services in a timely manner to notify them of a room from which a patient has been discharged in order for environmental services to prepare the room for the next patient.

SECURITY

The **security department**, also known as **loss prevention**, works to ensure the safety and security of patients, visitors, and health care facility staff. Although patients are discouraged from bringing cash and other valuables to the hospital, some still do. During the room orientation and personal belongings interview by nursing personnel, if it is determined that the patient has brought any valuables, the health unit coordinator will call the security department. The security department will then come to the patient's room, collect the valuables, have the patient sign for the valuables, and then take the valuables to a secure area until the patient is to be discharged, at which point the belongings will be safely returned to the patient.

Other duties of the security department include escorting visitors or staff to their vehicles during late night hours. Many security departments are equipped to jump start vehicles. They patrol the health care facility grounds, ensuring safety at all times. Usually, some police science course work is required before employment in this position. Figure 7-1 shows a security officer on rounds.

SOCIAL SERVICES

The social services department is staffed with social workers and department secretaries. The social workers provide a wide variety of services for patients. They are knowledgeable about the current assistance available from Medicaid and Medicare, from the Department of Aging, and from local and state assistance programs for the indigent.

The social services department plays a major role in the discharge of elderly patients and patients with special needs. Social workers have knowledge of support services and extended-care facilities. These services may need to be utilized by patients for

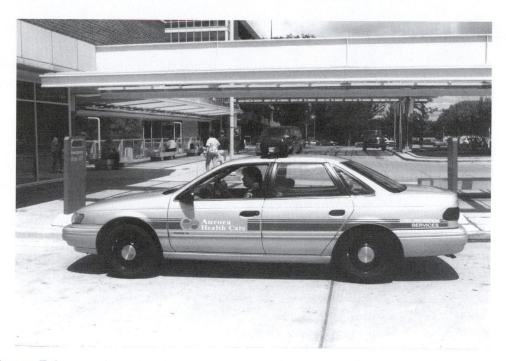

Figure 7-1 • *A security officer on rounds (Courtesy of Aurora Health Care)*

varying amounts of time, depending on their identified needs upon discharge. Social workers assist the patient and the patient's family with choosing a nursing home on the basis of location and financial obligations. Social workers make referrals and initiate contact with the nursing homes or long-term health facilities.

Another responsibility of a hospital social worker is to appear in court as a witness for guardianship, or durable power of attorney for health care, when the situation requires their expertise.

Social workers can assist patients with finding programs that give postdischarge support for drug or alcohol abuse. They work with home care agencies and places to contact for financial counseling.

PASTORAL CARE

Pastoral care, or **chaplain** services, are provided by employees or on-call ministers of various faiths who provide spiritual support when needed. They can often calm and assist patients and patients' families and friends in stressful and uncertain times. Hospital chaplains are usually available 24 hours a day for spiritual support. They make rounds in the emergency departments, intensive care units, and throughout the rest of the hospital. A service the health unit coordinator may provide is to contact the chaplain for situations, without being asked, for example when a patient has respiratory or cardiac arrest.

Chaplains provide support to the hospital staff as well. Staff members, for personal or professional situations, may consult them. Chaplains may also conduct services for the patients, family members, and staff routinely or on various religious holidays and during national incidents such as September 11, 2001, and war.

INDIRECT SUPPORT SERVICES

Indirect support services include the business office, computer services, education services, employee health, human resources, medical records, and public relations.

BUSINESS OFFICE

The **business office** has responsibilities for calculating the patient account and for sending and monitoring the patient's hospital bill. The business office also has specialists to assist patients in working out payment plans. This section is often referred to as patient financial services or financial counseling. This department is considered indirect support because all billing is done by U.S. mail or electronically. However, business office personnel are available during the daytime hours to answer billing questions. Health unit coordinators should have the phone extension of the business office and its location available in case they are asked questions about a patient's bill or how to contact the business office.

COMPUTER SERVICES

Whether a health care facility is large or small, rural or urban, computers are common in all aspects of health care. Much of the diagnostic equipment today, from clinical lab machines to large radiology scanners, is computerized. In addition, much of the patient's medical record is also computerized. Exam reports, history and physical reports, and consultation reports are all dictated and transcribed electronically. Physicians can even sign the reports electronically (called electronic signatures). There are also computer software programs that make the entire patient's record electronic. Everything from entering the patient's personal history and vital signs to ordering diagnostic exams and medication profiles and teaching records is computerized. Besides computers, there are fax machines and printers on the nursing units that the health unit coordinator uses throughout the day. The **computer services department** is responsible for ensuring that these computers enhance the role of health care. There are various roles of computer services.

Computer analysts and programmers analyze the current way the communication among departments is working and then write computer programs to enhance the process. The computer services department's help desk is the first place the health unit coordinator will phone when the nursing station's computers are not acting properly. If the help desk cannot assist the caller over the phone, they will contact site support. **Site support** personnel are people staffed by the health care facility to be on site to assist with software problems for a user. They also install, maintain, and repair the computer hardware. The computer services department offers valuable support to the hospital and ensures that patient care and treatment are not interrupted because of computer glitches.

EDUCATION SERVICES

It is imperative that health care employees stay current with their practice and the many changes affecting health care. Education services is responsible for assisting with orientation of new employees and offering continuing education to nursing staff and ancillary department staff. They offer general types of education sessions for employees, such as customer service, preceptor workshops, and introduction or updates to computers. More specific classes offered include critical care courses, electrocardiogram courses, and cardiopulmonary resuscitation (CPR) courses.

Community education is also a responsibility of the education department. Some examples of community education include cholesterol management, diabetes education, smoking cessation, and stress management.

EMPLOYEE HEALTH

The employee health department has the well-being of the individual employee as a main concern. Preventive care is especially important to health care workers because they deal with the public and are exposed to many illnesses. Employees must take every precaution to protect themselves. It is the employee health department personnel who administer and keep records of immunizations of the facility's employees.

The employee health department also has the responsibility to ensure that the health care facility is in compliance with regulatory agencies, such as the Occupational Safety and Health Administration (OSHA), which promotes safe working environments (Figure 7-2).

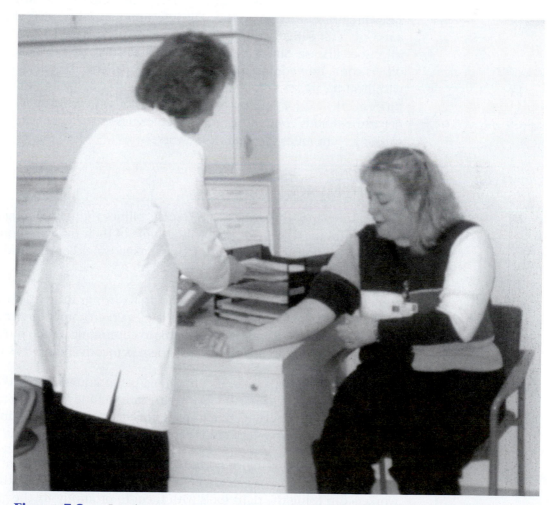

Figure 7-2 • *Employee health services (Courtesy of All Saints Health Care, Racine, WI)*

HUMAN RESOURCES, OR EMPLOYMENT DEPARTMENT

The **human resources**, or employment, department is responsible for finding the right person for the right job. Many jobs in the health care field require specialty education. Some positions may even require licensures or certification. In addition to interviewing a person for a position, human resources is responsible for knowing the qualifications of each position and for verifying that the applicant's credentials are current. The human resources department is also responsible for recommending cost-effective, market-priced, standard employee benefits to the health care facility's administration. Once the benefits have been determined, human resources is responsible for ensuring that the employees receive the earned benefits. Human resources must also be current with federal and state labor laws so as to advise appropriate administrative personnel regarding full compliance with the laws.

This is the first department you will have contact with to begin your health care career. It is important for you to make a good impression from the very beginning.

INFECTION CONTROL

The infection control department of a health care facility is responsible for educating patients and staff on how disease is transmitted and for teaching ways to prevent spreading infection and disease. The infection control nurse is charged with keeping a record of all patients admitted to the facility who have an infectious or possibly infectious disease. She or he must ensure that safety precautions are practiced when others come into contact with the infectious patient. Infection control is reviewed with health care staff on an annual basis. Health care facilities hold different opportunities every year for employees to review various safety features. The infection control department adds content regarding such things as the chain of infection and hand-washing techniques for health care workers.

MAINTENANCE

The maintenance department has responsibilities for maintaining and repairing the exterior and the interior of the facility. Some of their many responsibilities include painting, carpentry, floor repairs, fixing broken water coolers, and repairing a malfunctioning refrigerator, as seen in Figure 7-3.

Sometimes, maintenance must be called to fix things in a patient's room, such as a broken bed or a burnt-out light bulb. Here again customer service is very important. It is vital for the health unit coordinator to communicate the problem to the maintenance department accurately so the patient is inconvenienced as little as possible.

Heating, ventilation, and air conditioning, better known as **HVAC** is also part of the maintenance department. In large health care facilities, maintenance and HVAC may be separated. As the HVAC title implies, this department maintains, repairs, and replaces the heating units, ventilation units, and air conditioning units of the facility.

The health unit coordinator needs to know how to contact the maintenance departments and to be able to give them detailed information so that the maintenance workers can bring the right tools with them to promptly fix the given problem.

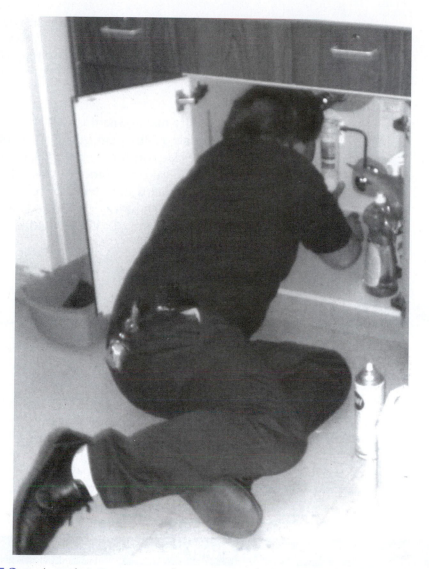

Figure 7-3 • *A maintenance employee at work* (Courtesy of All Saints Health Care, Racine, WI)

MEDICAL RECORDS

Medical records is also known as **clinical information services (CIS)** or the **hospital information management department (HIM)**. This department is responsible for storing medical records. Medical records clerks perform record analysis and coding procedures on patient records, coordinate release of information upon request, and tabulate data from medical records for research purposes. A medical records coder is responsible for ensuring that correct International Classification of Disease (ICD) codes are assigned to all applicable parts of the patients' charts.

The medical records department has many more responsibilities. They are responsible for ensuring that the patients' charts are complete, such as making sure all forms have a patient identification and all physician orders are signed before submitting the records to the business office for billing.

To provide historical treatment information, health unit coordinators contact the medical records department to retrieve records from past admissions for patients being readmitted to the health care facility. Upon discharge of a patient, the health unit coordinator gathers all parts of the patient's record and prepares them for the medical records department.

In small hospitals, quality management is part of the medical records department, whereas in large hospitals quality management may be a separate department. Quality management employees are consultants to medical and hospital staff. They are instrumental in reviewing and evaluating processes used throughout the care of patients. They advise the staff on quality and performance improvements. They assist in achieving goals of high quality and cost-effective patient care. They also ensure that the health care facility is complying with JCAHO and other external regulatory agency regulations.

PUBLIC RELATIONS

The public relations office is responsible for notifying the community of events the health care facility is offering to the community. Events may include health fairs, flu shots, and educational opportunities. Events within the health care facility may also warrant notification to the public. These events may include the installation of major diagnostic equipment, such as a gamma knife (not really a knife but a device that emits a highly focused beam of gamma radiation used to treat a disease process). Other major equipment may include high-tech MRI scanners or new cardiac catheterization laboratories. Health unit coordinators may contact public relations and ask for assistance publicizing a workshop or conference that they are planning to host.

TABLE 7-1 Support Services by Other Names

Admitting department	Patient access services	Patient registration	Bed placement
Environmental services	Housekeeping		
Security	Loss prevention		
Pastoral care	Chaplain services	Hospital ministries	
Business office	Patient accounts	Cashier	Financial counseling
Computer services	**Information services**		
Education services	Nursing education	Continuing education	Organization development
Human resources	Employment office	Personnel	
Maintenance	HVAC	Engineering	
Medical records	Clinical information services	Health information management	

The public relations department is also responsible for dealing with the media. They contact the media to inform the public about community and hospital events, and they are the department the media contact to get information, for example, if they find out a high-profile person was admitted.

SUPPORT SERVICES BY OTHER NAMES

Some hospitals are larger than others; some are more technically advanced than others; and some are more conservative than others. These are some of the reasons support services departments are known by various names. Table 7-1 lists the different names given to support service departments by various health care facilities.

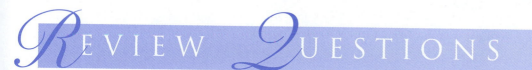

SUMMARY

In addition to diagnostic and therapeutic services, valuable services are performed by many different departments, all focusing on providing the best patient care. In the center of all this activity is the health unit coordinator. Whether the need affects the patient directly or indirectly, the health unit coordinator is a vital link to connect the department to the nursing station. The health unit coordinator needs to know whom to call, how to contact them in an expedient manner, and how to communicate the specific support that is needed. Here again is an example of how important the role of the health unit coordinator is to the nursing unit and patient care.

REVIEW QUESTIONS

1. Name three areas of responsibilities for the business office.

2. List four pieces of personal information the admitting department staff must request from a patient.

3. List the three areas of computer services.

4. Does the security department have responsibilities to both patients and staff?

5. List three functions of the medical records department.

6. Quality management is often part of what health care department?

7. Is it necessary for the health unit coordinator to be asked by the patient's nurse before calling a chaplain?

8. Social services can assist the patient with what information?

Match the terms in the left column to the definitions in the right column

9. Chaplain services

a. Occupational Safety and Health Administration

10. Information services

b. Another name for the security department

11. Human resources

c. Patient access services, another name for the medical records department

12. HVAC

d. The department that offers spiritual assistance to people in need

13. Loss prevention

e. The department that is responsible for interviewing and offering positions to qualified applicants

14. OSHA

f. Another name for the medical records department

15. PAS

g. A division of the maintenance department focusing on the heating, ventilation, and air conditioning of a health care facility

16. CIS

h. A division of computer services that assists with software and hardware needs

17. Site support

i. Another name for computer services

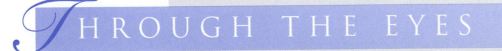

NAHUC CERTIFICATION EXAM

CONTENT AREAS

I. C. 2   Request services from support departments

THROUGH THE EYES

OF A HEALTH CARE PROFESSIONAL

Social workers rely on health unit coordinators for prompt, accurate, and complete notification of patients who are in need of financial or support service assistance. The more information health unit coordinators share with us the better prepared we are when we meet with the patient or family. Health unit coordinators and social services together provide a team effort to ensure a seamless transfer of a patient from one health care facility to another.

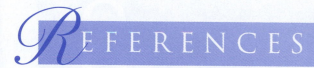

REFERENCES

http://www.naham.org.public/articles/index.cfm?Cat=12 Accessed February 3, 2003.

http://www.hcmachaplains.org

Chabner, D. (2001). *The language of medicine* (6th ed.). Philadelphia: Saunders.

Fischbach, F. (2000). *A manual of laboratory & diagnostic tests* (6th ed.). Philadelphia: Lippincott.

The Mosby medical encyclopedia (rev. ed.). (1997). New York: Mosby.

Simmers, L. (1998). *Diversified health occupations essentials* (4th ed.). Clifton Park, NY: Thomson Delmar Learning.

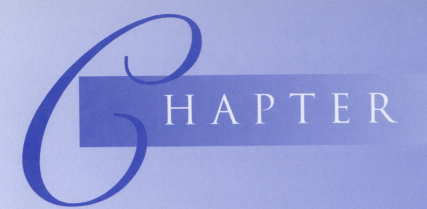

CHAPTER 8

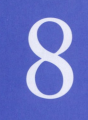

Administration

Learning Objectives

Upon completion of this chapter and review questions, the learner should be able to:

1. Describe the role of administration in health care.

2. Discuss leadership roles in health care.

3. Describe the challenges that face health care administration.

4. Identify how health care is meeting the challenges.

5. Describe three leadership styles.

Key Terms

administration The group of management people administratively responsible for the health care system.

chief executive officer The individual having overall responsibility for coordinating the health care system.

chief financial officer The individual having responsibility for the financial policies and procedures of the health care system.

director of nursing The individual having responsibility for the nursing departments and nursing department employees who deliver patient care.

governing board Also called hospital board, board of directors, or board of trustees; a group of people selected from the community to develop organizational and operational policy for the health care system.

leadership team The group of people who head the various divisions, departments, and units of the health care system; the administration.

middle management The group of managers between the employees and the leadership team.

mission statement A written statement of purpose that defines the essence of the health care system.

nurse manager A nurse who manages a patient care unit.

vision statement A written statement defining the health care system's future and the direction that will be pursued in achieving it.

Abbreviations

CEO Chief Executive Officer

CFO Chief Financial Officer

DON Director of Nursing

NM Nurse Manager

LEADERSHIP

Health care organizations require strong competent leadership to ensure a viable future in an increasingly competitive business climate. Hospital **administration** consists of people who have a strong business sense and futuristic vision for health care. The administrators need to provide leadership for a diverse group of health care workers. These health care workers watch the organization's leaders to be sure they are practicing what they require of others. In other words, the health care workers will model their behavior after what they see not what they hear. Health care leaders who require health care workers to provide positive customer service to all must, in turn, practice those customer service skills, acting as role models for the health care facility's employees. They must be the example for all to follow.

The size and type of administration depends on the size and type of the health care facility. Small facilities typically have a small administrative group. Privately owned for-profit facilities may have different missions and visions than do privately owned nonprofit organizations and the focus and way in which their administrative groups are organized and staffed could differ accordingly. The same holds true of facilities that are in the public domain, such as community, county, state, or federal government facilities. Whether the health care facility is located in a small community or a large metropolitan area will also influence the makeup and focus of the facility's administration.

CLASSIFICATION OF HEALTH CARE FACILITIES

Health care facilities can be defined by the customers (patients) they serve, by who owns the health care facility, or by the number of patient beds. When the patients they serve define health care facilities we look at the services the health care facility provides and the patients to whom they provide those services. For example, a cardiac health care facility provides services for patients with cardiac health issues. It may have patients with congestive heart failure, enlarged hearts, irregular heartbeats, and diseased hearts. The health care facility provides diagnostic tests, examinations, and required treatments using the most up-to-date equipment. These types of health care facilities often have patients referred from other health care facilities that are unable to provide the health care needed for the specific patient diagnosis.

Health care facilities may be classified by who controls them or who owns them. A facility may be privately owned or supported by the government. Government-owned health care facilities are supported by taxes and provide a variety of health care services. Some examples of federal government-owned facilities include military health care facilities, veteran's facilities, and U.S. Public Health facilities. State, county, and local governments may also own health care facilities. The government-owned facilities might serve one identified patient type or serve the general population.

Health care facilities that are classified as nongovernment vary as to ownership and control. Churches, organizations, and communities may own health care facilities. These facilities provide health care to the affiliates of the church or organization or the communities in which they reside.

Health care facilities may be privately owned and operated. These facilities may be for profit. A small group of investors may choose to run a health care facility, or many stockholders may own the facility. These facilities can provide general or specific health care services.

The size of the health care facility or number of patient beds is another way that health care systems are classified. This classification is difficult to use, because it no longer reflects the amount of business a health care system may be involved in owing to the fact that outpatient visits continue to increase and inpatient stays are decreasing.

No matter how a health care facility is classified, leadership in the health care setting is provided by a defined structure. The leadership defines that structure.

ADMINISTRATORS

All health care organizations have an administrator, an individual having overall responsibility for the organization. The administrator is responsible for making executive decisions and overseeing that the decisions are carried out. The administrator, staff, and governing board define the mission and vision for the organization. The administrator appoints members to various committees and attends functions both within and outside the health system as the official representative of the health system. The administrator often has the title of CEO (chief executive officer).

GOVERNING BOARD

The health care system's **governing board**, also called the hospital board, the board of directors, or the board of trustees, plays an important role in the health care system. Although their exact responsibilities vary from organization to organization, governing boards universally have three critically important responsibilities:

> To select and oversee the performance of the chief executive officer

> To oversee that the health care system is implementing and meeting its mission and vision

> To ensure that the health care system is operating in accordance with the policies as established by the governing board

Some boards may review the budget, approve expenditure requests for large projects and equipment, approve physician requests to be on the facility's staff, and keep abreast of issues of importance to the health system.

Members of the governing board are not health system employees. They are usually respected members of the community who have a strong interest in health care and its services. They are often community members having extensive senior management experience and knowledge in the financial and business world.

ADMINISTRATIVE TEAM

The day-to-day, nonclinical operation of the health system is managed by the health care system administration. This management includes such functions as managing the staff, receiving payments, purchasing materials and supplies, providing the patients with services, and providing the employees with services needed to provide for the patients. The CEO, who is hired by and evaluated by the governing board, heads the health care administration team, or **leadership team**. The administration team defines the management requirements in the health system. The size of the health care facility typically dictates the size and makeup of the administration team. For example, the amount of funds available to provide the wages for the administration team is determined by the health care facility's size. Small organizations having limited funds may be required to proportionately limit the size and makeup of administration team. The CEO builds the administrative staff from within. The administrative team changes as the health care facility changes; if the facility doubles in size, it is likely the team will increase in size.

In a health care facility of fewer than 50 inpatient beds you may see the following administrative team shown in Figure 8-1.

In a health care facility of over 300 inpatient beds you may see the following administrative team shown in Figure 8-2.

The members of the team perform the functions or competencies as defined. Let's look at some key members of the administrative team and their job descriptions.

HAPPY VALLEY HOSPITAL

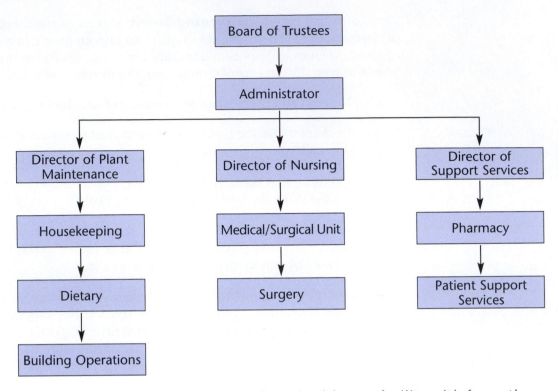

Figure 8-1 • *Organizational chart for a health care facility with fewer than 50 inpatient beds*

CHIEF EXECUTIVE OFFICER

The **chief executive officer (CEO)** is the administrator of the health care facility. His or her responsibilities include a wide variety of duties at the health care facility and in the community. The CEO is responsible for directing and coordinating the administrative team within the health care facility. This team is made of a diverse group of management employees such as accountants, registered nurses, physicians, engineers, and businesspeople. This team leads the health care workers by example. The CEO works closely with the physician staff at the health care facility. The physicians may be employees of the health care facility or they may have independent practices. The CEO provides reports to the governing board of the health care facility. These reports provide the governing board with information that they need to oversee the health care facility. The CEO plays an important role in the community by being the leader of the facility that provides health care to the community members and their families. This role is an important connection between the community and the health care facility. The community needs to know that the health care facility is a major player in the health of the community.

As an employee of the health care facility, the CEO has duties that must be fulfilled to meet the expectations of the defined position. Those duties could include coordination of the services of the health care system, building an effective management team,

Marquette General Health System Organizational Chart

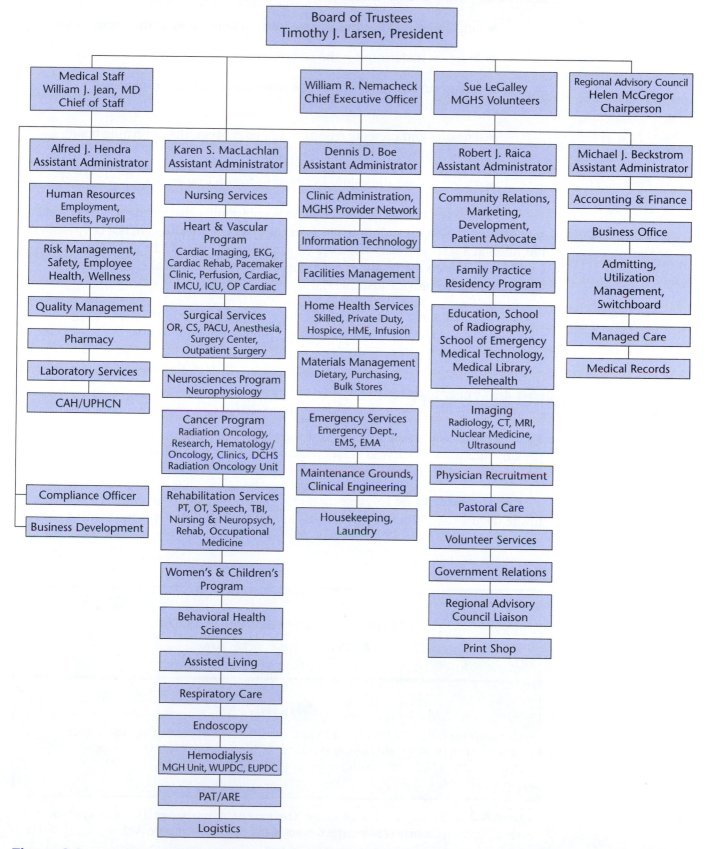

Figure 8-2 • *Organizational chart for a health care facility with more than 300 inpatient beds (Courtesy of Marquette General Health System, Marquette, MI)*

creating the mission and vision for the organization, and providing leadership. Consider the following as a job description for a health care system CEO:

◆ Implements and carries out the mission and vision of the organization.

◆ Provides leadership for the organization.

◆ Communicates the goals of the organization to the employees and community.

◆ Prepares and presents reports to the employees, the governing board, and the community.

◆ Demonstrates the ability to adjust to health care changes.

The role of the CEO has expanded to include community involvement. The community sees the health care administration as the leaders in health care not only locally but often at a state and national level. All communities wish to be able to provide health care close to home, and the communities look to the health care system administration to provide just that.

The mission statement approved by the governing board and implemented by the CEO provides insight into the organization's values and aspirations.

MISSION AND VISION STATEMENTS

Mission statements are usually created after careful thought and reflection to reflect the organization's beliefs and values (Figure 8-3). They state what the organization is all about, where it is going, and how it will get there.

Vision statements are an expression of where the organization wants to be in the future (Figure 8-4). Whereas mission statements typically are concerned with a time

---

Marquette General Health System
Mission, Vision and Values

Mission

Our *Mission* is to provide access to primary and tertiary health care services to improve the health status of the residents of Marquette County, the Upper Peninsula and the surrounding region.

Figure 8-3 • *Example of a mission statement from a health care system (Courtesy of Marquette General Health System, Marquette, MI)*

Marquette General Health System
Mission, Vision and Values

Vision

Our *Vision* is to provide quality, cost effective patient care services developed with excellence in patient care and customer service which will allow us to prosper as a business in order to invest in the health and well-being of the residents of the Region, partnering and collaborating with others whose goals align with ours.

Values

In order to accomplish our mission, we must strive to meet our *Values* of:

◆ *Competency:* People are our most important asset and are the source of our strength. Having the right people doing the right things at the right time improves our reputation and vitality.

◆ *Customer Service:* Excellence in patient care is the focus of everything we do. Our work must be done with our customers in mind, wherever possible, exceeding their expectations.

◆ *Quality:* Continuous quality improvement is essential to our service. To achieve customer satisfaction, the quality of our services must be a number one priority.

◆ *Safety:* Safety of our customer, staff, visitors, and others cannot be compromised.

◆ *Stewardship:* Our responsibility is to prudently manage and utilize our resources to improve the health status of the communities we serve.

◆ *Teamwork:* Employees, Medical Staff, Board and external partners comprise our Team and are key components to the success in meeting our mission. We must earn each others' trust and respect.

Figure 8-4 • *Example of a vision statement from a health care system (Courtesy of Marquette General Health System, Marquette, MI)*

period from the present to three years or so in the future, vision statements cover a period in the future, typically starting five years from the present. Vision statements are more idealistic and loftier than mission statements. A well-prepared mission statement and plan can be compared to a road map, whereas a well-planned vision statement is more like a compass. The vision statement indicates the general direction the organization wants to move—north rather than south.

The CEO will have as many senior management members on the administrative team as the organization requires. Some facilities refer to the senior management people as assistant administrators, vice presidents, or directors. Most facilities have a member of the administrative team who is responsible for the financial system in the health care system. That position is often labeled CFO (chief financial officer).

CHIEF FINANCIAL OFFICER

The **chief financial officer (CFO)** is responsible for advising the CEO and board of directors on the financial affairs of the health care system. The CFO is responsible for the budget of the health system, for depositing all money received, and for collecting all monies owed the health system. The CFO implements and carries out the policies for the financial business of the health care system, auditing and providing oversight to ensure that all areas adhere to the financial policies and procedures. The CFO oversees directly and indirectly the money paid out as well as the salaries of all employees, the vendors providing goods and services to the health care systems, and any other financial business the health care system requires to provide quality health care to its customers. Various management staff in the health care system can consult CFOs to plan hiring strategies for departments. Consider the following as a job description for a CFO:

◆ Is responsible for the procedures and policies related to the health system's financial process, including but not limited to annual financial reports and budgets.

◆ Generates all financial reports.

◆ Prepares and analyzes all financial reports for management and the board of directors.

◆ Monitors all financial transactions.

◆ Plans all audits, internal and external.

DIRECTOR OF NURSING

The CEO will have on the administrative team a nurse who is responsible for the nursing staff and nursing departments. That person may be titled **director of nursing (DON)**, chief nursing officer, director of patient care, vice president of nursing, or assistant administrator of the nursing division. Regardless of the title, the person who has this role is responsible for the nursing units and the staff that provides the clinical care to the patients of the heath care facility. The following example describes the responsibilities of a director of nursing:

◆ Creates and monitors the patient care delivery system for the facility.

◆ Ensures that policy changes are communicated to and practiced by the nursing staff.

◆ Demonstrates accountability for financial resources in assigned departments.

◆ Provides leadership to nurse managers consistent with the health system's mission and vision.

◆ Demonstrates a commitment to the health system by involvement in the community.

◆ Demonstrates the ability to manage change in the health care setting.

◆ Demonstrates the ability to work with government agencies.

The number of managers reporting to the DON varies from institution to institution—again, according to the size of the health care system. The health unit coordinator is usually a member of the nursing department and is either directly or indirectly supervised by the DON. The lines of authority are clearly defined by each health care facility.

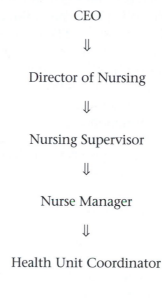

CEO

⇓

Director of Nursing

⇓

Nursing Supervisor

⇓

Nurse Manager

⇓

Health Unit Coordinator

NURSE MANAGER

The managers reporting to members of the administration team are often called **middle management**. They are the managers who supervise the workers. Not all health care systems require this management group. Remember, size and organizational structure are what decide management requirements.

A **nurse manager (NM)**, also called head nurse or patient care manager, is a member of middle management. It is the responsibility of the nurse manager to supervise the unit staff, evaluate the unit staff, recommend changes to administration, enforce the polices of the health care system, and perform other duties assigned by the administrative team. The nurse manager is the person responsible for the unit on which she or he is assigned. The nurse manager is responsible for staffing the unit with the correct number of clinical and nonclinical patient care providers for the safe delivery of patient care. In some health care facilities, the nurse managers are responsible for purchasing supplies, evaluating new products, teaching staff new procedures, being members of committees exploring new systems, and the unit's budget. All of these responsibilities have continued to expand as health care systems have expanded. The number of nonnursing responsibilities has continued to increase for nurse managers over the past several years. This increase has opened a door for the health unit coordinator, who is educated in providing these services for nursing units. The health unit coordinator is skilled in the nonclinical role on the nursing unit. The health unit coordinator can purchase supplies, assist with the budget, assist with staffing, and other clerical duties as assigned.

HEALTH CARE COSTS

Health care leaders are facing many challenges. One major challenge is the cost of health care. Health care is expensive, and the customers who use the health care systems are looking closely at what they are paying for and what they are receiving. The health care facility today must provide the best health care at the most affordable price. No longer is it a market where all the customers in a certain area use the neighborhood health care facility. Health care customers can go anywhere to acquire the care they need. It has become a market where the individual health care facilities compete for customers. What does the health care customer want? As do all customers, health care customers want value. Maximum value is defined as the maximum quality of care at the lowest cost. At a health care facility, the employees contribute significantly to the quality of health care provided to the patients by providing quality service. Good customer service comes from the bottom up and from the top down. Customers expect quality care and caring employees. This is an ongoing perpetual challenge for health care administrations.

Another ongoing challenge is keeping health care affordable. Patients are asked to contribute more out-of-pocket money to pay for health care costs as the cost of health care continues to rise. It is administration's goal to keep these costs as low as possible while still providing quality care for the patients.

Health care costs continue to rise because of many factors, many of which are beyond the capability of the health care facility to control. The government affects the cost of health care by paying for health care costs at a reduced rate for the elderly and poor, who make up a large number of health care users. Each year, the federal government requires health care facilities to meet certain standards that are costly to the facility. These standards are put in place to protect the patient.

STAFFING

The challenge of employing or staffing enough sufficiently skilled professionals to provide patient care is facing administrators across the country. This shortage of health care workers has become more evident as the aging population increases and increases its use of the health care systems. Although few careers are as fulfilling as careers in health care, fewer people are choosing health care careers as other careers offer increasingly interesting challenges, attractive working hours, and competitive wages. The challenge facing health care administrators is how to encourage people to enter, and stay in, a health care career.

Many health care systems are encouraging employees and students to choose those careers in health care that are facing the greatest shortages by offering various tuition reimbursement and incentive programs. Professions such as nursing, hospital pharmacists, respiratory therapists, and medical coders are currently facing shortages. The professional shortages can be specific to the geographical area.

COMMUNITY RESPONSIBILITIES

A challenge that is unique to the area that the health care facility serves is that posed by the community itself. How the health care facility is viewed in the community, what role it plays in the community, and what its leader's role in the community is are all questions that are vital to the health care facility's success.

Responses often include health care management initiatives and community education. One way health care facilities provide community education is by hosting lecture series for the community on current health care issues. Another way is by providing articles authored by local health care providers and published in the local media. Still another way is by publishing Web pages designed to provide health care consumers with accurate and current health information.

Health care facilities earn community goodwill and respect by doing such things as contributing personnel and resources to run diabetes screenings or providing a local health fair focusing on children's health. The health care facility's administration team works with the community, promoting health care services to the community and partnering in community projects that make the communities better places to live. For example, a health care system might offer flu immunizations free of charge to the community on specific days to promote a healthy community.

Being visible in the community that the health care facility serves has become a must for the administrative team members. These members can be seen at health fairs, giving presentations at local schools and colleges, belonging to local community groups, and being involved in volunteer activities. A small town has different requirements of its health care facility than does a large community, but all communities require the health care facility to be an active partner in the community.

Recruiting and retaining staff is everyone's job, but the administrative team knows that in order to offer quality care they must have quality health care providers on their staff. Incentives may be offered to employees if they can recruit staff for positions identified as hard to fill. Working closely with the employees at the health care facility is important for the administrative team. The employees are the mouth of the health care system. They share their ideas and experiences with each other. Providing employees with involvement in decision making increases employee morale. Encouraging employees to be on committees is an example of how this involvement may be accomplished.

When the employees of the health care facility are active community members they become positive and active advertisers for the health care facility. And, of course, health care workers may also be users of the health care system, which is an additional enticement for the facility's administration to encourage and to be supportive of their employees and their cultures.

It is the role of the administrative team to meet these community challenges while moving the health care system into the next decade. The challenges will not go away, and, in fact, if one challenge is met another one will move in to take its place. The administrative team works closely with the government both locally and nationally to lobby for what they believe is best for the health care system.

LEADERSHIP STYLES

There are many different leadership styles and examples of how those styles affect the health care system. It is good to consider the leadership style of the facility and how it affects the employees, the independent health care professionals who work at the health care facility, as well as the surrounding community that uses the health care facility. Let's look at the leadership styles that could be used in health care.

For years, it was believed that people dislike work and have to be closely supervised to correctly do what is required. It was also believed that people would do a good job only if they thought that if they did not they would be punished. Punishment could mean loss of job. The person at the top dictated what was to be done, and the middle managers did as they were told. Employees were watched closely to make sure things happened, for the most part, as planned. This management style is referred to as authoritative, autocratic, or dictatorial leadership. A health care system in which this style is used often has a high rate of employee turnover.

Participatory or team leadership is a leadership style that we see throughout the business world. It is easy to envision teams of employees working together, with someone leading the team to get the task or goal accomplished. In the health care setting, there are nursing teams, health care teams, physician teams, and dietary teams—all with a common focus of providing quality service to the patient who is the customer.

Team leadership encourages team members to interact and lend a helping hand to accomplish the task at hand. The team leader is usually a member of the senior or middle management group. In this setting, all employees are important team members and function for the good of the team. A group of people functioning as a team will invariably outperform a similar group of people working as individuals. The team members are motivated by each other and generally enjoy and take pride in the product of their group efforts.

Consider the following example. Mr. Smith is in an automobile accident. He is unable to eat without assistance. The dietary team makes sure that his food is easy for the patient care provider team to help Mr. Smith eat. The physical therapy team makes sure that Mr. Smith is up in the chair during mealtimes, planning his therapy so that he will be comfortable for mealtime. The teams work closely together through their team leaders.

Shared leadership is a leadership style in which all the group members share the leadership of the group. This style has value for employees in that it says that all employees can be leaders given the opportunity. Although one individual may be responsible for the group, employees feel that they can have input and all employees want to be recognized for the things they do well. Employees work well in settings in which they are appreciated.

Here is an example of shared leadership. In the nursing unit, a computer upgrade is to take place. The leader for this project will be the health unit coordinator. The health unit coordinator is the individual who will use the system most often and who currently uses the old system. The health unit coordinator will decide the training schedule and sign off the other employees when they are competent in using the new system. The following month, the staff will receive a new system for dispensing medications, and the leader for this project will be the unit pharmacist. Again, the leadership for the projects is shared within the unit or within the health care facility by targeting the leaders on the basis of established criteria. Shared leadership allows employees to value each other's strengths and encourage growth.

SUMMARY

Administration, the leaders of the health care facility, set the tone of the health care facility. They set the policies to which the staff adheres; they implement the mission and vision statements; they represent the beliefs and standards of the health care system; and they move the health care facility to the next level. The health unit coordinator is an important member of the facility, striving to carry out the mission of the health system. The health unit coordinator should be knowledgeable about the facility's administration team. The health unit coordinator interacts with members of administration on various levels, most commonly middle management. The leadership style of the facility permeates throughout the whole system and out into the community.

REVIEW QUESTIONS

1. Define administration

2. List three things that affect the administration in a health care facility

3. Describe two senior management positions in the health care facility.

4. List two different leadership styles.

Match the terms and abbreviations in left column to the definitions in right column.

5. Governing Board   a. Chief executive officer

6. CEO   b. Statement that describes the future of the health care system

7. Administration   c. A group of people selected from the community

8. Mission   d. Director of nursing

9. Vision   e. Statement that describes what the health care system is

10. Leadership   f. Chief financial officer

11. CFO   g. Group administratively responsible for the health care system

12. DON   h. The team leading the health care system

13. Middle management   i. The nurse who is a manager of a patient care unit

14. Nurse manager   j. The management between the employee and the administrative team

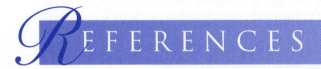

THROUGH THE EYES

OF A HEALTH CARE PROFESSIONAL

We, the staff on the patient care unit, see a member of the administrative team every day interacting with our staff members, our patients, and their families. They are a part of the health system; we are all a part of the whole. We make it happen every hour, every day, every year. We are there to provide health care to our community. Our administrative team supports us to do what we need to do to provide the best care possible to our patients.

REFERENCES

Porter-O'Grady, T. (1995). *The leadership evolution in health care.* Gaithersburg, MD: An Aspen Publication.

Powell, S. (1996). *Nursing case management: A guide to success in managed care.* Philadelphia: Lipponcott-Raven.

Sloane, R. M. (1999). *Introduction to health care delivery organizations* (4th ed.). Chicago: Health Administration Press.

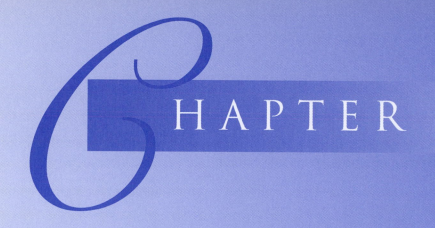

CHAPTER 9

Supplies and Service Management

Learning Objectives

Upon completion of this chapter and review questions, the learner should be able to:

1. Describe the supplies the health unit coordinator uses in the health care facility.

2. Discuss the health unit coordinator role in identifying and ordering supplies.

3. Identify two services the health unit coordinator coordinates.

4. List the three departments that are involved in the supplies and services that the health unit coordinator coordinates.

Key Terms

central supply A department within the health care facility that is responsible for the specific equipment rented or purchased by the patient; also called sterile processing and distribution.

daily charge A charge that is generated daily for a piece of equipment rented for that day.

in-service training Training conducted for the health care staff to provide the knowledge to use equipment correctly.

patient charges Charges generated to the patient bill for goods, services, or equipment purchased or rented.

purchase order Paperwork that is completed to process a request for a supply or service purchased from an outside vendor.

reusable equipment Equipment that a patient may rent for a given amount of time.

services The tasks performed for the benefit of the patients or to meet the requirements of other health care providers within the patient care department.

sterile processing and distribution Another name for central supply.

store room The room from which supplies can be ordered for the patient care unit or for the patient.

supplies One-time use and reusable items that are used in the profession of health unit coordinating and that are ordered from a different area or department.

Abbreviations

CS Central Supply

PO Purchase Order

SPD Sterile Processing and Distribution

SUPPLIES AND SERVICES

Health unit coordinators use supplies and services to meet the requirements and responsibilities of their jobs in their specific work areas. These supplies and services vary from health facility to health facility depending on the size of the facility, the patient population, and the health care providers. If the facility is an outpatient facility, it will require different supplies and services than an inpatient facility. For example, in an inpatient facility the pharmacy department would need to provide medications 24 hours a day, 7 days a week, 365 days a year. An outpatient facility, however, would be closed for a portion of the 24-hour day, and during the time the facility is closed no pharmacy needs would be generated, because there would be no patient population.

Supplies are defined as items used by the health unit coordinator in carrying out the requirements of the job. These items are either one-time use items or reusable items. **Services** are defined as tasks performed for the benefit of the patients or to meet the requirements of other health care providers within the health care unit. These supplies and services can be provided by outside vendors or departments within the health facility.

CLERICAL SUPPLIES

Nursing units have workstations that are set up to help the units' patient care staff efficiently complete their daily work assignments. There may be one workstation or several small workstations located in strategic places throughout the nursing unit. Health unit coordinators use the workstation to complete the majority of the daily work. The clerical supplies used in the workstation are organized so that the workflow is completed efficiently. Health unit coordinators use many clerical supplies to complete the requirements of their job. For example, health unit coordinators who are responsible for transcribing physician orders have to communicate the information in the physician orders to the individuals who are responsible for completing the order. Certain clerical supplies are required in this communication process. Writing instruments are one type of tool used to communicate. They are used for taking phone messages or documenting in the patient record. Examples of clerical supplies that the health unit coordinator may order include the following:

- Writing instruments (pens, pencils, markers)

- Paper chart forms

- Paper clips

- Tape

- Computer supplies

The health unit coordinator is responsible for ordering the supplies required by the department. These supplies include the supplies used by the staff for patients as well as the supplies used by the staff for the department needs. The health unit coordinator will have a defined time frame in which to order these items as well as a procedure on how to order. The health unit coordinator should have a system in place that alerts him or her to the fact that the supply of an item is low and the item will need to be reordered. The health care facility may have a designated supply order day, or supplies may be ordered on demand. The supply ordering system may be a paper system or a computer system. Health unit coordinators' job descriptions usually have a defined responsibility referring to supplies such as:

- Demonstrates how to order supplies for the department

- Maintains the supply inventory within established guidelines

The supplies that are ordered for the department will come either internally from a department within the health care facility or from an external vendor.

Some typical supply items one may find in a health care facility's storeroom are:

- Paper

- Note cards

- Calendars

- Paper cups

◆ Computer cartridges

◆ Phone books

◆ Message pads

The supply items found in the health care facility's storeroom are charged either to the patient care department or directly to the patient. Items charged to the patient care unit are the items that are required for the unit to function. Supply items that are used for many patients, rather than for just one patient, are also charged to the unit.

The health care system's storeroom should be easily accessible to all departments. In some health care facilities, the storeroom employees deliver the orders to the departments on a standard schedule. The **storeroom** carries supply items used by departments as well as items used by patients. This area of the health care facility would be responsible for supplying goods that are used by the ordering department. The storeroom carries a supply of these items to meet the needs of the health care facility.

OUTSIDE VENDORS

Outside vendors may be contracted by the health care facility to provide supplies and services. Outside vendors play an important role in providing supplies and services to the health care facility. They provide these services because it is not cost effective for the health care facility to provide them. In order to purchase goods or services from an outside vendor, the department requesting the goods or services fills out a **purchase order (PO)** and sends it directly to the outside vendor or to a department within the health care facility that processes the purchase orders. The department within the health care facility may be called the purchasing department. All purchase orders are sent to the purchasing department so that the ordering from outside vendors is centralized. Centralized ordering requires that one department be responsible for all the ordering within the facility. Benefits of centralized ordering include cost savings, decreased inventory, and easy access. The cost-saving benefit comes from quantity ordering, resulting in lower prices. Decrease in inventory means that the departments need to request only what they need and not use valuable space for storage. Access is easier when only one department is contacted versus contacting many individual outside vendors.

PATIENT SUPPLIES AND CHARGES

Specific patient supplies are ordered internally through the storeroom within the health care facility or externally through the purchasing department. The purchasing department may purchase the needed supplies locally or through vendors across the country. These items are either purchased by the patient through the health care system or rented by the patient to be used for a specific amount of time. If purchased, they may be considered part of the routine charge and bundled in with the daily room charge, or they may be items that are charged to the patient's account. Items that are used solely for one patient are charged to that patient. A **patient charge** is generated to the patient bill for those items. Usually, these are items that are used only once.

These items, if not used or disposed of, may be sent home with the patient. Each health care facility establishes a system to charge for the goods used whether they are charged to the unit or to the patient.

Charges that are bundled into a room charge may include items that all patients need to use during their health facility stay. For example, Mrs. Smith is admitted to room 3147 for a procedure. In the bedside stand, she finds the following items that are for her personal use: a box of tissue, a bar of soap, and a washbasin. During her health system stay, she will be provided with Band-Aids, tape, a water glass, and a patient rights and responsibilities booklet. She will be able to take with her on discharge things that she did not use completely, such as the tissue and soap. These items cannot be used for another patient, and, if not taken by Mrs. Smith, they would be discarded by the cleaning staff upon her discharge from the health care facility.

MANUAL CHARGE SYSTEMS

Systems developed to document use and to enter charges can be manual systems, computerized systems, or a combination of manual and computer entry. A manual system is a system in which a paper card is placed in the area close to the supplies that the patient care staff uses. The paper card is labeled with the patient name, room number, and other important information. Items that are chargeable to the patient have a sticker attached that the patient care provider removes and attaches to the paper card. The sticker indicates the patient use of the chargeable supply item. The paper card with stickers is periodically collected and immediately replaced with a new paper card, or it could be collected when the patient is discharged. The paper cards are sent to the department within the health care facility that enters patient charges so that the charge for the various items used by the patient can be entered on the patient bill. Items can also be charged to the department by having a paper card labeled "Surgical Unit Use" and having the staff place the sticker from the items used for the department on the card. The health unit coordinator is responsible for placing the new paper cards in the correct area so the patient care staff can place the stickers on the cards. The health unit coordinator sends the cards with stickers to the department responsible for entering the charges. Making sure the inventory is correct at defined times is also the responsibility of the health unit coordinator (Figure 9-1).

COMPUTERIZED CHARGE SYSTEMS

A computerized charge system is one that can be used throughout the health care system. In this system, the item that is charged to the patient contains a sticker with a universal code. The health care team member removing the item from the area scans this sticker and enters the patient identification code. This system requires that a scanning device be located near the supply area. The computer system posts this charge to the patient's bill and sends a message to the storeroom to refill the inventory in that department.

Items that are chargeable to a department rather than to a patient are handled by entering the department identification code instead of the patient's identification code. The health unit coordinator is responsible for educating the staff on the use of the system as well as for checking that the inventory is correct at the end of a defined time frame (Figure 9-2).

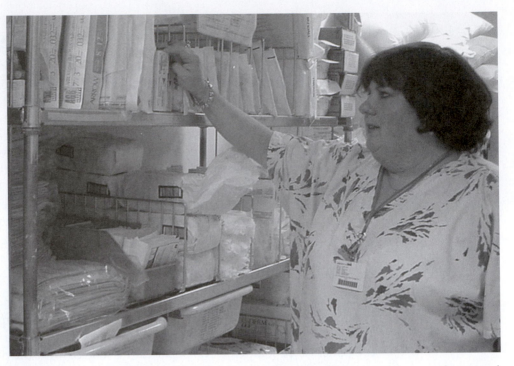

Figure 9-1 • *The health unit coordinator checks the supplies on the supply cart. (Courtesy of Marquette General Health System, Marquette, MI)*

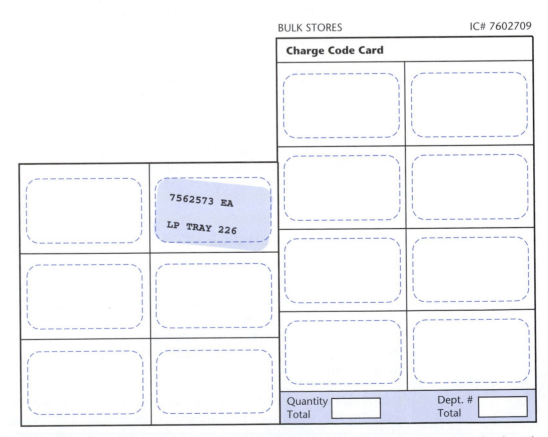

BULK STORES   IC# 7602709

Charge Code Card

7562573 EA

LP TRAY 226

Quantity Total

Dept. # Total

Figure 9-2 • *Stickers can either be scanned or the information can be hand entered into the computer system to charge the patient for items used during hospitalization.*
(Courtesy of Marquette General Health System, Marquette, MI)

COMBINATION CHARGE SYSTEMS

A combination manual-computerized system is similar to the paper system except that, after the health unit coordinator collects the patient-identified paper cards, instead of sending them to the department that enters in the charges the health unit coordinator directly enters the charges into the facility's computer system. In some systems, instead of having a sticker on each chargeable supply item, the health care provider withdrawing the supply item manually writes the item code onto the card. In this system, as in any system, it is important that the health care coordinator, upon collecting a card, immediately replace it to reduce the chance of a health care provider's neglecting to document the charge.

No matter what system is used for collecting and entering patient charges for supplies, the system must be easy for all members of the patient care team to use. The entering of patient charges for supplies must be accurate. Health care facilities often have procedures to ensure that supply charges are correctly entered (Figure 9-3).

Health care facilities have procedures to ensure that the health care staff members entering these charges are competent (have demonstrated how to correctly enter these charges). Charges are monitored and audits are performed by health care facilities to ensure that the supply charges are correct.

CENTRAL SUPPLY

Some supplies, called **reusable equipment**, that are used by patients are rented for a specific amount of time. These are usually items that patients would not want to purchase because they would not need to use them again. Other patients can rent these items or pieces of equipment after the equipment is cleaned according to the health care facility policies and procedures. These items usually are very expensive. The department that supplies these items for patients is called **central supply (CS)** or **sterile processing and distribution (SPD)**. The health unit coordinator requests these items by generating a charge by using a manual request (paper requisition) or a computer request. The patient is billed daily for the use of the equipment. These charges are called **daily charges**. Every day, the health unit coordinator must make sure that the supply charges for equipment are correct. Depending on the health care facility's charging system, the health unit coordinator will either enter a manual charge daily for the specific equipment or double-check that the computer charge is correct. Some computer charging systems automatically enter the charges daily until stopped. The health unit coordinator must be diligent in doubling-checking these charges. The following items are examples of items that central supply has available for patients to rent:

- ◆ Suction machines
- ◆ Feeding tube pumps (food pumps)
- ◆ IV pumps
- ◆ Specialty beds

It is very important that the charges be done correctly and that they are accurate because the patient health care bill reflects these charges (Figure 9-4).

MARQUETTE GENERAL HEALTH SYSTEM
Marquette, Michigan

RADIATION ONCOLOGY DEPARTMENT

SUBJECT: ENTERING CHARGES   PROCEDURE NO.: 723-054

EFFECTIVE DATE: 10/31/01

DISTRIBUTION: RADIATION DEPT.   REVISION DATE:

_____
Authorized by

1. If the date and/or initials have not been completed, return to appropriate person for completion before entering charges.

2. Log onto StanLan.

3. Press the F6 key.

4. Press the F1 key.

5. Press F1 key to select your patient.

6. Press F2 if the current account number is known, if not known press F3 and follow the on-screen instructions for entering the patient name.

7. Enter account number where shown on the screen.

8. Enter (??) where it asks for the patient type.

9. Press Enter twice.

10. Check to be sure the correct patient name is at the top of the screen.

11. Press F3 once you are sure you have the correct patient.

12. Then press the "control" and F3 key at the same time.

13. Type the first procedure code that is marked on the charge sheet.

14. Press enter.

15. Type in the quantity, then press enter.

16. Type in a second procedure code if there is one; if there is not one, press enter.

17. Enter the date (11302000), then press enter.

18. When it asks "Ordered by:" check the upper left hand corner to see what doctor appears there. If it is the correct doctor, press enter. If it is another doctor be sure to enter the correct doctor's code (4008—CD, 4009—PT).

19. Press F1.

20. If someone has written the word "complete" at the top of the charge sheet, be sure to mark the name, medical record number, and the date in which the patient completed on the "X-rays to be returned" log. This log gets sent up to radiology once the sheet is full.

21. Initial charge sheet after entering data.

Figure 9-3 • *An example of a procedure for entering charges (Courtesy of Marquette General Health System, Marquette, MI)*

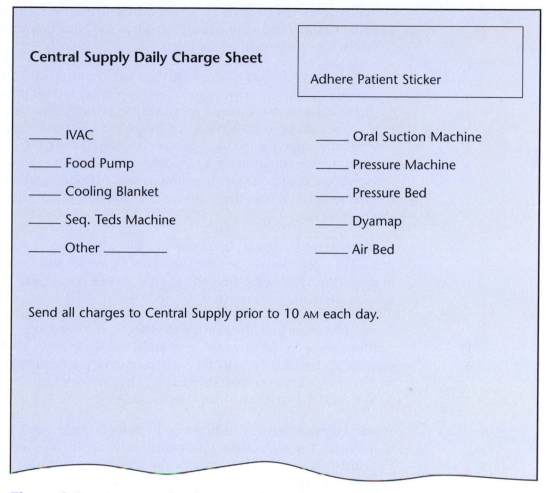

Central Supply Daily Charge Sheet

Adhere Patient Sticker

_____ IVAC

_____ Food Pump

_____ Cooling Blanket

_____ Seq. Teds Machine

_____ Other _____

_____ Oral Suction Machine

_____ Pressure Machine

_____ Pressure Bed

_____ Dyamap

_____ Air Bed

Send all charges to Central Supply prior to 10 AM each day.

Figure 9-4 • *An example of a central supply charge form used by the health unit coordinator*

It is important that health unit coordinators be familiar with patient equipment used in the health care facility. The health unit coordinator is involved in the process for ordering the equipment and generating the correct charges, and identifying the equipment is a key to generating the correct charge. **In-service training** conducted by the vendors of new equipment provides the health care staff with the knowledge to use the equipment correctly.

DEPARTMENT AND PATIENT SERVICES

The health unit coordinator requests services for the patient care unit. These services are important in the coordination of activities and may provide patients with assistance needed during their health system stay. Nonnursing departments and outside vendors are used to provide patients with services that the nursing care team members are not able to provide. These services may include activities that are done for a fee. The services are utilized by the patient care areas and by the patients. Services used by the patient care areas are services designed to facilitate the operation of the department and ensure that the area is performing to established standards. These standards are set by government agencies such as the Occupational Safety and Health Administration (OSHA) or accrediting agencies such as the Joint Commission on Accreditation of Health Care Organizations (JCAHO).

Nonnursing departments that provide daily services to a patient care area may include housekeeping, laundry services, and specialty services such as physical therapy services. Environmental services (housekeeping) may be provided by a health system department or by an outside janitorial service. The service includes the general housekeeping of the defined area: emptying the trash containers, cleaning the patient rooms and bathrooms, and keeping the common areas tidy. The service may also include cleaning the hallways, waxing the floors, hanging curtains, and performing other cleaning activities. It is the responsibility of the health unit coordinator to keep the work area at the workstation tidy.

Laundry services provide clean linen to each patient care area and remove the soiled linen. These services may be purchased from an outside vendor, or laundry may be done in the facility. The health unit coordinator may be responsible for notifying laundry services when linen is needed.

Some services are provided directly to patients who need services not provided by the nursing care team. Services such as physical therapy services, dietitian services, diabetes services, and similar specialty type services can be provided by other departments within the facility or by outside vendors. They are provided directly to the specific patient, and the service is charged to the patient.

Physical therapy services are provided to patients while they are inpatients as well as outpatients. The physician for the patient must order those services. The health unit coordinator transcribes the order for this service by contacting the physical therapy department to provide the service. The charge for this service is entered onto the patient bill after the service has been provided.

Some patients require a dietitian to provide nutritional services. These services are provided by a registered dietitian and charged to the patient's account. Dietitians provide a variety of services for patients, including meal planning, nutritional assessments, weight management programs, and recipe modifications.

Diabetes services are provided to patients who have diabetes. These services may also include information for family members and care providers. Diabetes services include insulin management, exercise education, diet instructions, and medication information. These services are provided to patients who are both inpatients and outpatients.

The services are an important part of the patient care plan. The health unit coordinator transcribes the orders for these services onto the correct forms and generates the charges when these services are completed.

SUMMARY

The health unit coordinator is responsible for ordering supplies and services for the patients and staff on the health care unit. Correctly ordering patient supplies and services is important because these are shown on the patient bills. The patient bill must be accurate and reflect only the supplies and services actually provided to the patient. The health unit coordinator contacts the various departments and vendors that supply the services and goods. It is important to receive these services and goods in a timely manner to provide the best possible care for the patients. Health unit coordinators are an important link in the acquisition of supplies and services needed to ensure quality patient care. They are also the link that acquires the goods and the services required by the department to provide that patient care, whether it is a new laundry cart or an overflowing toilet that needs to be repaired. The health unit coordinator knows whom to contact and how to contact the appropriate department efficiently to get the task completed.

REVIEW QUESTIONS

Match the term in the left column to the definition in right column.

1. Supplies

2. Services

3. Storeroom

4. Central supply

5. Reusable equipment

6. Patient charges

7. Daily charges

a. Tasks performed by another person(s) for the patient or department

b. A department within the health care facility that is responsible for the specific equipment rented or purchased by the patient

c. One-time use and reusable items that are used in the profession of health unit coordinating and ordered from a different area or department

d. Equipment that a patient may rent for a given amount of time

e. Charges generated to the patient bill for goods, services, or equipment purchased or rented

f. A charge that is generated daily for a piece of equipment rented for that day

g. The room from which supplies can be ordered for the patient care unit or for the patient

NAHUC CERTIFICATION EXAM

CONTENT AREAS

I. A. 12   Enter patient charges

I. C. 3   Request supplies and equipment

II. D. 1   Maintain a supply of chart forms

II. D. 2   Maintain stock of patient care supplies and equipment

II. D. 3   Maintain stock of clerical and desk supplies

II. D. 9   Arrange for maintenance and repair of equipment

II. E. 10   Reconcile patient charges/credits

II. E. 14   Inventory unit equipment

THROUGH THE EYES

OF A HEALTH CARE PROFESSIONAL

Correctly charging patient accounts for items used is an important part of the daily responsibilities of the health unit coordinator. Patients are careful to check their health care bills to make sure that they were not overcharged for items they did not receive. It is my job to process the charges accurately and in a timely fashion so that the patient receives the correct charges and the health system receives the correct fees for services and supplies provided.

The health care team depends on the health unit coordinator to have all the supplies needed for daily patient care as well as the supplies needed for the health care unit. Members of the health care team come to the health unit coordinator knowing that I will be able to locate the needed items either within the unit, within the health system, or by completing the necessary paperwork to get the items from an outside vendor. Knowing how to do this quickly and efficiently ensures that patients have what they need when it is needed. It is also important to keep a careful watch on our inventory so we are using our resources wisely.

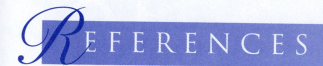

REFERENCES

Hegner, B. R. (2004). *Nursing assistant: A nursing process approach* (9th ed.). Clifton Park, NY: Thomson Delmar Learning.

Smith, S. (2000). *Clinical nursing skills* (5th ed.). Upper Saddle River, NJ: Prentice Hall.

CHAPTER 10

Healthy Environment and Safety

Learning Objectives

Upon completion of this chapter and review questions, the learner should be able to:

1. Define all key terms.

2. List three agencies involved in the regulation of health and safety.

3. List the departments within the health care facility involved in the enforcement and implementation of health and safety.

4. Describe incident reports.

5. Describe the term *code* as it is used in the health care facility.

6. Explain the health unit coordinator responsibilities in emergency situations.

7. Explain the health unit coordinator responsibilities regarding isolation.

8. Describe Standard Precautions.

Key Terms

crash cart A special cart containing life-saving equipment, including a defibrillator (pads used to deliver an electric shock to the heart) and equipment for establishing an airway (intubating).

incident report A document used to record any event within the health care facility that resulted or could have resulted in injury or loss.

isolation The process of containing and preventing the spread of microorganisms or germs that cause disease.

Material Safety Data Sheet A document that contains information about the type of chemical and how to protect oneself from the risks of using the chemical.

nosocomial infections Infections acquired by the patient while in the health care facility.

regulatory agency The term given to organizations outside the health care facility that control and monitor health and safety.

reverse isolation The process of protecting the patient from harmful organisms.

Abbreviations

APIC Association for Professionals in Infection Control and Epidemiology

ASHRM American Society for Health Risk Management

CDC Centers for Disease Control and Prevention

CNA Certified nursing assistant

DHHS Department of Health and Human Services

DOL Department of Labor

HICPAC Health Care Infection Control Practices Advisory Committee

HIPAA Health Insurance Portability and Accountability Act

IDSA Infectious Disease Society of America

JCAHO Joint Commission on Accreditation of Health Care Organizations

MSDS Material Safety Data Sheet

NIOSH National Institute for Occupational Safety and Health

OCR Office of Civil Rights

OSHA Occupational Safety and Health Administration

PPE Personal Protective Equipment

SHEA Society for Health Care Epidemiology of America

HEALTH AND SAFETY

The health and safety of the health care staff and the patients is a major concern of the health care facility. A health care facility is responsible for the safety of its staff and patients. It is such a concern that there are dozens of public and private agencies that govern and regulate health and safety. In this chapter, we will take a brief look at some of the agencies involved in health and safety. The departments that implement health and safety policies within the health care facility will be discussed, along with the health unit coordinator's responsibility for health and safety.

REGULATORY AGENCIES

Regulatory agency is the term given to organizations outside the health care facility that control and monitor health and safety. The regulatory agencies make and enforce laws and rules health care facilities must follow. Failure to follow the laws and rules not only makes the health care facility unsafe; it also can result in fines and loss of funding.

U.S. DEPARTMENT OF LABOR AND THE OCCUPATIONAL SAFETY AND HEALTH ADMINISTRATION

The U.S. Department of Labor (DOL) is a federal agency. The Occupational Safety and Health Administration (OSHA) is one of the important agencies within the DOL. The OSHA Web site states,

> OSHA's mission is to ensure safe and healthful workplaces in America. OSHA accomplishes its mission by establishing protective standards, by enforcing those standards, and by reaching out to employers and employees through technical assistance and consultation programs.

> . . . Top priority for OSHA are reports of imminent dangers—accidents about to happen; second are fatalities or accidents serious enough to send three or more workers to the hospital. Third are employee complaints. Referrals from other government agencies are fourth. Fifth are targeted inspections, such as the Site Specific Targeting Program, which focuses on employers that report high injury and illness rates and special emphasis programs that zero in on hazardous work. Follow-up inspections are the final priority.

> OSHA requires employers to maintain employee records of injuries and illnesses. About 1.3 million employers with 11 or more employees— 20 percent of the establishments OSHA covers—must keep records of work-related injuries and illnesses.

> OSHA issued an ergonomics guideline for the nursing home industry on March 13, 2003. To develop the guidelines, OSHA reviewed existing ergonomics practices and programs, state OSHA programs, as well as available scientific information. The guidelines, designed to prevent musculoskeletal disorders in the workplace, focus on practical recommendations for employers to reduce the number and severity of workplace injuries by using methods found to be successful in the nursing home environment.

DEPARTMENT OF HEALTH AND HUMAN SERVICES

The U.S. Department of Health and Human Services (DHHS) is another federal agency involved in the safety and health of patients. The DHHS Web site states,

> The Department of Health and Human Services is the United States government's principal agency for protecting the health of all Americans and providing essential human services, especially for those who are least able to help themselves. The Department includes more than 300 programs, covering a wide spectrum of activities. Some highlights include:
>
> ◆ Medical and social science research
>
> ◆ Preventing outbreak of infectious disease, including immunization services
>
> ◆ Assuring food and drug safety
>
> ◆ Medicare (health insurance for elderly and disabled Americans) and Medicaid (health insurance for low-income people)
>
> ◆ Financial assistance and services for low-income families
>
> ◆ Improving maternal and infant health
>
> ◆ Head Start (pre-school education and services)
>
> ◆ Preventing child abuse and domestic violence
>
> ◆ Substance abuse treatment and prevention
>
> ◆ Services for older Americans, including home-delivered meals
>
> ◆ Comprehensive health services for Native Americans
>
> HHS is the largest grant-making agency in the federal government, providing some 60,000 grants per year. HHS' Medicare program is the nation's largest health insurer, handling more than 900 million claims per year.
>
> HHS works closely with state, local, and tribal governments, and many HHS-funded services are provided at the local level by state, county or tribal agencies or through private sector grantees. The Department's programs are administered by 11 HHS operating divisions, including eight agencies in the U.S. Public Health Service and three human services agencies. In addition to the services they deliver, the HHS programs provide for equitable treatment of beneficiaries nationwide, and they enable the collection of national health and other data.

CENTERS FOR DISEASE CONTROL AND PREVENTION

The Centers for Disease Control and Prevention (CDC) is one of the major operating components of the DHHS. The CDC Web site states,

> It is recognized as the lead federal agency for protecting the health and safety of people—at home and abroad, providing credible information to enhance health decisions, and promoting health through strong partnerships. CDC serves as the national focus for developing and applying disease prevention and control, environmental health, and health promotion and

education activities designed to improve the health of the people of the United States.

CDC's mission is to promote health and quality of life by preventing and controlling disease, injury, and disability. CDC seeks to accomplish its mission by working with partners throughout the nation and world to monitor health, detect and investigate health problems, conduct research to enhance prevention, develop and advocate sound public health policies, implement prevention strategies, promote healthy behaviors, foster safe and healthful environments, and provide leadership and training.

Infectious diseases, such as HIV/AIDS and tuberculosis, have the ability to destroy lives, strain community resources, and even threaten nations. In today's global environment, new diseases have the potential to spread across the world in a matter of days, or even hours, making early detection and action more important than ever. CDC plays a critical role in controlling these diseases, traveling at a moment's notice to investigate outbreaks abroad or at home.

But disease outbreaks are only the beginning of [its] protective role. By assisting state and local health departments, CDC works to protect the public every day: from using innovative "fingerprinting" technology to identify a foodborne illness, to evaluating a family violence prevention program in an urban community, from training partners in HIV education, to protecting children from vaccine-preventable diseases through immunizations.

NATIONAL INSTITUTE FOR OCCUPATIONAL SAFETY AND HEALTH

An important part of the CDC is the National Institute for Occupational Safety and Health (NIOSH). The NIOSH Web site states,

> The National Institute for Occupational Safety and Health (NIOSH) is the federal agency responsible for conducting research and making recommendations for the prevention of work-related disease and injury. NIOSH is responsible for conducting research on the full scope of occupational disease and injury ranging from lung disease in miners to carpal tunnel syndrome in computer users. NIOSH is a diverse organization made up of employees representing a wide range of disciplines including industrial hygiene, nursing, epidemiology, engineering, medicine, and statistics. Although NIOSH and OSHA were created by the same Act of Congress, they are two distinct agencies with separate responsibilities. NIOSH is in the U.S. Department of Health and Human Services and is a research agency. OSHA is in the U.S. Department of Labor and is responsible for creating and enforcing workplace safety and health regulations. NIOSH and OSHA often work together toward the common goal of protecting worker safety and health.

OFFICE OF CIVIL RIGHTS

The Office of Civil Rights (OCR) is another agency of the HHS. The Office of Civil Rights oversees the Medical Privacy Standards, and the National Standards to Protect the Privacy of Personal Health Information, in turn, is under the auspices of the Office of Civil Rights. The privacy provisions of the federal law, the Health Insurance Portability and Accountability Act of 1996 (HIPAA), apply to health information created or maintained by health care providers who engage in certain electronic transactions, health plans, and health care clearinghouses. The OCR is the departmental component responsible for implementing and enforcing the privacy regulation. Additional information about HIPAA can be found in Chapter 11.

STATE DEPARTMENTS OF HEALTH

HHS oversees the state departments of health. Each state has its own government agency for public health concerns and the prevention and control of disease and injury. The range of a state public health department is broad. Services may include vaccinations to protect children against disease; testing to ensure the safety of food, water, and drugs; licensing to ensure quality health care in hospitals and nursing homes; investigations to control the outbreak of infectious diseases; collection and evaluation of health statistics to develop prevention and regulatory programs; and screening newborns for genetic diseases. Many of the members of the health care team must have a license to practice their profession in the state in which they work. The state's public health department controls the licensing of these professionals.

JOINT COMMISSION ON ACCREDITATION OF HEALTH CARE ORGANIZATIONS

The Joint Commission on Accreditation of Health Care Organizations (JCAHO) explains its mission in their Web site:

> Mission: To continuously improve the safety and quality of care provided to the public through the provision of health care accreditation and related services that support performance improvement in health care organizations. The Joint Commission evaluates and accredits nearly 17,000 health care organizations and programs in the United States. An independent, not-for-profit organization, JCAHO is the nation's predominant standards-setting and accrediting body in health care. Since 1951, JCAHO has developed state-of-the-art, professionally based standards and evaluated the compliance of health care organizations against these benchmarks.

> JCAHO accreditation is recognized nationwide as a symbol of quality that reflects an organization's commitment to meeting certain performance standards. To earn and maintain accreditation, an organization must undergo an on-site survey by a JCAHO survey team at least every three years. Laboratories must be surveyed every two years.

> JCAHO is governed by a 29-member Board of Commissioners that includes nurses, physicians, consumers, medical directors, administrators, providers, employers, a labor representative, health plan leaders, quality experts, ethicists, a health insurance administrator and educators. The Board of Commissioners brings to JCAHO countless years of diverse experience in health care, business and public policy. JCAHO's corporate members are the American College of Physicians, American Society of Internal Medicine, the American College of Surgeons, the American Dental Association, the American Hospital Association and the American Medical Association.

Benefits of JCAHO accreditation:

◆ Leads to improved patient care.

◆ Demonstrates the organization's commitment to safety and quality.

◆ Offers an educational onsite survey experience.

◆ Supports and enhances safety and quality improvement efforts.

◆ Strengthens and supports recruitment and retention efforts.

◆ May substitute for federal certification surveys for Medicare and Medicaid.

◆ Helps secure managed care contracts.

◆ Facilitates the organization's business strategies.

◆ Provides a competitive advantage.

◆ Enhances the organization's image to the public, purchasers and payers.

◆ Fulfills licensure requirements in many states.

◆ Recognized by insurers and other third parties.

◆ Strengthens community confidence.

JCAHO's standards address the organization's level of performance in key functional areas, such as patient rights, patient treatment, and infection control, and the standards focus not simply on an organization's ability to provide safe, high quality care, but on its actual performance as well. Standards set forth performance expectations for activities that affect the safety and quality of patient care. If an organization does the right things and does them well, there is a strong likelihood that its patients will experience good outcomes. JCAHO develops its standards in consultation with health care experts, providers, measurement experts, purchasers and consumers.

In 2003, JCAHO implemented its National Patient Safety Goals. JCAHO's Web site explains these goals:

Beginning January 1, 2003, all JCAHO-accredited health care organizations will be surveyed for implementation of the following recommendations— or acceptable alternatives—as appropriate to the services the organization provides. Alternatives must be at least as effective as the published recommendations in achieving the goals.

◆ Improve the accuracy of patient identification.

◆ Use at least two patient identifiers (neither to be the patient's room number) whenever taking blood samples or administering medications or blood products.

◆ Prior to the start of any surgical or invasive procedure, conduct a final verification process, such as a time out, to confirm the correct patient, procedure and site, using active—not passive—communication techniques.

◆ Improve the effectiveness of communication among caregivers.

◆ Implement a process for taking verbal or telephone orders that require a verification "read-back" of the complete order by the person receiving the order.

◆ Standardize the abbreviations, acronyms and symbols used throughout the organization, including a list of abbreviations, acronyms and symbols *not* to use.

◆ Improve the safety of using high-alert medications.

◆ Remove concentrated electrolytes (including, but not limited to, potassium chloride, potassium phosphate, sodium chloride > 0.9% from patient care units.

◆ Standardize and limit the number of drug concentrations available in the organization.

◆ Eliminate wrong-site, wrong-patient, wrong-procedure surgery.

◆ Create and use a preoperative verification process, such as a checklist, to confirm that appropriate documents (e.g., medical records, imaging studies) are available.

◆ Implement a process to mark the surgical site and involve the patient in the marking process.

◆ Improve the safety of using infusion pumps.

◆ Ensure free-flow protection on all general-use and PCA (patient-controlled analgesia) intravenous infusion pumps used in the organization.

◆ Improve the effectiveness of clinical alarm systems.

◆ Implement regular preventive maintenance and testing of alarm systems.

◆ Assure that alarms are activated with appropriate settings and are sufficiently audible with respect to distances and competing noise within the unit.

HEALTH CARE FACILITY DEPARTMENTS

In addition to the many outside regulatory agencies, there are departments within the health care facility that interpret and implement the many regulations set forth by the public and private agencies.

EPIDEMIOLOGY

The epidemiology or infection control department is responsible for infection control. The epidemiology department personnel may consist of a nurse, physician, epidemiologist, and medical technologist, or any combination of these. One of the main goals of the epidemiology department is to prevent and reduce **nosocomial infections**.

Nosocomial infections are infections acquired by the patient while in the health care facility. The epidemiology department investigates outbreaks of nosocomial infections in health care facilities, isolates sources of infection, implements corrective measures to limit the extent of infections, and helps to ensure that similar episodes are not repeated. The epidemiology department provides information and instruction to the health care team members.

The Association for Professionals in Infection Control and Epidemiology (APIC) Web site states,

> Infection control programs began to spring up in U.S. hospitals during the 1960s based on a recommendation by the Joint Commission on Accreditation of Health Care Organizations (JCAHO) in 1958 that hospitals appoint infection control committees. Since the committees could only give direction and other hospital personnel did not have the time or skills to perform the everyday duties required of an effective infection control program, a new health care profession was born—the infection control professional.

> As part of its hospital accreditation standards that stipulate key organizational structures and functions, JCAHO continues to prescribe the broad elements of infection control programs, but gives hospitals considerable latitude in designing their own programs.

> The Centers for Disease Control and Prevention (CDC) has provided much of the scientific and epidemiologic basis for infection control in the United States. Significant progress has been made in preventing and controlling nosocomial infections, thereby lowering the infection risk of patients in hospitals and other health care facilities. However, nosocomial infections continue to be a major source of morbidity and mortality, affecting more than 2 million patients annually in the United States. The estimated annual economic cost is more than $4.5 billion in 1992 dollars.

RISK MANAGEMENT

Risk Management is responsible for creating and maintaining safe environments with health care facilities. The American Society for Health Risk Management (ASHRM) Web site explains that health care risk management professionals are "responsible for the process of making and carrying out decisions that will promote quality care, maintain a safe environment, and preserve human and financial resources in health care organizations."

The risk management department is responsible for the review of all **incident reports**. An incident report is a document used to record any event within the health care facility that resulted or could have resulted in injury or loss (Figure 10-1). An incident includes accidents as well as thefts or errors in treatment. The incident report is not part of the patient's medical record. Some examples of incidents are:

◆ A visitor slips and falls in the hallway

◆ A health care team member sticks herself with a needle.

◆ A health care team member gives a patient the wrong medication.

◆ A theft occurs on the health care facility grounds.

TheBestMedicalCenter
INCIDENT REPORT

If patient, addressograph

| Last Name | First Name |

| Address | |

| City | State | Zip |

DESCRIPTION OF INCIDENT:

INCIDENT LOCATION

INCIDENT DATE & TIME

WITNESS(ES)

PROPERTY LOSS OR DAMAGE

Person Completing the Report

NOT A PERMANENT PART OF THE CHART, FORWARD TO SECURITY.

Figure 10-1 • *Incident report*

ENGINEERING/MAINTENANCE

Engineering, the department responsible for the health care facility's buildings and grounds, has significant responsibilities for ensuring a healthy and safe environment. They make certain that equipment is operating correctly. They are responsible for heating and ventilation and may be called when ventilation is an issue in isolation rooms. They are responsible for electrical and fire safety. A subdepartment of the engineering department is the Bio-Med department. Bio-Med is responsible for the patient monitoring equipment.

ENVIRONMENTAL SERVICES

Environmental services, or housekeeping, is the department responsible for the cleanliness of the health care facility. The environmental services department must know the hazards and identities of the chemicals they use. The environmental service personnel are instructed how to protect themselves and the patients from infection. For every chemical that is used within the health care facility, there should be a corresponding **Material Safety Data Sheet**. A Material Safety Data Sheet (MSDS) contains information about the type of chemical and how to protect oneself from the risks of using the chemical. This department would be notified of any spills that need to be cleaned.

EMPLOYEE HEALTH

The employee health department, or personnel health department, is responsible for the immunization of its employees. It is also responsible for keeping records of employee illnesses and injuries.

CENTRAL SUPPLY

The central supply department is responsible for the disinfection and sterilization of patient care items. They are responsible for knowing the proper techniques to ensure that patient care supplies and equipment are germ free.

SECURITY

The security department is responsible for the safety and security of staff, patients, and visitors. The security department would provide traffic control in an emergency situation.

HEALTH AND SAFETY COMMITTEES

Often, there are specific committees assigned to monitor health and safety issues. For example, there may be a patient falls committee or a medication error committee or a fire safety committee. Usually these committees are multidisciplinary, or made up of a variety of health care team members from throughout the facility. The health unit coordinator may be assigned to participate in a health or safety committee.

MANDATORY TRAINING

The health care facility employee must be aware of many health and safety guidelines. Because constant changes and improvements are made in health and safety, health and safety regulations are always changing. Because of the important nature of this information, the health care facility offers training. Health care facilities have health and safety training for all health care employees at least once a year. The health unit coordinator is expected to attend the mandatory training. An employee is required to attend mandatory training as a condition of employment. The health unit coordinator may also be responsible for posting and filing new and revised health and safety policies and procedures.

GENERAL SAFETY RULES

The health unit coordinator should adhere to the general safety rules that apply in the immediate work environment. These are commonsense safety rules. General safety rules may include:

- ◆ Know the proper use of equipment before using.

- ◆ Observe and report any broken or damaged equipment.

- ◆ Walk, don't run.

- ◆ Walk on the right side of the hall.

- ◆ Use caution near doors.

BODY MECHANICS

Body mechanics is the science of keeping the body in proper alignment during physical activity. It involves the use of good posture and using the strongest and largest muscles of the body to perform work. Health care team members who provide direct patient care must be careful not to injure themselves or others when lifting or moving a patient. Proper body mechanics helps the team members correctly use their physical strength. Health care team members who provide direct patient care should receive training in body mechanics. Although health unit coordinators do not provide direct patient care, they may do some lifting of supplies and equipment during the job.

The Cybernurse Learning Page for Certified Nursing Assistants (CNAs) lists several rules to help one use good body mechanics to lift and move residents or patients and heavy objects safely and efficiently:

- ◆ Stand in good alignment and with a wide base of support (spread your legs slightly apart).

- ◆ Use the stronger and larger muscles of your body. They are in the shoulders, upper arms, thighs, and hips.

- ◆ Keep objects close to your body when you lift, move, or carry them.

◆ Avoid unnecessary bending and reaching. If possible, have the height of the bed and overbed table level with your waist when giving care. Adjust the bed and table to the proper height.

◆ To prevent unnecessary twisting, face the area in which you are working.

◆ Push, slide, or pull heavy objects whenever possible rather than lift them.

◆ Use both hands and arms when you lift, move, or carry heavy objects.

◆ Turn your whole body when you change the direction of your movement.

◆ Work with smooth and even movements. Avoid sudden or jerky motions.

◆ Get help from a co-worker to move heavy objects or residents/patients.

◆ Squat to lift heavy objects from the floor. Push against the strong hip and thigh muscles to raise yourself to a standing position.

ERGONOMICS

Ergonomics is the science of fitting the job environment and equipment to the worker. When there is a mismatch between the physical requirements of the job and the physical capacity of the worker, work-related musculoskeletal disorders can result. For their own safety and comfort, health unit coordinators may want to assess the ergonomics of their immediate work area.

The American Federation of Teachers Web site for Ergonomics for Paraprofessionals lists the following healthy hints for office employees:

◆ Take frequent breaks from computer work. The National Institute for Occupational Safety and Health recommends that computer users work no more than 45 minutes at a time on a computer before taking a 15 minute break that can be used for doing non-computer work.

◆ Stand up, stretch and walk around before beginning another sedentary office activity.

◆ At least twice a day, take a few moments to do hand and finger exercises.

◆ If your computer workstation or desk is not adjustable, try putting the keyboard on your lap or raising your chair so that you are keying with your wrists in a neutral position. If your keyboard tray is adjustable, keep it in a low position.

◆ Try to position your monitor with the top a few inches below a point level with the top of your head.

◆ Keep your feet flat on the floor. If they dangle and don't reach the floor, try using telephone books or boxes as a footrest.

◆ Use accessories that will improve your comfort such as a document holder that will place hard copy at eye level, a lumbar pillow for back support or a footrest.

◆ Adding machines, calculators and typewriters should be placed on adjustable work surfaces.

◆ When collating materials, try to find a work surface that doesn't require you to bend over to do the job.

EMERGENCIES IN THE HEALTH CARE FACILITY

The health care facility provides a variety of types of health services to a variety of individuals. Health care facilities are organized to provide services in a timely and organized fashion. Despite careful planning and scheduling, services often must be provided for unplanned or emergency circumstances. Popular culture has adopted the use of the word *stat* in everyday conversation. The health care term *stat*, which is short for the Latin term *statim*, means immediate or with no delay. Many services and procedures in the health care facility are expected to be performed stat. Many emergencies that happen in and around the health care facility result in stat action from the health care team. The health unit coordinator must understand the types of emergencies and know how to respond in a stat manner.

EMERGENCY CODES

Emergencies in the health care facility are usually called *codes*. Different code terms are assigned to different emergencies. A code is a term given to an emergency situation. Code terms vary from facility to facility (Table 10-1). Codes are usually posted in the departments that provide patient care. Health care facilities have policies and procedures for each type of code. Codes are usually announced throughout the health care facility. Many health care facilities have a special emergency number to call for help.

TABLE 10-1 Sample Emergency Codes

Code	Meaning
Red	Fire
Blue	Cardiac arrest
Pink	Infant abduction
Green	Combative person
Gold	Bomb threat
Yellow	Disaster
Black	Tornado/weather

When the emergency number is called, the caller is routed immediately to the facility's switchboard or to the facilitywide intercom system. The type and location of the emergency are announced. The emergency is announced using the assigned code. When the code and location are heard throughout the health care facility, the appropriate health care team members can respond immediately.

The health unit coordinator should know the emergency codes in the facility. The health unit coordinator should also know how to immediately announce the code throughout the facility. Health unit coordinators should be familiar with the policies and procedures of each type of code so they will know what to expect and how to respond. In most emergencies, the health unit coordinator should remain at the central workstation, prepared to make calls and to follow instructions. The health unit coordinator should also have a current department census ready for unitwide or departmentwide emergencies.

Cardiac or Respiratory Arrest

A cardiac or respiratory arrest is an emergency situation that occurs when a patient's heart has stopped beating or the patient has stopped breathing, or both. This is a medical emergency. The patient is in danger of immediately dying. When either a cardiac arrest or a respiratory arrest is observed, the procedure is to immediately call for help and begin life-saving techniques as required. Qualified personnel on the scene will bring the nearest **crash cart**, a special cart containing life-saving equipment, including a defibrillator (pads used to deliver an electric shock to the heart) and equipment for establishing an airway (intubating). The health unit coordinator should be prepared to contact health care team members and order tests and supplies as directed. The health unit coordinator may also be expected to notify the chaplain or social service department for the patient's family and visitors.

Fire

A fire emergency occurs whenever smoke or fire is detected. Each department has policies and procedures in place in the event of a fire. The health unit coordinator should be prepared to assist in any way directed. Many health care facilities use the acronym RACE to help employees remember the protocol in case of a fire emergency.

> **R**escue/remove. Remove everyone from the area. If a fire occurs in a patient's room the staff should immediately remove the patient from the area. Patients are moved only if they are in immediate danger.
>
> **A**larm. The fire alarm should be activated. Fire alarm pull stations are located throughout the facility. Activating the fire alarm sets a fire action plan into motion. Firefighters receive the signal and initiate the emergency response. In most facilities, pulling the fire alarm will result in the automatic announcement of the type and location of the code. In addition, certain doors are automatically shut to contain the smoke or fire.
>
> **C**ontain. Once the room or area has been cleared of patients, the door must be closed, thus confining the fire, which enables the fire response team the time needed to arrive.
>
> **E**xtinguish or evacuate. When practical, and only when an employee has been properly trained in the safe and proper use of a fire extinguisher, should

TABLE 10-2 Classes of Fires and Extinguishers	
Fire	**Extinguisher**
Class A: Wood, paper, textiles, and other ordinary combustibles	A or ABC extinguisher: Uses water, water-based chemical, foam, or multipurpose dry chemical. A strictly Class A extinguisher contains only water.
Class B: Flammable liquids, oils, solvents, paint, grease, etc.	ABC or BC: Uses foam, dry chemical, or carbon dioxide to put out the fire by smothering it or cutting off the oxygen.
Class C: Electrical, live or energized electric wires or equipment.	ABC or BC: Uses foam, dry chemical, or carbon dioxide to put out the fire by smothering it or cutting off the oxygen.
Class D: Combustible metals (magnesium, titanium, potassium, etc.)	D: Uses dry powder or other special sodium-extinguishing agents.

extinguishing be attempted (Table 10-2). Evacuate if you are not comfortable using a fire extinguisher or if more than one extinguisher is needed. Each department should have the evacuation route posted.

Weather

There are times when the weather can cause an emergency situation within the health care facility. If the National Weather Services issues a weather advisory, it will be announced throughout the health care facility as an emergency code. The action plan for the weather advisory would then be enacted. In case of a tornado watch, the health unit coordinator may be responsible to help close window blinds, curtains, and doors.

Power Outages

Severe weather can result in power or telephone outages. The health unit coordinator should know the procedure for such emergencies. Health care facilities have a backup or relief generator or power system to supply electricity when the main source is down. However, the relief generator may not provide power to all areas of the health care facility. During a weather emergency, the incoming and outgoing phone lines may also be limited.

Disaster

There may be an external event or catastrophe that results in a disaster within the health care facility. Usually a disaster involves the anticipation of an emergent need for medical care for many people as a result of a large accident. A disaster might be the result of a moving vehicle accident involving many people, of an industrial accident or fire, or of terrorism. During a disaster, health care facility personnel are expected to report to emergency duty stations. The health unit coordinator should have an accurate up-to-date census and condition report because as many patients as possible may be discharged to make room for the incoming disaster patients.

Bomb Threat

A health care facility should have a policy in place for bomb threats. If a bomb threat is made by phone, the health unit coordinator may be the one who answers the call. The health unit coordinator would note and write down the time of the threat and the exact wording the caller uses. If the caller can be kept on the phone, the following questions should be asked in this order:

1. What time will the bomb go off?

2. Where is it?

3. What does it look like?

4. Why hurt us?

5. What kind of bomb is it?

6. Who are you?

Also helpful to note are the caller's voice and any background noises. The threat should be reported immediately to one's supervisor and the appropriate party listed in the policy.

Infant Abduction

A health care facility must be prepared for an infant or child abduction. Departments with children, such as the nursery and pediatrics, have a security policy in place. If an abduction is suspected, a code will be called. The security department may have a special plan for deploying its personnel and blocking all exits from the area until the child has either been found or the abduction has been found to be a false alarm.

ISOLATION AND INFECTION CONTROL

A health unit coordinator must understand the different types of **isolation**. Isolation is the process of containing and preventing the spread of microorganisms or germs that cause disease. Isolation protects the patients and the health care team. The health unit coordinator must be able to explain the varied isolation procedures to visitors. The health unit coordinator must be able to order the supplies needed for isolation. Personal protective equipment (PPE) may include gloves, masks, gowns, and eye shields. The health unit coordinator must know what type of information to communicate to other departments if the isolation patient is to be moved or transported to another area.

INFECTION CONTROL MEASURES

The Centers for Disease Control and Prevention (CDC) writes guidelines for infection control measures in hospitals. These measures include infection control measures involving:

- Handwashing and gloving

- Patient placement

- Transport of infected patients

- Masks, respiratory protection, eye protection, face shields

- Gowns and protective apparel

- Patient-care equipment and articles

- Linen and laundry

- Dishes, glasses, cups, and eating utensils

- Routine and terminal cleaning

All or some of the infection control measures above may be used, depending on the type of isolation required for the patient. Health care facilities have written policies and procedures for the different types of isolation.

TYPE OF ISOLATION

The type of isolation is determined by how the microorganism is spread. The CDC's Recommendations for Isolation Precautions in Hospitals, gives details about the types of isolation and their corresponding precautions. The CDC defines transmission-based precautions as "designed for patients documented or suspected to be infected with highly transmissible or epidemiologically important pathogens for which additional precautions beyond Standard Precautions are needed to interrupt transmission in hospitals. There are three types of Transmission-Based Precautions: Airborne Precautions, Droplet Precautions, and Contact Precautions. They may be combined for diseases that have multiple routes of transmission. When used either singularly or in combination, they are to be used in addition to Standard Precautions."

Reverse isolation is the process of protecting the patient from outside organisms rather than containing the patient's harmful organisms.

ISOLATION AND THE HEALTH UNIT COORDINATOR

Although health unit coordinators may never have direct contact with an isolation patient, they must consider the patient's isolation status while performing the health unit coordinator responsibilities. For example, when transcribing an order for a diagnostic exam, the health unit coordinator must communicate isolation status to the department that will be transporting the patient. When making room assignments for newly admitted patients, the health unit coordinator must consider the isolation status of patients in semiprivate rooms. The health unit coordinator must also know what types of personal protective equipment to order for the health care team members who do have direct contact with the isolation patient.

INFECTION CONTROL AND THE HEALTH UNIT COORDINATOR

Even though health unit coordinators may not provide direct patient care, they may be exposed to body fluids. Usually, this exposure is a result of having the responsibility for body fluid specimens being routed after collection. After a body fluid has been collected for testing, the direct patient caregiver may give the specimen to the health unit coordinator.

STANDARD PRECAUTIONS AND BIOHAZARD

Health unit coordinators must observe Standard Precautions anytime they come into contact with any body fluid. Standard Precautions are explained in the CDC's Recommendations for Isolation Precautions in Hospitals. The CDC states, "Standard Precautions apply to (1) blood; (2) all body fluids, secretions, and excretions *except sweat*, regardless of whether or not they contain visible blood; (3) nonintact skin; and (4) mucous membranes. Standard Precautions are designed to reduce the risk of transmission of microorganisms from both recognized and unrecognized sources of infection in hospitals." Standard Precautions are used for all patients regardless of their diagnosis. The precautions detail what the health care team members must do to protect themselves and the patients whenever they come into contact with blood, body, fluids, nonintact skin, or mucous membranes. Standard Precautions require that body fluids and medical waste be labeled and contained in the appropriate biohazard receptacle (Figure 10-2).

HAND HYGIENE GUILDELINES

Hand hygiene guidelines were developed by the CDC's Healthcare Infection Control Practices Advisory Committee (HICPAC), in collaboration with the Society for Healthcare Epidemiology of America (SHEA), the Association for Professionals in Infection Control and Epidemiology (APIC), and the Infectious Disease Society of America (IDSA). The *Hand Hygiene Guidelines Fact Sheet* states:

> Improved adherence to hand hygiene (i.e., hand washing or use of alcohol-based handrubs) has been shown to terminate outbreaks in health care facilities, to reduce transmission of antimicrobial resistant organisms, . . . and reduce overall infection rates.

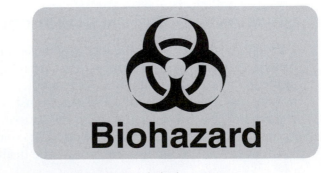

Figure 10-2 • *Biohazard warning label*

. . . In addition to traditional handwashing with soap and water, CDC is recommending the use of alcohol-based handrubs by health care personnel for patient care because they address some of the obstacles that health care professionals face when taking care of patients.

Handwashing with soap and water remains a sensible strategy for hand hygiene in non-health care settings and is recommended by CDC and other experts.

When health care personnel's hands are visibly soiled, they should wash with soap and water.

The use of gloves does not eliminate the need for hand hygiene. Likewise, the use of hand hygiene does not eliminate the need for gloves. Gloves reduce hand contamination by 70 percent to 80 percent, prevent cross-contamination and protect patients and health care personnel from infection. Handrubs should be used before and after each patient just as gloves should be changed before and after each patient.

When using an alcohol-based handrub, apply product to palm of one hand and rub hands together, covering all surfaces of hands and fingers, until hands are dry. Note that the volume needed to reduce the number of bacteria on hands varies by product.

Alcohol-based handrubs significantly reduce the number of microorganisms on skin, are fast acting and cause less skin irritation.

Health care personnel should avoid wearing artificial nails and keep natural nails less than one quarter of an inch long if they care for patients at high risk of acquiring infections (e.g., patients in intensive care units or in transplant units) . . .

SUMMARY

The health and safety of the health care staff and the patients are a major concern of the health care facility. A health care facility is responsible for the safety of its staff and patients. The U.S. government has various agencies such as DHHS, OSHA, and CDC to enforce and regulate health and safety. There are also private regulatory agencies such as JCAHO that work closely with health care facilities to improve health and safety practices. This chapter has listed many of the departments within the health care facility that work toward health and safety. Health care facilities seek to make improvements through continuous evaluation of incidents and performance and identifying opportunities to improve. It is the responsibility of the health unit coordinator to understand the roles of the regulatory agencies and departments that work toward maintaining and improving health and safety. Regulations change as improvements are made. New information becomes available, and previous information is outdated on a regular basis. The health unit coordinator is expected to know where to find the resources needed to follow the facility's health and safety policies and procedures.

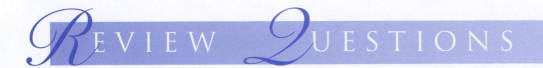

REVIEW QUESTIONS

1. List the department or agency that provides the following functions.

   a. Ensure equipment is functioning properly

   b. Provide and record employee immunizations

   c. A federal agency whose mission is to ensure safe and healthy workplaces

   d. A division of HHS whose mission is to promote health by preventing and controlling disease, injury, and disability

   e. Ensures cleanliness

   f. A division of HHS, responsible for implementing and enforcing the privacy regulation, HIPAA

   g. Responsible for the review of incident reports

   h. Department within the health care facility responsible for infection control

   i. Their mission is to improve care provided to the public through the provision of health care accreditation

   j. Would provide traffic control in an emergency situation

   k. The principal federal agency responsible for protecting the health of all Americans and providing essential human services

   l. Would sterilize surgical equipment

   m. Controls licensing for health care team professionals who are required to have a license to practice in their state

   n. Under CDC, agency responsible for conducting research on occupational disease and injury

2. List two cases in which completion of an incident report would be required.

3. List at least three tips for ergonomics for health unit coordinators.

4. What does the acronym RACE mean?

5. "The general rule for health unit coordinators in emergencies is to be prepared to respond as directed." Is this statement true or false?

6. "According to the CDC, frequent handwashing is the single most important measure to reduce the risk of transmission of organisms." Is this statement true or false?

NAHUC CERTIFICATION EXAM

CONTENT AREAS

II. F. 3   Communicate facility policies to visitors, patients, and staff (i.e., visiting hours, no smoking, etc.)

II. G. 1   Maintain a hazard-free work environment

II. G. 2   Maintain unit security

II. G. 3   Participate in emergency and disaster plans

II. G. 4   Respond to cardiac or respiratory arrests

II. G. 5   Initiate call to cardiac or respiratory arrests

II. G. 6   Comply with regulatory agency guidelines/rules

III. D. 2   Transport patient specimens, supplies, and medication using pneumatic tubes

IV. A. 1   Attend in-service training sessions

THROUGH THE EYES

OF A HEALTH CARE PROFESSIONAL

A hospital epidemiologist shares his thoughts.

As an epidemiologist, I have the opportunity to work with health unit coordinators throughout the hospital. When I visit the inpatient units, I rely on the health unit coordinators for the source of information I need for locating laboratory results, ordering isolation supplies, locating isolation signs and stickers, and locating the patients on their units that have been placed on isolation precautions. Although she make not have direct contact with the patient, the health unit coordinator helps the control of infection in a variety of ways. When ordering tests for the patients, she understands the importance of communicating isolation information to the department that will see the patients. When accepting body fluid specimens, she makes sure the patient care staff has placed the specimen in the correct biohazard container. And, like all health care staff, she understands the role of proper hand-washing techniques in the control of infection.

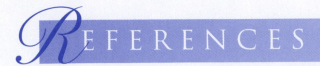

REFERENCES

American Federation of Teachers (AFT). Ergonomics for Paraprofessionals and School-Related Personnel. *http://www.aft.org/psrp/* Accessed January 2004.

American Society for Health Risk Management (ASHRM). About ASHRM. *http://www.hospitalconnect.com/ashrm/aboutus/aboutus.html* Accessed December 2003.

Association for Professionals in Infection Control and Epidemiology (APIC). About APIC. *http://www.apic.org/orgn/history.cfm* Accessed January 2004.

Centers for Disease Control and Prevention (CDC). About CDC. *http://www.cdc.gov/aboutcdc.htm* Accessed January 2004.

Centers for Disease Control and Prevention (CDC). Hand Hygiene in Health Care Settings. *http://www.cdc.gov/handhygiene* Accessed July 2004.

Centers for Disease Control and Prevention (CDC). Recommendations for Isolation Precautions in Hospitals. *http://www.cdc.gov/nicidod* Accessed July 2004.

Cyber-nurse Page's Learning Center for CNAs. Body Mechanics. *http://www.cyber-nurse.com/page/mech.htm* Accessed December 2003.

Joint Commission on Accreditation of Health Care Organizations (JCAHO). Facts about JCAHO. *http://www.jcaho.org/about+us/index.htm* Accessed December 2003.

National Institute for Occupational Safety and Health. (NIOSH). About NIOSH Research and Services. *http://cdc.gov/niosh/about.html* Accessed December 2003.

Occupational Safety and Health Administration (OSHA). OSHA's Mission. *http://www.osha.gov/oshinfo/mission.html* Accessed December 2003.

U.S. Department of Health and Human Services (DHHS). What We Do. *http://www.hhs.gov/news/press/2002pres/profile.html* Accessed December 2003.

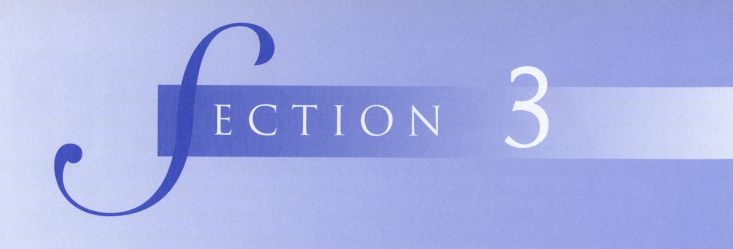

SECTION 3

Management of Information

Confidentiality

Learning Objectives

Upon completion of this chapter and review questions, the learner should be able to:

1. Define *confidentiality*.

2. Describe ways to protect patient confidentiality verbally.

3. Discuss ways to protect the confidentiality of the patient's written record.

4. List five ways to protect the computerized records.

5. Discuss various aspects of the Health Insurance Portability and Accountability Act (HIPAA).

6. List the 11 areas of concern that health unit coordinators must always keep in mind to ensure patient confidentiality.

7. Differentiate a civil case from a criminal case.

Key Terms

accountable   An obligation or willingness to take responsibility; to account for one's actions.

confidentiality   The act of not telling certain information to anyone but another authorized person.

deposition   Testimony under oath by a witness that is written down or recorded for use in court at a later date.

due care   The duty to have adequate regard for another person's rights.

ethical   Conforming to proper professional behavior.

expert witness   A person requested to testify under oath because of the person's education, profession, specialized experience, or superior knowledge of a subject.

felony A crime more serious than a misdemeanor and punishable by imprisonment for more than one year or death.

liable Obligated according to law.

misdemeanor An offense that is less serious than a felony and that may be punished by a fine or sentence to a local jail for less than one year.

morals Rules or habit of conduct based on standards of right and wrong.

negligence Failure to exercise the care a prudent person usually exercises.

respondeat superior Latin, "Let the master answer."

responsibility Being able to answer for one's conduct and obligations.

tort A private wrong or injury, other than breach of contract, for which the court will provide a remedy.

Abbreviations

CDC Centers for Disease Control and Prevention

DHHS Department of Health and Human Services

H & P History and Physical

HIPAA Health Insurance Portability and Accountability Act of 1996

PHI Private Health Information

WHO World Health Organization

HEALTH CARE AND CONFIDENTIALITY

Confidentiality is synonymous with secretiveness or privacy. One of the most important responsibilities of the health unit coordinator is to maintain confidentiality of the patient's records.

A patient and caregiver need to establish a rapport with one another. This rapport will make it easy to ask questions and agree on treatment for maintaining a healthy way of life for the patient. The very first thing that caregivers do to establish that rapport is gain the trust of the patient by assuring him or her that all the information discussed regarding the patient's condition and treatment will be kept confidential. Figure 11-1 is a sample of how some health care providers inform their patients of the practice of confidentiality.

The patient needs to provide a complete history and physical, or **H & P**. A history and physical includes information from the patient including health, work, environment, and social factors both past and present. Family history is an important part of the

TheBestMedicalCenter
Fresno, California

Sample
Notice of Confidentiality Practices

Our goal at TheBestMedicalCenter is to offer you services to keep you healthy. During the performance of these services, we collect, create, use, and share information about you.

We are dedicated to keeping your health information private. As required by the federal Health Insurance Portability and Accountability Act of 1996 (HIPAA) we provide you with this information in this notice.

We may use and disclose your health information to appropriate persons, authorities, and agencies, as allowed by federal and state law.

The following purposes require your written permission:

Regarding Your Treatment
As we treat you, we may need to use and share information with other health care providers such as consulting physicians, pharmacists.

Regarding Payment of Treatment
We may use your health information and disclose it to insurance companies or employer health plans, and to others in order to receive payment for your bill.

Reminders and Information Sharing
We may use your health information to remind you of an appointment or tell you about treatment options or health products and service that may be of interest to you.

We may use or disclose your personal health information without your written permission for the following purposes:

Hospital Directory
When you are hospitalized we may keep brief information about you in our directory. Unless you tell us otherwise we may disclose your room number and phone number along with general health condition such as "stable" or "good" to anyone who asks for you by name. We disclose your religious affiliation to clergy, even if they do not ask for you by name.

Family and Friends for Care and Payment
Unless you state otherwise and in emergency situations, we may disclose information to your family members, relative or others who are helping care for you or helping you pay your medical bills.

Other reporting situations not requiring your written permission include:

> Death and Disaster Relief Efforts
>
> Health Care Oversight and Law Enforcement
>
> Legal Proceedings and Military, National Security, Law Enforcement Custody
>
> Organ, Eye, or Tissue Donation and Public Health
>
> Research and Reporting Victims of Abuse or Neglect
>
> Required by Law

Other Restrictions
State and federal law may have more requirements than HIPAA on how we use and disclose your health information. State statutes listed.

You have the right to ask us in writing for a list of places or persons to whom your health information was disclosed within the past six years.

Figure 11-1 • *Confidentiality statement*

patient's history. This historical information could include very personal information such as child abuse, alcoholism, or mental health disease. The patient must be assured that all information regarding his or her past and present will be kept confidential. The health unit coordinator must ensure that the patient's charts and chart reports are never left in an area to which the public has access.

In all health care settings, the health unit coordinator is the custodian of the patient's charts. A custodian is one who guards, protects, or maintains items or persons. The health unit coordinator protects the patient's chart by knowing the people who have access to the chart. The health unit coordinator will become familiar with the various doctors, nurses, and other caregivers who have responsibilities with the charts. **Responsibility** is being able to answer for one's conduct and obligations. Handling confidential patient information is a large responsibility. A health unit coordinator who sees an unfamiliar person looking at a chart is responsible to find out who the person is and whether the person is authorized to look at the patient's chart. An easy approach would be for the health unit coordinator to ask if the person needs help in finding some information.

The health unit coordinator guards and protects the records by knowing where the patients' charts are at all times, such as when the chart accompanies the patient to another department within the facility or if a physician is using the chart in a dictation room. There are various tools or sign-out sheets to assist the coordinator in knowing where the charts are at any given time. See Figure 11-2 for an example of such a sign-out form.

The health unit coordinator has access to all the patients' charts in a given unit and thus to all the information within the patients' charts for every patient in the unit. A workstation may have from 6 to 50 patients, depending on the type of unit and facility. Although health unit coordinators have access to the patient's entire chart, they should not read the entire chart unless it is pertinent to the role at that time. For example, a history and physical is dictated by a physician, typed, and sent to the workstation to be filed in the chart. The act of filing requires the health unit coordinator to look at the patient's name and the type of document to know in which chart and where in the chart to file the document. There is no reason for the health unit coordinator to read the history and physical. Maintaining confidentiality is an **ethical** (professionally correct) thing to do. Health unit coordinators also realize that maintaining confidentiality is also the **moral**, or right (versus wrong), habit to develop.

VERBAL CONSIDERATIONS

Health care workers must take every precaution to keep all patient information confidential. At the health care system where this author is currently employed, there are signs in all the elevators stating "Remember where you are, patient confidentiality is important." These signs remind all hospital employees to think of patient confidentiality at all times. Health unit coordinators are asked numerous questions regarding the patients. Information regarding patients should be discussed only with those employees who are caring for the patient. The discussion should be limited to the care of the patient. Health unit coordinators should refer all inquiries about the patient's care and progress to the nurse who is caring for the patient at that given time. Health care employees must keep their voices quiet when discussing patient care, activity, and information. Family members or friends of a patient may be just around the corner of the area in which the patient is being discussed.

PATIENT TRANSPORTATION LOG

Date

	W/Chart	Cardiac Ser	CT	DX	US	MRI	Pulmonary	PT	OT	Other
Patient name & room # Time– off unit Time returned										
Patient name & room # Time– off unit Time returned										
Patient name & room # Time– off unit Time returned										
Patient name & room # Time– off unit Time returned										
Patient name & room # Time– off unit Time returned										
Patient name & room # Time– off unit Time returned										
Patient name & room # Time– off unit Time returned										
Patient name & room # Time– off unit Time returned										
Patient name & room # Time– off unit Time returned										
Patient name & room # Time– off unit Time returned										

Figure 11-2 • *Transportation log, departmental sign-out sheet*

Most health unit coordinators are responsible for sharing information about how to contact patients by giving the room number or phone number of the patient's current room. This type of responsibility varies from facility to facility, so one needs to be sure to read, know, and adhere to the employer's policies and procedures. Many areas throughout health care facilities are public, such as elevators, cafeterias, and parking structures. Patients must never be discussed in these public areas. Patients must never be discussed after work hours. All health care employees need to fight the urge to go home and tell family and friends about celebrities or neighbors who are being cared for in the facility.

TELEPHONE CONVERSATIONS

Health unit coordinators need to know to whom they are speaking when using the telephone. The caller can be asked to identify himself or herself early in the conversation. When family members or friends of patients call, refer them to the nurse who is caring for that patient at the present time. Limited patient information may be given over the telephone to other health care providers. An example would be when a doctor's office calls requesting additional insurance information. A health unit coordinator who is not sure of the identification of the caller should request a call-back phone number and return the call after properly identifying the caller.

The health unit coordinator can share patient information with other departments within the health care facility over the telephone. Ancillary departments may call requesting information to assist them in scheduling a test or procedure for a patient. The transport department may call to verify that the patient is in the room and ready to be taken to another department.

RELEASING AND SHARING RECORDS

There are times when the patient's medical records need to be shared. Patient records need to be shared with other health care facilities when a patient is being transferred to a specialty hospital or long-term facility. Patient records need to be shared with insurance companies or other payers of health care bills. The vast amount of communication technology today makes sharing records quite simple, for example by using computers, scanners, copiers, and fax machines. All health care workers must ensure that these very important and personal records do not end up in the wrong place. Dialing a wrong fax number, perhaps because of haste in dialing, is a simple thing to do, but it could result in a terrible error.

When a patient is transferred from a hospital or medical center to a specialty hospital or long-term facility, certain medical records should accompany the patient. These records will give the receiving facility information regarding the history of the injury or condition as well as the treatment the patient has been receiving. The records will also give the patient's current condition and physician orders for treatment. The *original* medical records should *never* leave the health care facility's premises. Copies of the pertinent forms and records should be made to accompany a patient who leaves for any reason. Health care facilities have patient's sign release forms before they copy and share records with outside caregivers. The health unit coordinator must ensure that the release form is signed and filed in the chart before copying any part of the patient's record (Figure 11-3). Health unit coordinators need to know and follow their facility's rules regarding copying and releasing records.

TheBestHospital
RELEASE OF MEDICAL INFORMATION FORM

1. **Patient Full Name** _____

2. **Date of Birth** _____ / _____ / _____

   Address _____

   City/State _____

3. **Health Information to Be Disclosed:**

   Laboratory Reports—specify report and date _____

   Radiology Reports—specify report and date _____

   Billing Records _____

   Other _____

4. **Purpose of Disclosure** _____

5. **Persons/Organizations Authorized to Release Information:**

   Name of Health Care Provider _____

   Address _____

   City _____ State _____ Zip Code _____

6. **Persons/Organizations Authorized to Receive Information:**

   Self _____

   Name of Health Care Provider _____

   Address _____

   City _____ State _____ Zip Code _____

7. **Signature of Patient/Legal Representative**

   _____ Date _____

8. **Witness** (when applicable) _____

You are not obliated to authorize a disclosure of your health information. You may limit the amount of information as you wish.

You have the right to inspect or copy the health information to be released for this authorization.

You have the right to receive a copy of this consent form.

You have the right to refuse to sign this authorization.

You have the right to revoke this authorization.

Figure 11-3 • *Release of medical information form*

At times, it is necessary to share health information with the federal government in order to track disease. An example is SARS (severe acute respiratory syndrome), which broke out in the Republic of China in February 2003 and spread to Vietnam, Singapore, Toronto, and the United States and killed more than 200 people in just a few months. In such cases, the Centers for Disease Control and Prevention (CDC) and World Health Organization (WHO) must be informed of all disease instances to track and share ways to prevent the spread of these types of communicable diseases. In these types of cases, the health care facility's medical records department may track and release such records. Always refer to the facility's policies.

COMPUTERIZED PATIENT RECORDS

Computers are in every hospital and health care facility, but the extent to which computers are used varies. Some health care facilities use the computer to keep track of which patients are in which beds and patient test results; some facilities use computers to enter charges for services rendered; and some facilities enter test requests to in-house departments. More sophisticated computer systems will have the all patient information and documentation online; in other words, the facility has completely computerized patient records. Health care employers must limit the amount of information an employee can access via the computer. All users are given individual logins and passwords. These logins will allow the individual to gain access to the appropriate computer conversations and data to complete their duties. These computer systems also track which employees are using which patients' charts throughout the day. It is extremely important to always log off the computer before leaving the computer, even if just for a short walk around the unit. In that short period of time, any number of unit employees—nurses, nursing assistants, doctors—can see an "open" computer and sit down and start working on that computer. When one person does not log off and another person starts working on the computer, the name and signature of the first user will appear on all the work processed by the second person. There is a saying that a computer password should be used like a toothbrush; use it often, change it often, and never share it with anyone.

Current technology makes it easy for an integrated health care system to use one computer network to share patient information. For example, the BestHealthSystem is made up of two hospitals and four clinics providing health care within a 50-mile radius. Computer systems make it possible for the following scenario to occur. Monday, Latoya Nyumen became very ill and was seen in TheBestMedicalCenter. She was treated and sent home. On Wednesday, while Ms. Nyumen was at work, she became very ill again and needed to be taken to the nearest hospital. She was taken to the TheBestHospital. When she entered the TheBestHospital her personal information was already in the computer system and showed her records from Monday's visit at TheBestMedicalCenter. Consequently, less information was needed from Ms. Nyumen, saving time and duplication of documentation in her chart. Ms. Nyumen was treated and released. She was also instructed to follow up in two weeks at her doctor's office at the TheBestClinic.

Two weeks later, Ms. Nyumen arrived for her appointment with Dr. Kumar at the TheBestClinic on West Street. Dr. Kumar's office was able to find all previous information about Ms. Nyumen's illness and treatment of two weeks ago via the computer in just a matter of moments. Having this information enabled Dr. Kumar to provide care that was consistent with what was recommended at TheBestMedicalCenter.

Section 3

You can see that no matter where this patient went within TheBestHealthSystem, her records were available. As the scenario shows, an employee of a health care system that has an integrated computer system has access to patient information anywhere within the entire system. All of this sharing of health information has caused the public to fear that their health records are not being kept confidential. The public have asked their politicians to write laws ensuring health record confidentiality.

GOVERNMENT RESPONSIBILITIES

Worldwide governments have many concerns about maintaining confidentiality with all of this advanced technology. The European Union (EU) has addressed the issue; Canada has addressed the issue; and the United States has addressed the issue.

In the United States, **HIPAA**, the Health Insurance Portability and Accountability Act, was enacted in 1996 to provide continuous insurance coverage for persons who lost or changed jobs. *Standards for Privacy of Individually Identifiable Health Information*, better known as *Privacy Rules*, were added to HIPAA to protect individuals' health information. These standards, addressing privacy and confidentiality, are directed at health care providers including insurers, pharmacies, and doctors. Seven key areas regarding patient protection in the 1996 HIPAA privacy act are:

1. *Access to medical records.* This ensures that the patients may see or obtain copies of their medical records and request corrections if they find any errors or mistakes.

2. *Notice of privacy practices.* This states that health care providers must notify patients of how their personal medical information will be used and must inform patients of their rights under this privacy act. This notification is usually done in the form of a one-page pamphlet designed by the provider and given to the patient.

3. *Limits on use of personal medical information.* At times, the provider may need to share information to provide the best possible care. However, if the provider is requested to share medical information with the patients' life insurer or bank or with a marketing firm or other outside business not related to the care needed, the patient has to sign a specific authorization to allow such a release.

4. *Prohibition on marketing.* This restricts the use of patient information for marketing purposes. In other words patient lists may not be shared or sold to marketing firms.

5. *Stronger state laws.* Some states within the United States had laws regarding medical record privacy before these federal standards were enacted. However, the state laws varied from state to state, and not all states had laws. This stipulation says that if the state law is stricter than the federal guideline, the state law has precedence.

6. *Confidential communications.* This rule states that patients may request that their health care providers take steps to ensure that their communications with the patient are confidential. For example, the providers might be

asked to phone the patient at home instead of at a place of employment and not to leave test results on a message machine. This rule also affects a health care facility's list, or directory, of all patients currently admitted. The directory may include the patient name, the room, the general condition of the patient (not including specific medical information) and the patient's religious affiliation. It is now required through HIPAA that the facility inform patients of such a list and give patients the option to restrict the information that can be given out or have their names and information deleted from the list. The health unit coordinator may be responsible for informing the patient and updating the list.

7. *Complaints.* This covers information as to where to file a formal complaint and whom to contact.

HEALTH CARE ENTITIES' INDIVIDUAL POLICIES

The national standards to protect private health information (PHI) require the health plans and providers to individually establish their own policies and procedures for enforcing the standards. However, their policies and procedures must include the following:

1. *Written privacy procedure.* Health care employers must determine how much patient information is given to each employee on the basis of the employee's position or responsibilities. The security level and limits for patient information access must be defined for each position. All of this must be included in a written policy. Health unit coordinators in general have access to all parts of a patient's chart, whereas nursing assistants have access to only the vital signs portion of the patient's chart.

2. *Employee training and privacy officer.* All health care team members must become knowledgeable about their employer's policy and procedures regarding PHI. To protect themselves, employers educate employees regarding patient confidentiality. Most employers review these policies annually and have the employee sign a confidentiality statement. Signing such a statement means the employee will not share any information about a patient with anyone else unless it is work related. This statement is extremely important for health unit coordinators to understand because, as previously discussed, health unit coordinators have access to all health medical records.

3. *Public responsibilities.* Health care facilities use their professional judgment to decide on what they will share with the public. Some of the circumstances that may require public disclosure are emergency situations, notification to the public regarding the identification of a deceased body, cause of death, and research.

4. *Equivalent requirements for government.* This basically means that the rules apply to both public and private health care entities. It needs to be stressed that all these policies and procedures must be in writing, and health unit coordinators must keep current with federal, state, and employers' policies on patient confidentiality.

OUTREACH AND ENFORCEMENT

The Office of Civil Rights within the U.S. Department of Health and Human Services (DHHS) oversees and enforces these federal regulations. There are considerable written and technical materials to assist health care entities in becoming knowledgeable about these standards. The five elements of the outreach and enforcement efforts are:

1. Guidance and technical assistance materials. The Department of Health and Human Services must provide written information such as a Web site, regarding these standards.

2. Educational offerings such as conferences and seminars.

3. Information line toll-free numbers.

4. Complaint investigations. When complaints are filed, the Office of Civil Rights, under the DHHS, will investigate to ensure that patients' privacy rights are being protected.

5. Civil and criminal penalties. Depending on whether it is a civil or criminal offense, monetary penalties range from $100 to $250,000. These penalties are imposed on individuals as well as employers. Health unit coordinators must know and follow the policies of their employer.

LEGAL AWARENESS

The legal system is in place to protect the innocent. In the course of a day, everyone makes mistakes. However, in health care a mistake may have lasting consequences for the patient and family. When a patient is harmed by a health care provider's mistake, the affected party may seek punishment for the offender and may ask to be compensated for discomfort or disability. For a better understanding on how the law works, let's look at the following.

Civil cases are crimes against persons. Criminal cases are crimes against the state or federal government. A crime is a wrongful act that the state or federal government has identified as a crime. **Felony** crimes are generally considered serious crimes, whereas **misdemeanors** are lesser crimes. **Torts** are wrongful acts that injure or interfere with a person or property. Torts are the most common medical-related cases. All health care professionals are held to the ethics and standards of care as defined by the various state and federal government entities. Health unit coordinators are **accountable**, which means they accept the obligation or are willing to take responsibility for their actions. Health unit coordinators need to practice **due care** when handling patient records. Health unit coordinators are **liable**, or obligated by law, for their **negligence** (failure to exercise the care a prudent person usually exercises).

Experienced health unit coordinators may be requested to be an expert witness. An **expert witness** may be requested to testify under oath because of the person's education, profession, specialized experience, or superior knowledge of a subject. Before a court appearance, a **deposition**, or testimony under oath that is written or recorded for use in court at a later time, may be taken.

The health care employer may also be held accountable according to **respondeat superior** ("Let the master answer"). Respondeat superior goes into effect only if the employee made the error while following the job description and the policies and procedures of the facility. For example, if a health unit coordinator takes laboratory results that were given incorrectly over the phone and shares them with the patient's nurse and a wrong treatment begins, the health unit coordinator will be accountable for taking and sharing this information *only if* the employer's policy is that only nurses should take lab results over the phone. However, if the employer's policy is for the health unit coordinator to take results over the phone and the health unit coordinator has been trained to take the results, respondeat superior would go into effect because the health unit coordinator followed policy and took the results as they were given by the laboratory personnel.

Health unit coordinators' job descriptions state that the health unit coordinator should fax requested patient records to a physicians' office. When medical records are faxed, many outcomes may result:

1. The automatic dial feature of the fax machine malfunctions and dials a private business instead of the physicians' office.

2. The health unit coordinator misdials, and the records are received by a business office.

3. The health unit coordinator faxes the positive result of the HIV test, which was not requested.

4. While faxing the records, the health unit coordinator notices that this patient lives two doors down from her parents, and, on her break, she phones her parents to inform them of their neighbor's hospitalization.

Let's consider the legal effects of each of the above situations. In cases 1 and 2, there should be no legal issues. All medical faxes should be accompanied by a notice that the facsimile transmission contains confidential information and if the recipient is not the intended receiver state and federal laws restrict this information from being shared and the sender should be notified immediately. In case 3, tort has occurred. Although the confidentiality statement mentioned for cases 1 and 2 also applies here, the HIV results were not requested, and, because of the nature of the information, a private wrong did occur—negligence. In case 4, the health unit coordinator violated the federal standard and the employer's confidentiality policy and breached the ethics of professional health unit coordinators.

SUMMARY

Health unit coordinators handle a great deal of patient information. It is imperative that all communication be handled confidentially. Maintaining confidentiality is important not only to the patient but also to the other health care providers and the health care facility. Health unit coordinators must carefully observe the following points to ensure such confidentiality.

◆ Know who is accessing the patients' records.

◆ Know where the patient records are at all times.

◆ Read only the parts of the patient record that pertain to the task at hand.

◆ Keep records out of the sight of the public.

◆ Discuss patient information only when it pertains to patient care.

◆ Discuss patient information quietly.

◆ Know to whom you are giving information over the telephone.

◆ Always send copies of the chart forms; never send original chart forms outside of the health care facility.

◆ Always log off the computer before leaving your work area.

◆ Stay current with state and federal regulations regarding PHI confidentiality.

◆ Know and follow your employer's policies and procedures for handling PHI.

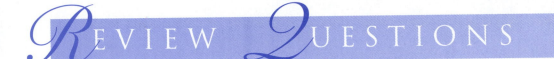

REVIEW QUESTIONS

1. Define confidentiality.

2. Describe ways to protect patient confidentiality verbally.

3. Discuss ways to protect confidentiality of the written patient record.

4. List five ways to protect computerized records.

5. Discuss various aspects of HIPAA.

6. List the seven professional standards to meet legal and ethical requirements.

7. Differentiate a civil case from a criminal case.

NAHUC CERTIFICATION EXAM

CONTENT AREAS

I. C. 4 Request patient information from external facilities

II. H. 1 Screen telephone calls and visitor requests for patient information to protect patient confidentiality

II. H. 2 Restrict access to patient information (i.e. charts, computer)

IV. B. 1 Review job related publications (e.g., NAHUC Standards of Practice, journals)

IV. B. 2 Review facility-specific publications, memos, policies

THROUGH THE EYES

OF A HEALTH CARE PROFESSIONAL

Confidentiality is a very important part of the health unit coordinator's role. When people call on the telephone looking for information on family and friends, it is the health unit coordinator who needs to know exactly who the caller is before giving any information or forwarding the call to another caregiver. Another part of the confidentiality role is to make sure forms, lists, and communication boards are kept out of the sight of people who approach the desk with questions. The health unit coordinator plays a big role in maintaining confidentiality of all patient information.

REFERENCES

http://www.cdc.gov/nc/dod/sars Accessed May 1, 2003.

http://www.hhs.gov/gov/news/facts/privacy.html Accessed May 1, 2003.

http://www.hhs.gov/ocr/hipaa/ Accessed May 1, 2003.

Flight, M. (1998). *Law, liability, and ethics for medical office professionals* (3rd ed.). Clifton Park, NY: Thomson Delmar Learning.

CHAPTER 12

Patient Rights and Responsibilities

Learning Objectives

Upon completion of this chapter and review questions, the learner should be able to:

1. List five patient rights.

2. Differentiate between Power of Attorney for Health Care and a Living Will.

3. Identify at least two government agencies that oversee managed care.

4. Discuss patient responsibilities.

Key Terms

advance directive A legal document, executed (signed) by a competent person, that gives direction to health care providers about treatment choices in certain circumstances.

Durable Power of Attorney for Health Care The means by which an individual may appoint another person to make decisions about health care needs.

living will The means by which an individual may express his or her wishes about life-sustaining treatment if he or she should become terminally or irreversibly ill.

Abbreviations

AD Advance Directive

AMA Against Medical Advice

CMS Center for Medicare and Medicaid Services

DHHS Department of Health and Human Services

EMTALA Emergency Medical Treatment and Active Labor Act

JCAHO Joint Commission on Accreditation of Health Care Organizations

THE IMPORTANCE OF PATIENT RIGHTS AND RESPONSIBILITIES

Patients have certain rights and responsibilities when they are admitted to a health care facility. It is important for patients to know and acknowledge their rights and responsibilities in order to take an active part in their care and treatment. It is also important for the health care staff to know these rights and respect them. It is equally important for the health care staff to be knowledgeable about the patients' responsibilities so they may help educate and inform patients of their responsibilities as well as encourage patients to carry out their responsibilities.

ADVANCE DIRECTIVES

One right that patients may exercise even before the need for hospitalization arises is the right to make decisions about their care should they become unable to act on their own behalf during hospitalization. People often have strong convictions about the type and duration of health care treatment they might receive under certain conditions. To clearly state their convictions, people may complete an **advance directive (AD)**. An advance directive is a legal document, executed (signed) by a competent person, that gives direction to health care providers about treatment choices in certain circumstances. There are two forms of advance directive. One is a special type of power of attorney that is called a **Durable Power of Attorney for Health Care**, or simply a Medical Power of Attorney. The other type of advance directive is a **living will**, which expresses the person's wishes regarding life-sustaining treatments.

POWER OF ATTORNEY

An ordinary power of attorney is a legal document that authorizes an individual (the principal or grantor) to designate another person to act as his or her "attorney-in-fact" (or agent) and to do certain things for the principal. For example, assume that a developer is very interested in a piece of property you own. However, you and your spouse are leaving tomorrow for a long-planned trip to Europe. The sales contract will have to be signed while you will be in Paris. How will you be able to get the contract signed while you are climbing up the Eiffel Tower? The answer is simple: sign a power of attorney, which will authorize a trusted friend, business associate, or lawyer to act as your attorney-in-fact, or agent, to negotiate any last-minute details and to sign the contract for you. In this example, the power of attorney will expire after the sales contract has been signed by your designated agent, who is the attorney-in-fact. You would probably have the power of attorney document written so it will expire after a certain date or after you return from your trip, even if the sales contract is not signed. This ordinary type of power of attorney is commonly used in business, financial, and commercial situations. It allows the agent, or attorney-in-fact, to enter into contracts, negotiate, and settle matters for the principal.

An ordinary power of attorney expires if the principal or grantor becomes incompetent or dies. The theory behind this limit is that, if the principal could not do the transaction on his or her own then the attorney-in-fact, or agent, should not be allowed to do it either. So if you have the misfortune to fall off the Eiffel Tower and die before your agent completes the deal, your agent no longer has the authority to act for you. Although this limitation makes good sense in business and commercial situations, it often makes little sense in health care situations, when people want their wishes carried out even if health circumstances preclude them from acting on their own. A special type of power of attorney is used in these circumstances. It is a power of attorney that will endure even if the principal is incapacitated and cannot make decisions on his or her own. This form of power of attorney is called either a Durable Power of Attorney for Health Care or a Medical Power of Attorney. The two terms refer to the same document. A Durable Power of Attorney for Health Care enables people to make decisions about their care should they be unable to act in their own behalf. This type of power of attorney is called *durable* because it endures even if the patient is not able to make decisions for himself or herself.

DURABLE POWER OF ATTORNEY FOR HEALTH CARE

A Durable Power of Attorney for Health Care, or a Medical Power of Attorney, is the means by which an individual appoints another person to make decisions about future health care needs should the individual be unable to do so. This other person, who will be acting as the patient's agent, could be a family member or a close friend or just someone who truly understands the person's wishes regarding health care. However, because of the potential for conflict of interest, health care providers may not be given Power of Attorney to act on behalf of their patients.

The Durable Power of Attorney for Health Care will be implemented only if a patient's physician and one other physician concur that the patient is not competent or is unable to make or express decisions regarding health care. A Durable Power of Attorney for Health Care must be in writing. When a patient has a completed Durable Power of Attorney for Health Care and enters a health care facility, this document should be given to the nurse or health unit coordinator upon admission to be part of the patient's record throughout the stay.

LIVING WILL

The second type of advance directive is a living will. It is also called a Declaration to Physicians. A living will allows an individual to express his or her wishes about life-sustaining treatment if he or she should become terminally or irreversibly ill. An individual who makes a living will states that, if he or she has a terminal incurable condition or is in a persistent vegetative state, the individual does not want his or her life to be prolonged by extraordinary means or by artificial nutrition and hydration.

People who are terminally and incurably ill are those who will die soon, for example, people in the last stages of cancer or heart disease. Those in a persistent vegetative state are very often accident or stroke victims.

A living will is simple to fill out and, in most states, only requires the signature of two witnesses, neither of whom is related to the individual, and a notary public. Health care providers, including health unit coordinators, may not legally witness a living will. A living will becomes effective only when the individual (patient) can no longer direct his or her health care and is not expected to recover. Unlike the Durable Power of Attorney for Health Care, the living will does not give anyone else the right to make health care decisions on the patient's behalf, but gives directions regarding what artificial means should and should not be used to prolong the patient's pain and demise, as seen in Figures 12-1 and 12-2.

USE OF ADVANCE DIRECTIVES

Although it is not required that patients have either a Durable Power of Attorney for Health Care or a living will, they are both widely accepted as being in the best interests of the patient and of the health care facility. These advance directives provide the health care facility and its caregivers with information that will help in carrying out the sincere convictions and beliefs of the patient regarding his or her treatment.

An attorney may be helpful in writing a Durable Power of Attorney for Health Care or a living will, but an attorney is not necessary. Most physicians' offices and health care facilities have forms and instructional materials to assist patients in completing advance directives. It is not necessary that both a Durable Power of Attorney for Health Care and a living will be completed, because a Durable Power of Attorney for Health Care takes precedence over a living will.

Copies of Durable Power of Attorney for Health Care forms and of living wills should be given to the primary physician and kept as a permanent part of the patient's hospital record. Upon receipt of these documents, the health unit coordinator should file them in the patient's current chart according to hospital protocol.

AGENCIES PROVIDING HEALTH CARE OVERSIGHT

The **Department of Health and Human Services (DHHS)** and **Centers for Medicare and Medicaid Services (CMS)** are two federal agencies that oversee various aspects of health care. They have introduced legislation to ensure that all patients, regardless of race, religion, sex, national origin, or source of payment, receive the same health care rights. An example of this type of legislation is the Emergency Medical Treatment and Active Labor Act (EMTALA). This act states that all patients must be seen and receive treatment from an emergency room regardless of the means of payment.

Legislation in many states addresses the right of patients to information concerning diagnosis, treatment, prognosis, and self-care education. State legislation may also address the right of the patient to know which physician is primarily responsible for giving care. This right explains why many health care facilities require staff to wear name tags or badges with both the employee's name and the employee's title.

SAMPLE DURABLE POWER OF ATTORNEY FOR HEALTH CARE

—————————————————————

I, _____, hereby appoint:
(name)

_____
(name, home address and telephone number of agent)

as my health care agent to make any and all health care decisions for me, except to the extent that I state otherwise.

This Durable Power of Attorney for Health Care shall take effect in the event I become unable to make my own health care decisions. My health care agent and any alternate health care agent shall have the authority to make all health care decisions regarding any care, treatment, service, or procedure to maintain, diagnose, treat, or provide for my physical or mental health or personal care. My health care agent and any alternate agent shall also have the authority to make decisions regarding the providing, witholding or withdrawing of life sustaining treatment pursuant to state laws.

Optional Instructions:

If the health care agent I appoint is unable, unwilling or unavailable to act as my health care agent, then I appoint:

_____
(name, home address and telephone number of alternate agent)

Signed this _____ day of _____, _____.
   (day)   *(month)*   *(year)*

Signature_____

Statement by Witnesses (must be 18 or older)

I declare that the person who signed this document appeared to execute the durable power of attorney for health care willingly and free from duress. He or she signed (or asked another to sign for him or her) this document in my presence.

Witness _____
                              (Sign and Print name)

Witness _____
                              (Sign and Print name)

(This is a sample document and not intended for use)

Figure 12-1 • *Durable Power of Attorney for Health Care*

SAMPLE LIVING WILL

_____

INSTRUCTIONS	

If I should have an incurable or irreversible condition that will cause my death within a relatively short time, and I am no longer able to make decisions regarding my medical treatment **or** if I should become permanently unconscious, I direct my attending physician, pursuant to state laws, to withhold or withdraw treatments that only prolong the process of dying and are not necessary to my comfort or to alleviate pain.

With regard to artificially supplied nutrition and hydration, I specifically direct that
(*check the option desired*):
    ( ) artificial nutrition be withheld after consultation with my attending physician.
    ( ) artificial hydration be withheld after consultation with my attending physician.

(*check the option desired*):
    ( ) artificial nutrition may *not* be withheld.
    ( ) artificial hydration may *not* be withheld.

Other directions:

I direct my attending physician, pursuant to the state laws, to follow the instructions of

_____
(name of proxy)

whom I appoint as my Health Care Proxy to make medical treatment decisions on my behalf, including whether life-sustaining treatment should be withheld or withdrawn.

Signed this _____ day of _____, _____.
                (day)   (month)   (year)

Signature _____

The declarant voluntarily signed this writing in my presence

Witness _____

Witness _____

(This is a sample document and not intended for use)

Instructions (side column):

CHECK THE OPTION THAT REFLECT YOUR WISHES ABOUT ARTIFICIAL FEEDING & HYDRATION

ADD PERSONAL INSTRUCTIONS (IF ANY)

PRINT THE NAME OF YOUR PROXY

SIGN AND DATE THE DOCUMENT AND PRINT YOUR ADDRESS

YOUR WITNESSES MUST SIGN AND PRINT THEIR ADDRESSESS

© 2004 LAST ACTS PARTNERSHIP

Figure 12-2 • *Living will* (Reprinted with permission ©2004 Last Acts Partnership, Washington, DC. All rights reserved.)

Patients have the right to examine and receive an explanation of their bill regardless of the source of payment. This means that even if the hospital bill is paid in full by private insurance or Medicaid, patients should receive an explanation of charges appearing on their financial statement if requested.

Accrediting agencies such as the Joint Commission on Accreditation of Health Care Organizations (JCAHO) have standards to be followed by accredited health care facilities regarding patient's rights. Health care providers realize that these rights not only provide guidelines for the patient but, when followed, also improve patient outcomes. A good example of such as standard is the right of the patient to be included in decision making and involvement in his or her care. Patients have the right to refuse treatment after being informed of all consequences. Such a refusal is often referred to as **AMA**, or against medical advice.

Some other guidelines for patient rights according to the JCAHO include the following:

◆ The right of reasonable access to care

◆ The right to consideration and respect for personal values and beliefs

◆ The right to participate in ethical questions that arise in the course of care, including issues of conflict resolution, withholding resuscitative services, forgoing or withdrawal of life-sustaining treatment, and participation in investigational studies or clinical trials

◆ The right to security, personal privacy, and confidentiality of information

JCAHO goes on to say that hospitals must have a method for informing and educating patients of their rights and that patients shall receive a written statement regarding their rights.

PATIENT RESPONSIBILITIES

Patients also have responsibilities to ensure safe care. The major responsibilities of patients are:

◆ To provide complete and accurate information about current symptoms, past illnesses, hospitalizations, and medications to the health care provider

◆ To follow the plan of treatment developed by the primary physician

◆ To ask questions if they do not understand the information or instructions given regarding their care and to accept responsibility for consequences if they refuse or do not follow their health care provider's directions

◆ To fulfill their financial obligations

Health care facilities typically provide a summary of all of the patient rights and responsibilities. Figure 12-3 is an example of a health care facility patient information brochure. This summary of patient rights and responsibilities is often given to patients

PATIENT Rights

Aurora Health Care wants you to know you have rights as a patient, including the right to make decisions about your health care. An Ethics Committee is available to support those making difficult health care decisions. The patient rights policy outlined here is provided for under Wisconsin law.

Care Decisions

1. You have the right to the information you need to make decisions about your medical care.
2. You have the right to refuse treatment, to the extent permitted by law, and to be informed of the medical consequences of your action.

Advance Directives

3. You will receive information about Advance Directives, including, but not limited to, the Living Will, the appointment of a surrogate health care decision-maker, and the Power of Attorney for Health Care.
   - You will have an opportunity to formulate an Advance Directive.
   - Your Advance Directive will be made a part of your permanent medical record.
   - The terms of your Advance Directive will be followed by the staff, to the extent allowed by law.
4. You will receive care regardless of whether you have formulated an Advance Directive.

Provision of Care

5. You have the right to considerate, safe and respectful care. This includes:
   - The right to medically necessary treatment regardless of race, religion, sex, national origin or sources of payment for care.
   - The right to have a family member or a representative and your physician notified promptly of your admission to the hospital.
   - The right to information concerning diagnosis, treatment, prognosis and self-care education from your health care provider, presented to you in ways you can understand.
   - The right to information from your physician about planned procedures and treatment so that you may give informed consent.
   - The right to be free from restraints of any form that are not medically necessary or for safety of the patient or others.
   - The right to every consideration of your privacy concerning your medical care.
   - The right to expect that all communications and records concerning your care are confidential.
   - The right to know the identity and professional status of those providing care to you and to know which physician is primarily responsible for your care.
   - The right to consult with a specialist at your request and expense.
   - The right to be informed by your physician of any ongoing care requirements following your discharge from the hospital.
   - The right to obtain information concerning the relationship of the hospital to other health care and educational institutions involved in your care.
   - The right to appropriate assessment and management of your pain.
   - The right to know the process the hospital follows concerning documenting, reviewing and resolving complaints.
   - The right to know what hospital rules and regulations apply to your behavior as a patient.
   - The right to obtain information about advocacy organizations for protective services.
   - The right to expect unrestricted access to communication. In instances when restrictions are necessary, the patient will be included in the decision to impose restrictions.
   - The right to protective services.

Explanation of Your Bill

6. You have the right to examine and receive an explanation of your bill regardless of source of payment.

Complaints

7. The people of Aurora are striving to find better ways to provide health care. We value your feedback. If you have a concern, please contact any staff member. you also may contact a manger or administrator, who will resolve the complaint or submit the issue to our grievance process for resolution. You also have the right to file a complaint by contacting:

   Health Services Section
   Bureau of Quality Assurance
   P.O. Box 2969
   Madison, WI 53701-2969
   Phone (608) 266 8084
   Fax (608) 266 1518

Figure 12-3 • *Patient rights and responsibilities (Courtesy of Aurora Health Care, Milwaukee, WI) (continues)*

Aurora Health Care®

PATIENT
Rights &
Responsibilities

PATIENT
Responsibilities

Providing Information

1. You are responsible for providing complete and accurate information about your current symptoms, past illnesses, hospitalizations, medications and other matters concerning your health.

2. You are responsible for notifying your physician or nurse about any unexpected change in your condition.

Following Instructions

3. You are responsible for following the treatment plan developed by the physician who is primarily responsible for your care. This plan may include instructions by nurses and other health care personnel as they carry out the physician's orders.

4. You are responsible for notifying your physician or nurse immediately if you do not understand instructions or feel you cannot follow them. The hospital will make every effort to adapt the treatment plan to meet your specific needs and limitations.

Accepting the Consequences of Not Following Instructions

5. You are responsible for your actions if you refuse treatment or do not follow your physician's instructions.

Asking Questions

6. You are responsible for asking questions when you do not understand what you have been told about your care or what you are expected to do.

Acting With Consideration & Respect

7. You are expected to be considerate of other patients and hospital staff by not making unnecessary noise, smoking, or causing distractions. You are responsible for respecting the property of other persons and that of the hospital.

Financial Obligations

8. You are responsible for assuring that the financial obligations of your health care are met as promptly as possible.

www.AuroraHealthCare.org

05 402760 (10/01) ©AHC

Figure 12-3 • *continued*

by the hospital staff upon admittance. Other health care facilities include it as part the admission packet in the nursing unit. Then the health unit coordinator or nurse gives it to the patient upon the patient's arrival in the nursing unit. It is important that patients understand that they are being treated equally and conscientiously regarding their rights. It is also important that patients understand their responsibilities so they can contribute in a positive manner to the outcome of their health care treatment.

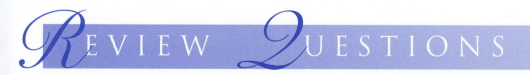

SUMMARY

An advance directive is a means by which people can make known the type of health care treatment they want. One type of advance directive is a Durable Power of Attorney for Health Care. It lets an individual appoint another person to make decisions about the individual's health care treatment should the individual be unable to do so.

A second type of an advanced directive is a living will. A living will is the means by which an individual may express his or her wishes concerning life-sustaining treatment in the event he or she becomes terminally or irreversibly ill. It is important that health care facilities accurately file advance directives in the patient's chart.

Patients have other rights, which are mandated by federal agencies such as the Department of Health and Human Services and the Centers for Medicaid and Medicare Service. Individual states also have laws and regulations covering patient rights. The Joint Commission on Accreditation of Health Care Organizations has guidelines that, when followed, ensure the rights of the patient and improve the outcomes of their treatment. Health unit coordinators should be aware of all of the patient's rights and responsibilities.

Health care facilities usually provide patients with a summary of patient rights and responsibilities. Health unit coordinators should maintain a sufficient supply of these summaries, ordering replacements as required.

REVIEW QUESTIONS

1. Define Durable Power of Attorney for Health Care.

2. Define living will.

3. Explain the health unit coordinator's responsibilities when a patient brings an advance directive to the health care facility.

4. List five patient rights.

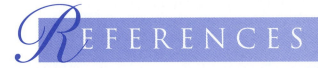

AHUC CERTIFICATION EXAM

CONTENT AREAS

II. H. 3   Assist with Advance Directives documentation

HROUGH THE EYES

OF A HEALTH CARE PROFESSIONAL

Today, patients know more about health care and their rights than ever before. The health unit coordinator must have that same knowledge and familiarity of the employer's policies regarding these rights and responsibilities in order to answer questions. By knowing and having a caring attitude for the patients' rights and responsibilities, the health unit coordinator is demonstrating the same attitude the health care facility strives to promote.

EFERENCES

http://www.aspe.os.dhhs.gov/asmnsimp/PVCREC2.HTM Accessed April 10, 2003.

http://www.hhs.gov/news/facts/privacy Accessed May 3, 2003.

http://www.hhs.gov/ocr/hippa Accessed May 3, 2003.

Patient Care Record

Learning Objectives

Upon completion of this chapter and review questions, the learner should be able to:

1. Discuss four legal aspects of the patient care record.

2. Describe how to maintain a legible patient care record.

3. Define ownership of the patient care record.

4. Discuss three reasons why a health care facility may choose a computerized patient care record over a paper patient care record.

5. Discuss the custodial responsibilities of the health unit coordinator for the patient care record.

6. List eight standard chart forms.

7. List three supplemental chart forms.

8. Define "thinning" and "stuffing" a patient care record.

Key Terms

account number Another term for financial number.

admission agreement A form the patient or guardian signs agreeing to the admission, treatment, and payment for services performed. This can be a separate form or found on the reverse side of the face sheet.

chart holder A binder that holds a patient's health care documents together during a health care stay.

discharge planning communication form A form all health care providers use to communicate and document discharge planning and postdischarge plans.

face sheet A form on which personal data and the patient's specific identification number are recorded, and at times contains the admission agreement.

financial number A unique number assigned to a patient each time she or he is admitted or has work done at a health care facility.

graphic sheet A form on which a patient's vital signs are documented and graphed.

history and physical A note recorded by a physician or physician's assistant documenting a patient's history, including health, work, environment, and social factors and a complete physical evaluation including medications and drug allergies.

medical record number A set of numbers assigned once to a patient to be used to locate chart documents.

medication administration record A form used to document every medication administered to a patient during a health care stay.

physician order sheet A form on which physicians request all diagnostic tests and treatments, including diet and medications, for a particular patient.

progress notes A form physicians and other health care professionals use to document a patient's progress during a health care stay.

standard chart forms Forms found in all patient care records.

supplemental forms Forms added to a patient care record as needed to document specific treatments.

Abbreviations

H & P History and Physical

I & O Intake and Output

MAR Medication Administration Record

MRN Medical Record Number

PATIENT CARE RECORD

Keeping track of all of the information regarding the care and treatment of patients is crucially important. Patients may be treated and cared for by multiple health care providers, with each one relying on the other members of the health care team. Patients may receive treatment in several locations and departments within the health care facility, in their room, and sometimes in even a totally separate facility. All of the health care providers need rapid, easy, and reliable access to certain patient information and records.

Others, besides the direct care providers, also need to have certain information and records. The health care facility's accounting department needs information in order to calculate accurate charges. Insurance companies need certain information regarding the care and treatment of a patient in order to accurately process insurance claims and reimbursements. Both state and federal governments also have record-keeping regulations.

Health care facilities use a data and record-keeping system in which all of the information required for the care and treatment of a patient is kept in one location convenient to the caregivers providing care and treatment to the patient. All of the information is contained in one single binder or container. Having all of the patient information at a single location and in a single unified source makes it easy for all the health care providers involved in a patient's care to locate notes and information. This patient data recording and retention system is commonly called the patient care record or the patient's chart. Other names that are sometimes used for the patient care record are:

◆ Medical chart

◆ Medical record

◆ Patient's record

◆ Health care record

◆ Health record

◆ Computerized patient record

No matter what term is used for the patient care record, it is a very important record for the patient and health care team members.

The patient care record has numerous purposes:

◆ It provides communication among the physician, the nursing staff, and all other health care providers during a health care stay.

◆ It is a record of the patient's personal and medical history.

◆ It is a recording of all care and treatment provided to the patient during the health care stay.

◆ It documents care and treatment for insurance purposes.

◆ It is a legal document.

This chapter will detail the many different forms that make up a patient care record. The patient care record begins in the patient access, or admitting, department. It is the patient access department personnel who are responsible for gathering important identification information regarding the patient. Some of this information includes:

◆ The patient's full name

◆ The patient's address

- The patient's phone number

- The phone number of person to contact in case of an emergency

- The patient's birth date

- The patient's Social Security number

- The name of the admitting physician

- The name of the referring physician

- The reason for admission

- Insurance information

- The name of the patient's employer

All this information is entered into the hospital's patient registration computer system. This system generates various paper forms used for patient identification throughout the health care stay. The items used for patient identification consist of a name band, an imprinter plate or patient stickers, and patient name labels, or stickers. These tools are shown in Figures 13-1, 13-2, and 13-3.

When all of the patient's identification forms reach the unit workstation, it is the health unit coordinator's responsibility to assemble the patient's chart.

Some health care facilities have the patients go directly to their room, and the health unit coordinator obtains the personal information from the patient or an accompanying family member in the patient's room. The health unit coordinator then enters the data into the health care facility's computer system and the forms are printed out.

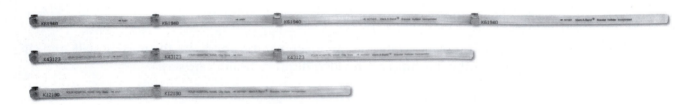

Figure 13-1 • *Patient name bands (Permission to use this copyrighted photo of Ident-A-Band® Insert Bracelet has been granted by the owner, Hollister Incorporated.)*

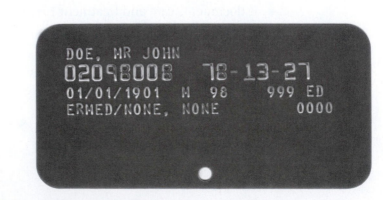

Figure 13-2 • *Imprinter plate*

These types of health care facilities usually use bar-coded sticky labels instead of imprinter plates to identify all the patient forms. Bar-coded forms are used because of the rapid and simplified data-tracking capability they provide in conjunction with computers. Figure 13-4 is an example of a computerized bar-coded label.

CHART HOLDERS

A **chart holder** holds all the patients' documents together during a health care stay. A chart holder can be thin or thick; it can open at the top or on the side (see Figure 13-5). These documents are separated by preprinted dividers and organized

> James F. Smith   01-02-65
> 11-22-33
> 987654555
> Dr. Joseph F. Edwards
> Inpt

Figure 13-3 • *Patient name label (sticker)*

> DOE, JONATHAN E.
> DOB 11-22-55   78-13-27
> 12345671   IP   M.
> HANSON, JAMES

Figure 13-4 • *Bar-coded patient label*

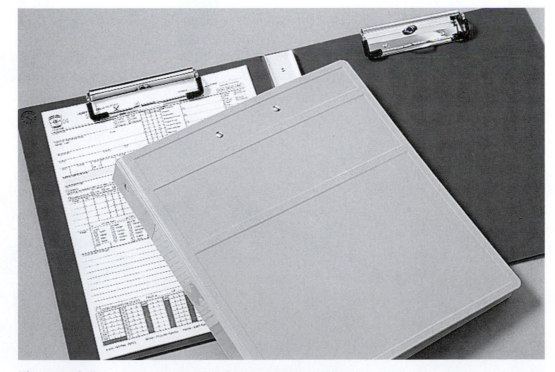

Figure 13-5 • *Chart holder (Courtesy of Carstens, Inc.)*

according to the health care facility's policy. An example of preprinted dividers is shown in Figure 13-6.

STANDARD PATIENT CARE RECORD FORMS

The patient care record consists of eight **standard chart forms**. Standard chart forms are defined as forms found in every patient care record. Table 13-1 provides the titles of these standard chart forms, explains their purpose and origin, and tells the number of each type usually found in a patient care record.

Data Base

The data base is a form that nurses use to document and share information received during an admission interview with the patient. It contains information regarding the patient's past and present physical conditions and social situation.

Face Sheet

The **face sheet** is used by many health care facilities to assist in providing quality care. It is called a face sheet because it is usually the first sheet of a patient care record. It can also serve as an **admission agreement**. It lets health care providers, with a

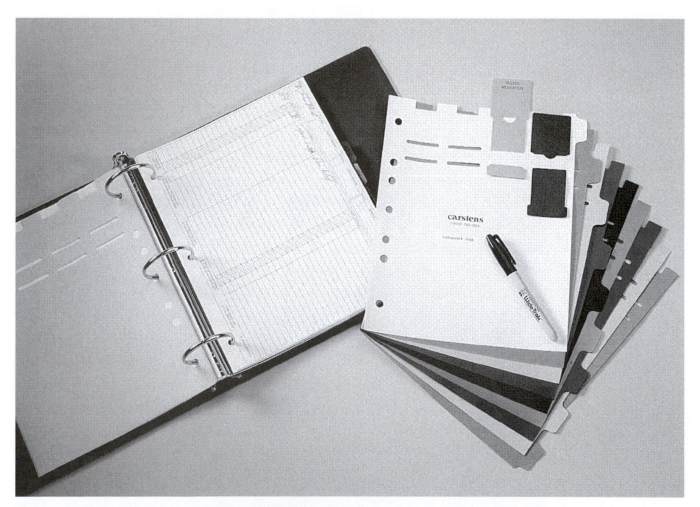

Figure 13-6 • *Chart dividers (Courtesy of Carstens, Inc.)*

TABLE 13-1 Standard Chart Forms

Name of Form	Purpose of Form	Department That Originates Form	Typical Number of Forms Found in a Patient Care Record Chart
Data base	Provides a concise place for nurses to document patient's past and current medical history.	Nursing unit	One
Face sheet/ admission agreement	Records patient personal data and identification number.	Patient access	One
Discharge planning communication form	Provides a standardized form for all health care providers to document discharge planning.	Nursing unit	One
Physician order sheet	Document for diagnostic and treatment orders to be written.	Nursing unit	Two or three
Progress notes	Document on which physicians and other health care providers write about the patient's progress.	Nursing unit	Two or three
Graphic sheet	Document and graph the patient's vital signs.	Nursing unit	One
History and physical	Document that physicians use to record the patient's health, work, environment, and social factors as well as a current physical assessment.	Nursing unit	One
Medication administration record (MAR)	A document to record every medication administered to a patient during a health care stay.	Nursing unit	Three
Supplemental forms	Forms added to the chart for documentation on an as-needed basis.	Nursing unit	One

quick glance, determine helpful and needed information. A face sheet is shown in Figure 13-7. The face sheet is a record of all the personal information gathered by the staff during the admission process as well as a medical record number and a case or financial number.

Medical Record Number

The clinical information services department, also called the medical records department, assigns the medical record number. The **medical record number** is often referred to as the **MRN**. This number identifies a patient and remains the same every time the patient is admitted or has services provided at that specific health care facility. An example of one of the many services that might be provided is presurgical laboratory tests. Clinical information services files all patient care records according to the MRN. When patients are readmitted to a health care facility, the previous patient care records are sent to the workstation to be used for reference and continuity of care. Clinical information services uses a medical record number instead of names to provide a safe way of filing patient care records, especially for patients with common names such as Smith and Jones. Many imaging departments also use the medical record number to file the images for all patients, both inpatients and outpatients.

Financial Number

The **financial number**, or **account number**, is separate from the medical record number and is usually longer. It is assigned to the patient by the patient access department. This number is used to charge the patient for services rendered during the health care stay. Assigning a number different from the medical record number ensures that the numerous charges health care can generate will be accurately entered for each patient stay at the facility.

Discharge Planning Communication Form

In some cases, the patient may require additional equipment and care to continue the recovery process at home. The **discharge planning communication form** provides one location for all health care providers to communicate and document the progress each service is planning. Having one document in a single known location enables all health care providers to communicate and document the care each is planning to provide. A discharge planning communication form is illustrated in Figure 13-8.

Physician Order Sheet

Physicians use the **physician order sheet** to document their orders regarding the diagnostic tests, examination, medication, treatments, diets, and other health care the patient is to receive. Other health care professionals may also write orders on the physician order sheets. The policies and procedures of the health system as well as the scope of service practiced by the health care professional determine who is allowed to write orders on the physician order sheet. As can be seen in Figure 13-9, this form is quite plain, leaving room for the many different orders the physician will write throughout the patient's stay. The entries on this form generate most of the work for a health unit coordinator.

TheBestMedicalCenter
Hometown, USA

INPATIENT ADMISSION FACESHEET

PATIENT NAME   *GUARANTOR*

MRN: 50-30-70-90
CASE # 98765432

ADMIT DATE
05/05/2004

PAICIENT, POLLY   PAICIENT, POLLY
4321 S. CHERRY LANE   4321 S. CHERRY LANE
SUNNY CITY, USA   SUNNY CITY, USA
     DOB: 10/20/1950   SSN: 111-22-4444

MARITAL STATUS: M   GUAR EMPLOYER
RACE 4-2   LANG: SPANISH   CBA COMPANY
RELIGION: CATH   OCC: CLERK
                                             9876 W. WASHINGTON AVE.
                                             SUNNY CITY, USA

                                        CONTACT
                                        CATE, ANGELA
                                        PH# 141-242-3434
                                        5677 CHESTNUT ROAD

31 DAY READMIT: N
INJ: NOT AN INJURY

CHIEF COMPLAINT: ILL

ALLERGIES: **FISH**

PRIMARY INS: IN HEALTH   SUBSCRIBER RELATION: SELF
P.O. BOX 864   PAICENT, POLLY
DUNES, USA   EMPLOYER: CBA COMPANY
POLICY #879605954433   9876 W. WASHINGTON AVE.
GROUP #465329   SUNNY CITY

ADMIT PHYSICIAN: 73421 KEI KUMAR
ATTEND PHYSICIAN: 89700 HATTIE BROWN
PCP   89700 HATTIE BROWN

ADVANCE DIRECTIVES WITH PATIENT

Figure 13-7 • *Face sheet*

```
St. Luke's Medical Center
Milwaukee, Wisconsin

Patient Admitted from: Home _____ N.H. _____

Other: _____

D/C needs anticipated at this time: No _____ Yes _____

Primary D/C Contact Person: _____

Relationship: _____ Phone: _____
```

DATE	PROBLEMS/PLAN/OUTCOMES	SIGNATURE/PAGER

SS/js:3657w   **DISCHARGE PLANNING COMMUNICATIONS**   05-164200 (Rev. 1/90)

Figure 13-8 • *Discharge planning communication form*
(Reprinted with permission of Aurora Health Care, Milwaukee, WI)

Aurora Health Care®
Milwaukee, Wisconsin
☐ St. Luke's Medical Center   ☐ Hartford Memorial Hospital
☐ Sinai Samaritan Medical Center ☐ _____
☐ West Allis Memorial Hospital

PHYSICIAN'S ORDERS   ①

When no number shows in the circle, change forms

PLEASE USE BALL POINT PEN

Formulary approved equivalent will be dispensed unless
the words "**NO SUBSTITUES**" are written.

Date / Time of Order	CHECK ALLERGIES BEFORE WRITING MEDICATION ORDERS

White Copy - CHART / Yellow Copies - PHARMACY

PHYSICIAN'S ORDERS

05402460 (6/99)

05402460

Figure 13-9 • *Physician order sheet (Reprinted with permission of Aurora Health Care, Milwaukee, WI)*

Progress Notes

The physician and other health care professionals use the **progress notes** to document the progress the patient is making during the health care stay. In some health care facilities, nurses also document their care, treatment, and observation of the patient on this form, as you can see in Figure 13-10. If the nurses do not use the progress note, they have a separate form called the nurses' notes.

Graphic Sheet

The **graphic sheet** is used to document the vital signs of patients. Vital signs include temperature, pulse, respiration rate, and blood pressure. All this information is recorded in graph form to allow easy reading and assessment. Some health care facilities have the nurses and nursing assistants bring the vital signs to the workstation for the health unit coordinator to chart and graph on the graphic sheet, as shown in Figure 13-11. In facilities that have computerized patient records, the nurse or nursing assistant enters the vital signs into the computer.

History and Physical

The physician may write or dictate the patient's **history and physical (H & P)** after interviewing the patient and completing a physical evaluation of the patient. If the H & P is dictated, it is then typed up by the transcription department and sent to the workstation to be filed into the patient's chart by the health unit coordinator. Figure 13-12 (page 201), shows a sample history and physical form.

Medication Administration Record

Health care professionals such as nurses and respiratory therapists use the **medication administration record (MAR)** to document every medication given to the patient. Some health care facilities have the health unit coordinator transcribe the medication ordered for a patient by the physician onto the medication administration record. The nurse then can easily find the medication name on the MAR form and chart that the medication was given and when it was given. Other health care facilities have medications listed on the medication administration record via a computerized process. Listing the medications on the MAR as soon as the physician's order is written results in a more efficient method for the nurse to chart than does having the nurse transcribe the medication and then sign out the given medication. Figure 13-13 (page 202) shows a medication administration record form.

Supplemental forms

Supplemental forms are forms added to the patient's chart as needed. Some common supplemental forms are:

◆ The anticoagulant therapy sheet records test results pertaining to the anticoagulants that patients are receiving (Figure 13-14 [page 203]).

◆ The diabetic record records blood sugar monitoring results (Figure 13-15 [page 204]).

◆ The intake and output form is where all nursing personnel record all food and drink the patient takes in as well as measurements for any elimination of urine, stool, or vomit (Figure 13-16 [page 205]).

Aurora Sinai Medical Center ®

PATIENT PROGRESS NOTE

Date/Time	Focus	D = Data A = Action R = Response

05200000

PATIENT PROGRESS NOTE

Figure 13-10 • *Progress note* (Reprinted with permission of Aurora Health Care, Milwaukee, WI)

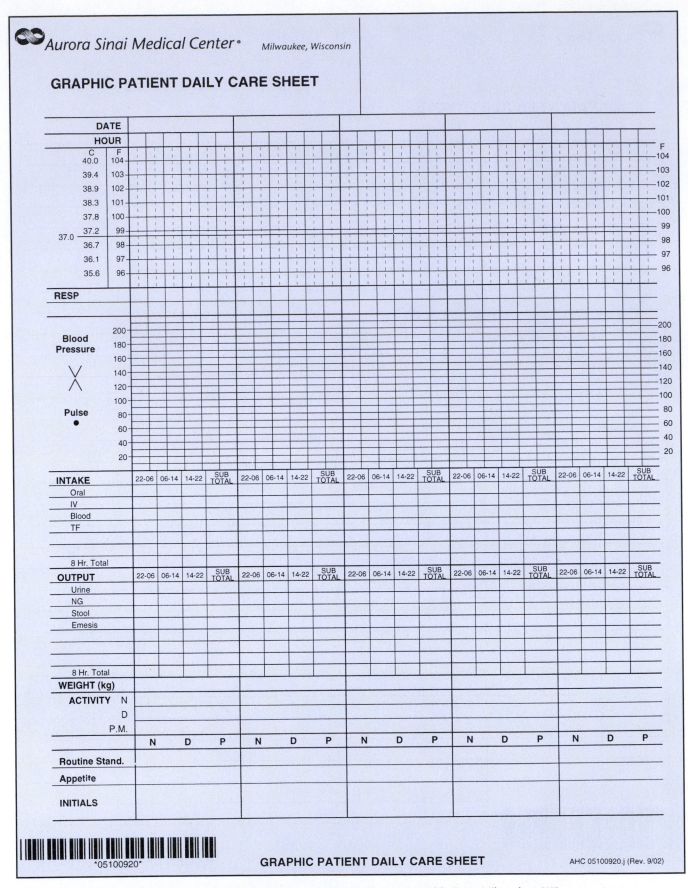

Figure 13-11 • *Graphic sheet (Reprinted with permission of Aurora Health Care, Milwaukee, WI)*

TheBestHospital

HISTORY AND PHYSICAL REPORT

Date and Time report was generated

Date of Admission:

Chief Complaint

Allergies

History of Present Illness

Past Medical History

Physical Exam

   HEENT

   NECK

   CHEST

   ABDOMEN

   EXTREMITIES

Medications

Social History

Assessment & Plan

Dictated by Dr. Sample   date and time.

Patient Name and Room Number

Figure 13-12 • *History and physical form*

ALLERGIES:	DATE	DATE	DATE	DATE	DATE	DATE	NON-RECURRING MEDICATIONS DRUG DOSE, ROUTE	GIVEN BY
SCHEDULED MEDICATIONS						TIME		

DIAGNOSIS: CHF
MD: RED, JOSEPH

CASE NO.: 87658765
MRU:
AGE:

VALENTINE, AL
ROOM:

Figure 13-13 • *Medication administration record (Reprinted with permission of Aurora Health Care, Milwaukee, WI)*

Aurora Sinai Medical Center® Milwaukee, Wisconsin

ANTICOAGULANT THERAPY SHEET

AGENT: ____________________

DATE / TIME	PTT		
	SECONDS	BOLUS	DRIP

AGENT: ____________________

DATE / TIME	PROTIME (Control 12.0)	
	SECONDS	DOSAGE

ANTICOAGULANT THERAPY SHEET

AHC 05300310.j (04/02) Front

Figure 13-14 • *Anticoagulant therapy sheet (Reprinted with permission of Aurora Health Care, Milwaukee, WI)*

St. Luke's Medical Center
Milwaukee, Wisconsin

DIABETIC RECORD

TO COMPARE SIMULTANEOUS LAB AND ACCU-CHEK VALUES,
MULTIPLY ACCU-CHEK VALUE X 1.11. IF LAB VALUE IS <100 mgldl,
ACCU-CHEK VALUE X 1.11 SHOULD BE WITHIN ± 15 mgldl.
IF LAB VALUE IS >100 mgldl, ACCU-CHEK VALUE X 1.11 SHOULD BE
WITHIN ± 15%.

Chemstrip bG lot # _____   Control lot # _____

BLOOD GLUCOSE IN MG/DL					DIABETIC MEDICATION					URINE TESTS		
											KETODIASTIX	
DATE	HOUR	LAB	ACCU-CHEKbG METER	VISUAL CHEM-STRIP bG	INITIALS	HOUR	INSULIN/ORAL HYPOGLYCEMIC AGENT	INJEC-TION SITE	DOSE	INITIALS	HOUR	GLUCOSE	KETONES

INITIALS	SIGNATURE		INITIALS	SIGNATURE		INITIALS	SIGNATURE

DIABETIC RECORD

Rev.
05-613000

Figure 13-15 • *Diabetic record (Reprinted with permission of Aurora Health Care, Milwaukee, WI)*

Aurora Sinai Medical Center

24 HOUR INTAKE/OUTPUT WORKSHEET

05100820 (Rev. 5/95) - 61

STANDARD OF MEASUREMENTS (in CC's)

Styrofoam Cup - 8 oz.	240	Jello w/ Fruit	90	Graduated Water Cup-16 oz 480
Soup Bowl	180	Jello, Plain	120	D.B. Grape/Prune Juice 90
Coffee Cup	220	Ice Cream	90	D.B. Apple/Pineapple Juice 120
Juice	120	Sherbet	90	Popsicle 80
Milk	240	Creamer	15	30cc = 1oz.
12oz. Soda Can	355			16cc = 1 Tbsp.
				4cc = 1 Tsp.

Name:

Room:

Date:

	Time	INTAKE						OUTPUT					
		Oral	IV	Blood Product	Enteral	Enteral Flush	Other	Urine	Stool/ Ostomy	NG/ G.Tube	Emesis	Drains	Other
NIGHTS													
TOTAL													

		Oral	IV	Blood Product	Enteral	Enteral Flush	Other	Urine	Stool/ Ostomy	NG/ G.Tube	Emesis	Drains	Other
DAYS													
TOTAL													

		Oral	IV	Blood Product	Enteral	Enteral Flush	Other	Urine	Stool/ Ostomy	NG/ G.Tube	Emesis	Drains	Other
EVENINGS													
TOTAL													

05100820 (Rev. 5/95) - 61

24 HOUR INTAKE / OUTPUT WORKSHEET

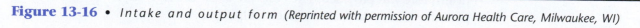

Figure 13-16 • *Intake and output form (Reprinted with permission of Aurora Health Care, Milwaukee, WI)*

Dictated Reports

Other forms that are included in a patient's chart can be categorized as dictated reports. All diagnostic examination results are dictated, typed, and sent to the workstation to be filed into the patient's medical record. Some of those reports include consultation reports, cardiac reports, imaging reports, and therapy notes.

Computerized Patient Care Record

Some health care facilities have computer systems that allow all of the data for the forms to be entered into a computer right at the bedside. There are many advantages to computerized charting. For instance, the information can be entered from any computer terminal, immediately, whereas with written documentation there may be a delay in getting to the chart if the patient and chart are in another department where the patient is having a diagnostic exam performed. The computerized chart is always available. Most computer systems allow multiple users to be in one chart at the same time. Reading computerized records and reports is easier than reading manually prepared records because the format is always the same no matter who documents. In addition, computers use color to highlight critical values.

OWNERSHIP OF THE PATIENT CARE RECORD

The forms, or the actual paper that the patient care record is made up of, are the property of the health care facility. The chart itself and the documents inside it never leave the health care facility. The information in the patient care record, however, belongs to the patient. This means that if the patient asks to see the content or parts of the chart, it can be shown to the patient according to the health care facility's policies and procedures.

LEGIBILITY AND LEGAL ASPECTS OF THE PATIENT CARE RECORD

Because the patient care record is a legal document, it must be maintained in an acceptable manner. All health care providers must follow certain rules for these legal documents:

- Writing must be legible.

- Information must be accurate.

- No erasures or Wite-Out can be used.

- All entries need to signed with the full name and title of the documentor.

- The date and time of the documentation must be recorded.

- Patient care records for court proceedings usually are needed years after the health care was provided. The best way to ensure legibility after an extended period of time is to write in black ballpoint ink.

All health care team members should practice writing legibly. Health unit coordinators should practice marking and initialing all orders according to their employer's policy. Excess markings on the forms, such as brackets and unnecessary lines, clutter the form and make the record less legible.

CORRECTING ERRORS ON THE PATIENT CARE RECORD

The proper way to correct an error is to draw one single line through it, write your initials, time and date the error, then document the correct information. It is very important not to obliterate, write over, or cover over any error. If an error is covered so that no one can read it, it will be impossible to explain at a later time.

CUSTODIAL RESPONSIBILITIES FOR THE PATIENT CARE RECORD

As discussed in Chapter 11, a custodian is one who guards, protects, or maintains the patient care record. Maintaining a patient care record may include processes known as thinning, or splitting, and stuffing.

Thinning, or *splitting*, a patient care record means to pull out certain forms from a chart holder because the record has become too large or cumbersome to handle. Each health care facility has established rules for thinning the record, including which forms may and may not be thinned, how many days of current forms should be kept, and where and how the removed forms should be kept. Most policies require documentation to be included somewhere in the chart stating that the chart was thinned, by whom, and when.

Here is an example of a hospital policy for thinning charts:

Never thin any physician order sheets.

Never thin a face sheet, advance directive [see Chapter 12], or history and physical.

Never thin any laboratory or imaging reports.

Leave at least 5 days' worth of the most current progress and graphic notes.

Write your name and the current date on a label and affix it to the inside of the patient care record after thinning.

Send the thinned chart forms to medical records, or place the forms in a file cabinet on the unit according to facility policy.

Stuffing the chart refers to placing blank forms into the chart so the physician and health care providers have a place to document things such as orders and progress notes. Stuffing charts ahead of time helps the caregivers because they have the necessary forms at hand and saves the health unit coordinator from having to interrupt other activities in order to provide a needed form.

Another custodial duty is to ensure that all previous patient care records, thinned records, and medication administration records are included with the current patient care record when a patient is transferred to another unit. When the patient is discharged, the health unit coordinator must ensure that all of these records are sent to the clinical information services department.

SUMMARY

The patient care record is an important communication tool for all the health care team. It is an important record of all of a patient's medical care and treatment during a health care stay. The health unit coordinator must have a good understanding of the various documents that make up a patient care record. It is a responsibility of the health unit coordinator to know the employer's policies and procedures for ensuring that the chart has the most current documents filed in the appropriate order so that all health care providers can easily access the information.

REVIEW QUESTIONS

1. Who owns the patient care record?

2. To correct an error on a patient chart form, what should you never do?

3. List eight standard chart forms.

4. Discuss three reasons why a health care facility may choose a computerized patient care record over a paper patient care record.

5. List three custodial responsibilities of the health unit coordinator for the patient care record.

6. To thin a chart is to do what to the patient care record?

7. List three supplemental chart forms.

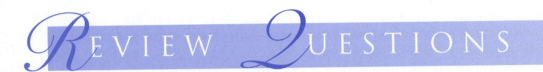

NAHUC CERTIFICATION EXAM

CONTENT AREAS

II. D. 4 Maintain patient charts by thinning and adding forms as needed

II. D. 5 File forms and reports

II. E. 5 Graph and chart information onto appropriate forms

II. E. 9 Perform quality assurance on charts (i.e. verify that chart forms are filed and labeled correctly, all orders have been transcribed, allergies are noted in appropriate places, prepare incident reports, etc.)

THROUGH THE EYES

OF A HEALTH CARE PROFESSIONAL

Since the medical record is not in the hands of the health information management department while the patient is receiving care, the traditional HIM role responsibilities in several areas fall on the health unit coordinator.

Record Integrity/Timeliness: The HUC is responsible for gathering all components of the medical record and assembling them in an organized manner to provide easy and prompt access to clinicians. This is a never-ending process, as test results and dictated reports are constantly arriving on the unit and need to be filed promptly.

Patient Rights: Confidentiality and privacy issues are coordinated through the health unit coordinator. Callers want to know of patients' presence and hear of the patients' condition. Physicians' offices call for information to be faxed for ongoing care needs.

Continuity of Care: The health unit coordinator needs to serve the HIM role in sending information to other facilities whenever patients are being transferred or considered for transfer.

Streamlined Record Keeping: If the record keeping is done well by the health unit coordinator, the processing of the record postdischarge is more efficient for the health information management staff. Less time is spent looking for missing documents, documents in wrong records, missing thinned portions, and old records.

We really do appreciate the health unit coordinators. (Cathy Ptak, Clinical Information Services Director, Aurora Health Care)

REFERENCES

Flight, M. (1997). *Law, liability, and ethics for medical office professionals* (4th ed.). Clifton Park, NY: Thomson Delmar Learning

LaFleur, M. (1998). *Health unit coordinating* (4th ed.). Philadelphia: Saunders.

CHAPTER 14

Admission, Transfer, and Discharge

Learning Objectives

Upon completion of this chapter and review questions, the learner should be able to:

1. Describe how a patient is admitted to a health care system.

2. List the three common types of admissions.

3. Describe the three common types of patient.

4. Describe three types of transfer.

5. Describe the health unit coordinator role in discharging a patient.

Key Terms

admission process   The process of admitting a patient into the care of the health care system.

against medical advice   Leaving the health care facility without permission of the admitting physician.

direct admission   An admission to a health care facility when the patient does not stop in the admitting department or the emergency department but is brought directly to the patient care unit or department.

discharge   The process of dismissing a patient from the care of the health care system.

Emergency Medical Treatment and Active Labor Act An act the U.S. Congress passed in 1986, requiring hospitals and ambulance services to provide care to anyone needing emergency treatment regardless of citizenship, legal status, or ability to pay.

length of stay How long the patient can stay in the health care facility, determined by the diagnosis.

patient consent form A form the patient or guardian signs agreeing to the admission, treatment, and payment for services performed.

patient data base A form that contains health information about the patient that is used by the health care team.

registration The process of entering a patient's personal information into a health care facility's records and file system.

scheduled admission An admission that is arranged before the patient arrives in the health care facility; a planned admission for the patient and the health care facility.

transfer The process of moving a patient from one location to another location.

unscheduled admission An admission that is not scheduled or arranged before admission.

Abbreviations

AMA Against Medical Advice

EMTALA Emergency Medical Treatment and Active Labor Act

LOS Length of Stay

ADMISSION PROCESS

In order for a person to receive care in a health care facility, the admission process must be completed. The **admission process** is the process of admitting a patient into a health care facility. The admission process used is unique to the health care system. The health care facility staff begins the admission process by registering the patient. **Registration** is the process of entering a patient's personal information into a health care facility's records and file system.

The registration program may be computerized. Registration computer programs are integrated with the other computer programs and systems used in the health care system. Information can be hand entered into one computer program and will then pass into another computer system without having to be re-entered. In the health care system, the staff person responsible for entering this information into the registration program may be called an admitting clerk, a health unit coordinator, or an emergency department clerk.

ADMISSION

Admission is the term used to define the processes used to admit a patient into the health care system. All patients who enter into the health care system must be registered into the health care registration system. Registration is a component of the admission process. This process can be started before the patient's physical admission by contacting the patient either by telephone or computer to collect the needed personal information. If this is the method used, the patient or responsible guardian will provide the information to the heath care facility staff. The information requested will be:

- The correct spelling of the patient's name

- The patient's telephone number

- The patient's address

- The patient's insurance company and policy numbers

- The telephone number and name of the next of kin to be contacted in case of emergency

- The patient's employer

- The sex of the patient

- The name of the family physician

- The name of the referring physician

- The name of the admitting physician

- The patient's Social Security number

- The patient's birth date

- Other identifications the health care facility may use to differentiate same-name patients

All of this information will then be entered into the computer system, which will generate information and forms needed by the various departments in order to correctly process the admission upon the patient's arrival at the health care facility. An especially important form containing all the demographic information unique to the individual patient is called the face sheet (refer to Chapter 13). See an example of a face sheet in Figure 14-1. During this process, a unique number is generated for the patient for this admission. This number is called the account number, the billing number, the financial number, or the encounter number. This number is used for this admission and for this patient only. It is an identifier linked to the specific patient and admission. It will be used in the computer programs to order services. Because patients could have more than one account in a health care system, it is very important to choose the correct account when entering information and charges to a patient account. The patient will also be assigned a medical record number. This number is assigned to an

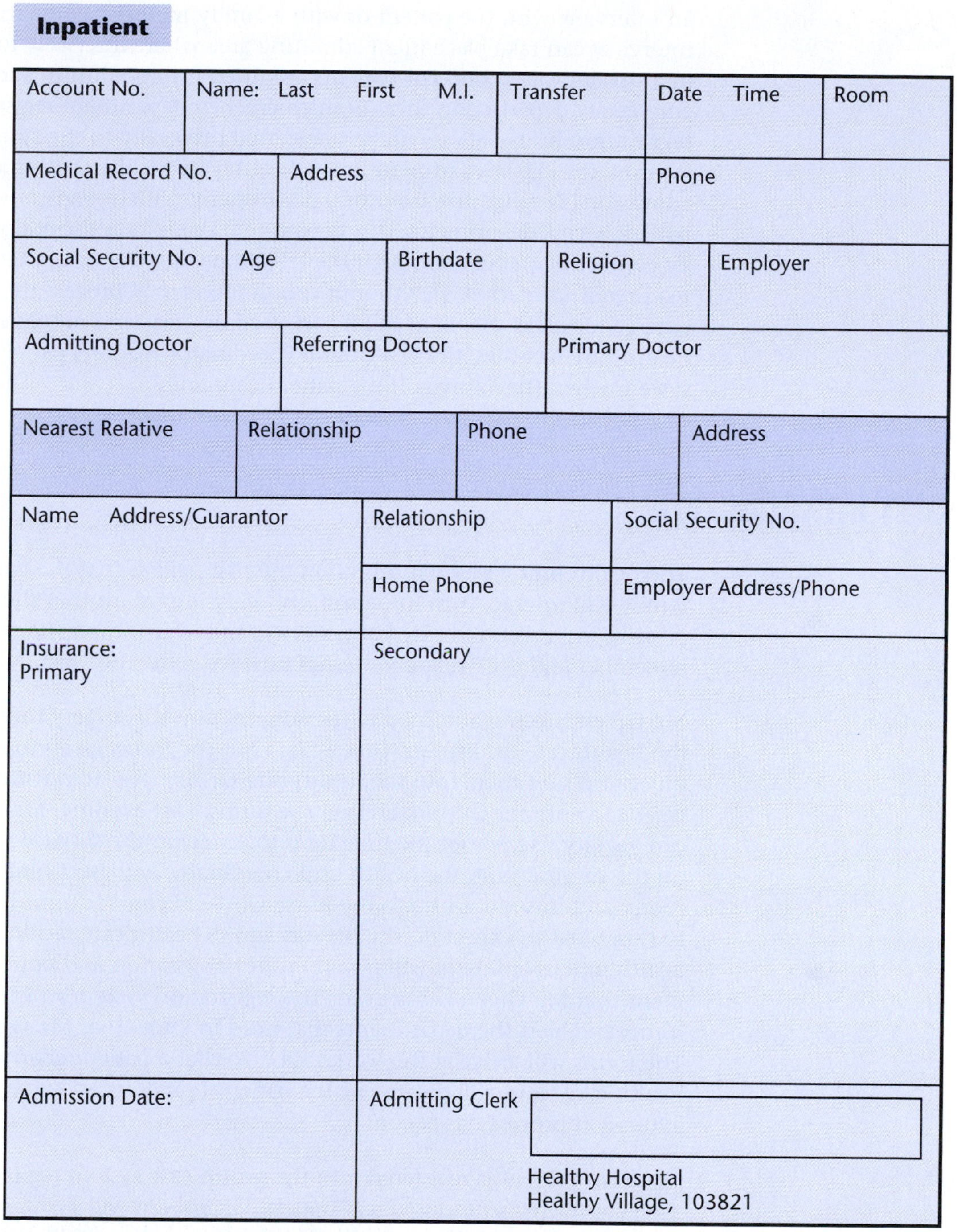

Inpatient

Account No.	Name: Last First M.I.	Transfer	Date Time	Room

Medical Record No.	Address	Phone

Social Security No.	Age	Birthdate	Religion	Employer

Admitting Doctor	Referring Doctor	Primary Doctor

Nearest Relative	Relationship	Phone	Address

Name Address/Guarantor	Relationship	Social Security No.
	Home Phone	Employer Address/Phone

Insurance: Primary	Secondary

Admission Date:	Admitting Clerk

Healthy Hospital
Healthy Village, 103821

Figure 14-1 • *Face sheets contain patient information used by the health unit coordinator to process orders.*

individual only once. The medical record number will not change with additional admissions. It is used as a reference number for filing and retrieving records. It is used to keep all the patient's medical records together over time, and is unique to one patient only.

When a patient is unable to be contacted before admission, or if the admission is unplanned, the registration forms may be completed in the health care facility during an interview with the patient or with a family member, companion, or guardian. The interview can take place in an admitting area where interview rooms are available or in a patient care room. For patients admitted into the health care system through an emergency department, there is an emergency department registration process. This registration information will be transferred internally to the systems that require the information. The department in the health care facility that processes the majority of admissions is called the admitting department, patient registration department, or patient access department. This department completes the majority of the registrations by contacting patients through the telephone and the computer systems to collect the required information. Health unit coordinators may process the patient registration in emergency areas as well as in physician clinic areas and outpatient areas. In some health care facilities, the health unit coordinator registers patients into the computer system when they arrive on the patient care unit.

UNIT INTRODUCTION

The health unit coordinator is often the first person that the patient and the patient's family will interact with in person. It is very important that the first impression be a positive impression for the patient and family. First impressions are what people remember and it is what determines how welcome they feel. An example follows.

Mr. Green is being admitted to the surgical unit for surgery today. Before coming to the health care facility, Mr. Green filled out the forms given to him by the physician's office and sent them into the health care facility. The admitting clerk called him last week to verify the information on the forms. Last evening, Mr. Green called the health care facility to find out the time he is to arrive on the surgical unit. When he arrives on the surgical unit, the health unit coordinator will greet him, show him to his room, and introduce him to the nurse who will care for him. The nurse will explain to him what to expect during his stay in the health care facility, his plan of care. The health unit coordinator will return to the workstation and notify the admitting department that Mr. Green has arrived. The registration system will then create the required forms and alert the departments that need to know that Mr. Green has been admitted. The forms will arrive at the workstation so that a patient chart can be created. The health care team will document the patient's progress and activities. The clerical admission process has begun.

Once the patient is registered into the health care system registration program, it is then considered a processed registration. The patient will sign a **patient consent form** either in person or electronically. This form gives the health care facility permission to treat the patient and to bill the patient's insurance company or the patient if the patient has no insurance coverage. The form may also provide permission for the health care facility to submit the patient's health information to the insurance carrier, to provide data to a research study, and to share the patient's health information with other physicians employed in the health care facility. Each patient consent form is unique to the health care facility (Figure 14-2).

MARQUETTE GENERAL HOSPITAL, INC.
Patient Admission Consent Form

Name of Patient	Medical Record & Account Number

1. Knowing that I have a condition requiring hospital and medical treatment, I do hereby voluntarily consent to such routine and/or emergency diagnostic procedures and hospital care by Marquette General Hospital, Inc. as is deemed necessary by my physician (or his designees) or by staff of the hospital, and do hereby voluntarily consent to such medical treatment by my physician or physicians (or by his or their designees) as is deemed necessary.

2. I am aware that the practice of medicine and surgery is not an exact science and I acknowledge that no guarantees have been made to me as to the results of said hospital care and medical treatment which I have authorized.

3. Recognizing that I have a condition requiring hospital and medical treatment and understanding that I may be harboring an infectious disease such as Hepatitis B or Human Immunodeficiency Virus (HIV) which could endanger the health of individuals accidently exposed to my blood or bodily fluids, I do hereby voluntarily consent to such routine diagnostic procedures and hospital care by Marquette General Hospital, Inc., as is deemed necessary by my physician (or his designees) or by the staff of the hospital. I further understand that any test results will become part of my medical record, and as such its confidentiality is protected by Federal Law.

4. I authorize you to release to my insurance company, to the agency assuming responsibility for cost of hospitalization or continuing care, or to the physician or hospital providing subsequent treatment or hospitalization any and all information which you possess relative to my disability for which I was confined within and treated for at Marquette General Hospital.

5. I am aware the hospital maintains a safe for storage of my money and/or articles of value. I, the patient or responsible party, assume full responsibility for items which I retain. The hospital assumes no liability for loss of or damage to articles not desposited in the safe.

6. It is understood that the hospital is a teaching institute and that unless the hospital is notified to the contrary in writing, the patient may participate as a teaching subject in the medical/nursing programs of the institution.

7. *"I hereby authorize Marquette General Hospital that, upon inquiry as to my general condition, it may release at its discretion my name, address, age, sex, reason for admission, general nature of injury and my general condition.* **I understand that I have the right to request that Marquette General Hospital not disclose this information in whole or in part."**

AGREEMENT OF PAYMENT
In consideration of the services rendered, the undersigned does hereby expressly agree to pay and guarantee in full any and all charges for hospital services rendered and materials furnished to or for the patient by Marquette General Hospital, Inc., Marquette, Michigan.

ASSIGNMENT OF BENEFITS AND RELEASE OF MEDICAL INFORMATION
Agreement and authorization of the reverse side of this form.

This form has been fully explained to me and I certify that I understand its contents:

_____   _____
Signature   Date

_____   _____
Relationship of Other than Patient

Patient Unable to Sign Because:_____

_____   _____
Witness   Date

D:\IC MGH\PtAdmConsent.pmd Rev. 6/29/98, 4/01/03   MRUR-subApprove:4/01/03

Item# 760252

Figure 14-2 • *Patient consent form (Courtesy of Marquette General Health System, Marquette, MI)*   *(continues)*

MARQUETTE REGIONAL MEDICAL CENTER
ASSIGNMENT OF BENEFITS
<u>RELEASE OF MEDICAL INFORMATION</u>

I authorize the Hospital and each physician/provider who treats/treated me, to release to any party responsible for payment, for the patient's information from the medical records as are required in order for the Hospital and/or physician/providers to obtain direct payment and to any participant in audits of such payments. This authorization to release information for purposes of payment, includes all records, including those records protected under the regulation in Code 42 of the Federal Regulations, Part 2, and Michigan Public Act 258 of 1988 of Alcohol and Drug Abuse and Treatment, records of psychological services, and records of social services, including communications made by the patient to a physician/provider, social worker or psychologist as well as treatment for serious communicable diseases, including Acquired Immune Deficiency Syndrome (AIDS), HIV infection, AIDS Related Complex, and Hepatitis. This authorization is effective only so long as necessary to obtain complete payment or reimbursement. **I understand that I am financially responsible to each physician/provider for charges not covered by my insurance plan.** In the event that I am transferred from this Hospital to be treated or cared for at another hospital, extended care, or other facility, including each of the hospitals and subsidiaries of the Hospital, I hereby consent and direct that medical and other information be released by the Hospital as may be necessary or useful in my obtaining such further care and treatment. I further authorize the release of my name and social security number to the manufacturers of a "permanently implantable device", if required by the applicable law.

_____   _____
Signature of Patient or Authorized Representative   Date

_____   _____
Witness   Date

<u>MEDICARE AUTHORIZATION</u>

I CERTIFY that information given by me in applying for payment under Title 18 of the Social Security Act is correct, I authorize any holder of medical or other information about me to release to the Social Security Administration or its intermediaries or carriers any information needed for this or related Medicare claims. I request payment of authorized benefits be made in my behalf. **I understand I am responsible for any health insurance deductibles and co-insurance payments.**

_____   _____
Signature of Patient or Authorized Representative   Date

_____   _____
Witness   Date

<u>ACKNOWLEDGEMENT</u>

The Notice of Privacy Practices for Marquette General Health System has been made available to me for my review. I understand that I may request a copy of the notice or obtain a copy from their website at www.mgh.org at any time.

_____   _____
Patient/Representative Signature   Date

Figure 14-2 • *continued*

TYPES OF ADMISSION

There are three basic types of admission to health care facilities. They are a scheduled admission, an unscheduled admission, and a direct admission.

SCHEDULED ADMISSION

The **scheduled admission** is a planned admission. The patient has been requested to arrive at the health care facility by the admitting physician, and the facility has prepared for the patient's arrival. The physician's office staff has a procedure for scheduling admissions for health care facilities where the physician has privileges to practice medicine. After the physician's office has completed their procedure to schedule the patient to the health care system for admission, the admitting department staff complete their admission procedure. At this point, the admitting department will create a list of all the scheduled admissions for each nursing unit within the health care facility for the day. This scheduled admission list is created from the information provided by the various physicians' offices. Each physician's office staff communicates with the admitting department on an ongoing basis. The scheduled admission list will be provided to each nursing unit or department either the night before the scheduled admission or the morning of the admission. From this list, which will include the patient's name, date of birth, sex, admitting physician, and diagnosis, the health unit coordinator, along with the other members of the nursing care team, will determine the patient's room assignment. The room assignment is based on availability. If the patient is being assigned to a semiprivate room, compatibility factors with a potential roommate will be considered. A semiprivate room is a room shared by two patients of the same sex. The health unit coordinator, who monitors the whereabouts of all the patients on the nursing unit, is aware of the open beds on the patient care unit at all times. Often, the health unit coordinator will have an updated written census showing what beds are open for new patients.

UNSCHEDULED ADMISSION

Unscheduled admissions are patients admitted to the health care facility who did not plan to be admitted. They were not scheduled through any physician offices before being admitted, nor did they appear on any lists created and provided to the nursing units. Usually, unscheduled admissions are emergency patients. Emergency patients who either come to an emergency department with health concerns or go to their physician's office with health concerns are unscheduled admissions if they must be admitted to the health care facility. These health concerns are serious, and the patient must be admitted to the health care facility to be treated. It would unsafe for them to not be admitted. Unscheduled admissions are still coordinated through the admitting department. The admitting staff will contact the nursing unit to request a bed for an unscheduled admission. After the health unit coordinator receives the request from admitting, she or he will consult the nurse manager, or the nursing care team, to select the best available bed placement for the unscheduled admission. Unscheduled admissions to large health care facilities can also come as unscheduled admissions from smaller outlying health care facilities that cannot provide the care or services that the patient requires. These are called direct admissions.

DIRECT ADMISSION

Patients who are admitted as **direct admissions** are not scheduled in advance and they are not seen by a physician on the health care staff before being admitted to a patient care area. Direct admissions are requested for patients of outlying health care facilities. These patients are admitted directly to a patient care bed, bypassing the admitting department or the emergency department. They are transported directly to a unit. Emergency medical service workers most often transport the patient in these situations. Before transport, the attending physician must call the receiving physician to request services. The health facility requesting the transfer will contact the admitting department after the receiving physician has accepted the patient so that the receiving nursing unit can be alerted to the fact that a direct admission will be admitted to that area. The health unit coordinator will provide the admitting department with the assigned bed for the patient. Often, the call alerting the staff on the nursing unit that the patient will soon be arriving will come directly from the emergency medical service team who is transporting the direct admission patient.

ADMISSION ON THE PATIENT CARE UNIT

Once the patient arrives on the patient care unit, the health unit coordinator alerts the departments that need to know that the patient has arrived. This notification can be accomplished by calling the admitting department or by completing a process in the computer program. Departments that need to know that the patient is admitted to the health care facility may include the following:

Department	Reason the Department Needs to Know
Switchboard	Phone calls can be directed to correct room
Dietary	Food requests can be sent to correct room
Business office	To begin the billing process
Bed control	Bed is now occupied
Ancillary services	Services can begin (labs drawn, x-rays taken)
Pharmacy	Medications can be sent to the patient as ordered

Patient chart forms will be created so that the health care providers can document the care that will be provided. The health unit coordinator is responsible for getting the patient charts prepared for this process. Whether the chart is paper or electronic, the health unit coordinator must prepare the chart and input the correct information, following the procedure used in the health care facility. All chart forms must be identified as to the patient they represent. There are three common methods for specifying the patient on the forms. A label containing the patient identifying information can be placed on the chart forms; an imprinter can imprint the information on the chart forms, or a computer program can place the patient identifying information on the forms. Health care facilities use one of these procedures for admitting a patient (Figure 14-3).

MARQUETTE GENERAL HOSPITAL

NURSING PROCEDURES

Procedure: Admission of a Patient	**Procedure No.:** A-003
Distribution: All Nursing Departments	**Effective Date:** January 1988
Authorized By:	**Revision Date:** 5/91; 11/91; 2/92; 7/92; 3/94; 12/95; 3/97; 3/98; 4/00; 8/02

PURPOSE: To acclimate the patient to the hospital environment in a method that will make him/her comfortable and relieve anxiety.

To gather information about the hospitalized patient that will aid in the development of the treatment plan.

EQUIPMENT: Patient Database
Stethoscope/thermometer
Scale
Patient gown/pajamas
Additional ID bands as indicated

PROCEDURE	POINT OF EMPHASIS
A. PATIENT'S ARRIVAL ON UNIT	
1. Introduce patient/family to healthcare providers and orient to room and unit. Place patient ID bracelet on patient.	Verify the patient identify by asking patient his name and date of birth and compare to ID bracelet. If patient unable to state name, ask family or caregiver familiar with patient.
2. Encourage patient to place valuables into safe. Check appropriate box on Patient Database.	Every attempt should be made to send money/valuables home with family member(s).
3. Fill out clothing list when admitting patient to Psych Unit.	
4. To put valuables in hospital safe:	
a. Put items in labeled "Patient's Valuable Envelope."	Document envelope's contents with patient/family.
b. Hand carry <u>unsealed</u> envelope to the Admitting Office.	Admitting staff will recheck contents and seal the envelope.
c. Attach white copy from envelope to Discharge Summary.	

Figure 14-3 • *An example of an admission procedure (Courtesy of Marquette General Health System, Marquette, MI)*

(continues)

A-003-2 – Admission of a Patient

PROCEDURE	POINT OF EMPHASIS
d. Give pink copy to the patient.	
5. Assist patient with changing into gown / pajamas.	
6. Orient patient to the environment by explaining and demonstrating the use of the call light and the bed controls.	
7. Provide fresh water unless contraindicated.	
B. RESPONSIBILITIES OF RN/GN	
1. Complete Patient Database, including Physical Assessment(s) and appropriate addendums.	Refer to Nursing Procedure C-008A.
2. Obtain information regarding Advanced Directives.	Reassure patient that it is his/her choice to exercise the right to formulate an advanced directive. An advanced directive will be initiated only if the patient is declared unable to participate in medical decisions according to specific criteria.
3. If patient <u>has</u> written Advanced Directives:	All patients should be made aware of hospital policy regarding accepting or refusing treatment and advanced directives.
a. Check appropriate box on Database.	
b. Obtain a <u>copy</u> for the medical record.	Return the original to the patient.
c. Make sure the document is dated, signed by patient, and witnessed by <u>two</u> individuals.	Hospital personnel may not act as witnesses.
d. Give copy to the unit clerk to flag with special sticker.	The flag will alert physicians and other staff of the patient's wishes.
e. If unit clerk not available, flag copy and place in chart.	
f. If document is not with the patient, request that a copy be provided as soon as possible. Document advanced directive intent on progress notes.	The advanced directive will remain a permanent part of the chart.
g. Review the advanced directives with patient for current decisions.	
4. If the patient <u>has</u> <u>not</u> formulated advanced directives:	

Figure 14-3 • *(continues)*

A-003-3 – Admission of a Patient

PROCEDURE	POINT OF EMPHASIS
a. Check appropriate box on Patient Database.	All hospital patients should be made aware of the hospital policy regarding accepting or refusing treatment and the right to formulate advanced directives.
b. Provide patient with information on formulating an advanced directive (written material, video, or resource staff), if patient agreeable.	
c. If patient wants to complete, send referral to Social Work.	
d. Check appropriate box indicating that information was provided.	
e. Check appropriate box on database if patient is unable to understand information (sedated, unconscious, mentally impaired, etc.). Ask a family member or legal guardian the above questions. Document explanation of the situation in the nurse's notes, if applicable.	
5. Make sure appropriate armbands have been applied to patient's wrist.	Allergy; Spot the Dot.
6. Record allergies. See procedure.	Complete allergy record.
7. Make sure that patient allergies have been addressed on physician's order sheet before sending yellow sheet to the Pharmacy.	Pharmacy will not dispense medications for a patient without allergy status identified.
8. If patient brought medication(s) to the hospital and meds cannot be sent home:	
a. Fill out information on Patient's Medication Receipt envelope following instructions.	Verify contents with patient/family then seal envelope.
b. Tear off stub and attach to Discharge Summary sheet.	
c. Put envelope in Pharmacy pick-up basket.	
9. Using information gathered during admission, formulate Nursing Plan of Care.	Refer to Nursing Procedure C-008.
10. Initiate "Spot the Dot" if the patient is at high risk for falls.	Refer to Spot the Dot Procedure S-003.
11. Make sure patient's height and weight are entered in the computer.	Can be done by unit clerk.
12. In case of an emergency admission, when the patient arrives unaccompanied, check to see if the	Ask unit clerk to make notification.

Figure 14-3 • *(continues)*

A-003-4 – Admission of a Patient

PROCEDURE	POINT OF EMPHASIS
family has been notified.	
13. Notify physician of patient's arrival and obtain orders, if applicable.	Ask Unit Clerk to make notification.
14. Initiate STAT treatments and/or medication orders.	
15. If the patient is admitted with an IV line already established, note date of insertion on IV Flow Sheet in Comments Section.	Will facilitate changing the line at 72 hours.
C. RESPONSIBILITIES OF THE UNIT CLERK	
1. Label forms necessary for patient's chart(s).	
2. Assemble chart(s) in correct order in labeled binders.	
3. Fill out Kardex cards if appropriate.	
4. Label Bulk Stores and Pharmacy cards as indicated.	
5. Log patient in the appropriate book(s).	
6. Record allergy information (specific known allergies or NKA) on med sheets, Kardex, front of chart(s), armband, and allergy record.	Record in red ink.
7. Notify physician of admission.	
8. Transcribe orders to appropriate forms.	Refer to Nursing Procedure N-001.
9. Place flagged copy of patient's Advanced Directives behind the Physician's Progress Notes.	

END

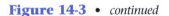

Figure 14-3 • *continued*

The **patient data base** is a form that contains information about the patient (Figure 14-4). The nursing staff completes this form by asking the patient, or patient's family, key questions to provide information needed for quality patient care based on the patient needs. The patient data base form is completed and filed in the patient chart. The health unit coordinator will refer to this form for needed information as documented on the form. For example, the patient's height and weight, current medications, allergies, native language, and other information the health care facility requires can be found on the form.

MARQUETTE **G**ENERAL
HEALTH SYSTEM
PATIENT DATA BASE

PATIENT LABEL

☐ **See ER Record** for allergy, medication, and health history information.
IF < age 18 complete pediatric box.

Wt._____ kg.
Ht._____ cm.

Date:_____ Time:_____ From: _____
Legal Guardian_____ phone_____ relation _____
Contact/care giver_____ Relation _____
Home Phone_____ Work Phone _____

☐ Valuables in Safe
☐ Pt./family declined to place
valuables (money, jewelry) in safe
☐ States no valuables

Reason for admission/chief complaint/expectation _____

ALLERGIES	☑ OLD RECORDS	REACTION

Allergies Listed on Band ☐
Latex Allergy: ☐ Yes ☐ No   Latex Allergy Band ☐

HOME MEDICATIONS: Prescription/Nonprescription/Herbal

☐ Sent Home	☐ Sent to Pharmacy	☐ None Brought
		Last Dose

Health History
☐ May use MD's H&P if on chart and <30 days old
☐ No changes/problems since last admit
OR ✓ changes below:

	Self Yes No	Family Yes No	
Neurological Disorders/Seizures	☐ ☐	☐ ☐	
Heart/Circulation	☐ ☐	☐ ☐	
Hypertension	☐ ☐	☐ ☐	
Bleeding Problems	☐ ☐		
Kidney/Urological Disease	☐ ☐		
Cancer	☐ ☐	☐ ☐	
Arthritis	☐ ☐	☐ ☐	
Diabetes/how long	☐ ☐	☐ ☐	
Lung Disease	☐ ☐		
GI Disease	☐ ☐		
Tobacco/how long/how much	☐ ☐		
Infectious Disease–i.e. HIV/HEP/TB/MRSA	☐ ☐	☐ ☐	
Recent Infections—cold/flu/diarrhea	☐ ☐	☐ ☐	
Infection with Drug Resistant Organism	☐ ☐	☐ ☐	
Emotional Problems	☐ ☐		
Alcohol/Drug Use/Amount	☐ ☐		
History Anesthesia Problems	☐ ☐	☐ ☐	
Significant/Previous Pain	☐ ☐		
Other Pertinent Illnesses/Surgeries	☐ ☐		

Cleared from MRSA   ☐ Yes   ☐ No
☐ No previous health problems   ☐ Family Hx Unknown
Do you have any reason to believe you are pregnant? ☐ Yes ☐ No
LMP_____
Dates of last vaccines influenza_____ Pneumovax_____
Other:_____

COMPLETE AS AGE APPROPRIATE: Infant/Pediatric/Adolescent/Special Needs Patients *(up to 18 years of age)*
Developmental Age: ☐ Infant ☐ Pediatric ☐ Adolescent   Grade in School _____   Social Work Notified ☐
Developmental Milestones appropriate for age? ☐ Yes ☐ No   Describe _____
If No,   Presently enrolled in Programs *or* referral sent: ☐ Specialty clinic ☐ ISD ☐ Early On
Is your child immunized? ☐ Yes ☐ Unsure, no.   If <u>no or unsure</u> provide immunization schedule & free immunization clinic locations ☐
Last immunication (date/type) _____ (Refer to MICR Database)
Do you have concerns/problems regarding your child? _____
Daily Routine ☐ Daycare ☐ Preschool ☐ School. Child's diet _____ ☐ Cup ☐ Bottle ☐ Breast
☐ Potty Trained Word for potty _____ Routine nap/sleep time _____ Head Circ. (<1yr) _____cm.
Psych/Social/Emotional Needs: What comforts your child when he/she is afraid, tired, lonely? _____
How would you like to be included in child's treatment/care? _____

Date/Time	RN Signature	Init.	Date/Time	RN Signature	Init.	Date/Time	MD Signature	Init.

D:\IC MGH\PtData.pmd 3/96, Rev. 2/04 MRURsub-Approve: 8/22/03

ITEM # 760361

Figure 14-4 • *The patient data base must be filed in the patient chart when it is completed.*
(Courtesy of Marquette General Health System, Marquette, MI)

(continues)

PATIENT DATA BASE Pg. 2 Of 3

KEY: Check those that apply

Other Health Problems / Concerns	With Pt.

☐ Speech_____   Aids_____ ☐
☐ Hearing_____   Hearing Aid ☐ Rt. ☐ Lt. ☐
☐ Vision_____   ☐ Glasses ☐ Contacts ☐
☐ Dentures_____ ☐ Upper ☐ Lower ☐
☐ any special therapy that you wish continued:
Explain:_____

FUNCTIONAL DEFICITS

☐ **Infants/Pediatric/Special Needs Pt.:** Does not meet developmental milestones in areas of gross motor & cognitive skills for chronological age (see policy 600-507) **And/or** recent change in assistive device.

☐ **Adolescents/Adults:** Note current and 3 month history or level of assist with the following activities of daily living.

I = Independent   D = Dependent

	Current	Prior 3 Mths		Current	Prior 3 Mths
Bathing			Feeding		
Dressing			Assist Device		
Toileting					

☐ Cane ☐ Walker ☐ Crutches ☐ Commode ☐ Other_____
☐ PT/OT/Speech consult requested from MD, if change in ADL or Pt. dependent prior to this admission but no previous rehab therapy initiated.   ☐ **No Consult Sent**

REHAB TO COMPLETE IF CONSULTING

Home/discharge destination description _____
Occupation _____
Leisure/Community Activities _____
Important Pt. Activities Post Discharge _____
Pt. Input _____
Family Support _____

DISCHARGE PLANNING: ≥ 1 checked Send Referral

☐ Financial concerns related to this hospitalization
☐ Lack of necessary equipment or aids
☐ Inability to perform household activities ADL/treatment plan
☐ S.O. Concerns
☐ Additional resources requested
☐ Presently using other health professional
☐ Other social concerns: _____
☐ **Social Service Consult Sent**   ☐ **No Consult Sent**

ADVANCED DIRECTIVES/CHAPLAIN/PATIENT RIGHTS

☐ Patient Rights/Responsibilities/Advance Medical
  Directive Handout (Item # 760786) given.
Does the Pt. have an Advance Directive? ☐ Yes   ☐ No
If **YES**: ☐ Directive on Chart.
       ☐ Directive not available – intent/substance
         is documented in the progress notes and
         Social Work consult sent.
If **NO**:   ☐ Materials (Designation of Patient Advocate
         Form & Durable Power of Attorney for
         Healthcare) offered and accepted.
       ☐ Above Materials Declined
       ☐ Patient requests help in filling our advance
         directive. Social Work notified.
☐ If status unknown due to Pt. condtion Social Work notified.

Chaplain requested and notified ☐ Yes   ☐ No
Religion:_____
Any cultural practices we should be aware of: ☐ Yes ☐ No
If Yes, explain;_____

PATIENT LABEL

SKIN RISK – If traction or decube present, initiate skin care measures *and* automatic ET referral. If ≥ 2 checked, initiate skin care measures and ET referral.
☐ Cannot verbalize discomfort ☐ Poor Nutrition
☐ Skin always moist   ☐ Diabetic
☐ ↑ Friction ☐ Red Skin   ☐ Ulcers
☐ Complete Bed Rest
☐ Other skin problems_____
☐ **ET referral sent**   ☐ **No Consult Sent**

FALLS / RISK

History of previous falls or lower extremity amputee or ≥ 3 checked Pt. at high risk – initiate Fall Prevention Program *(SPOT THE DOT).*
☐ **Infants/Pediatric/Special Needs Pt.** < 5 yrs. and/or behavior outside of developmental milestones.
☐ > 70 years of age
☐ Impaired memory/judgment/confusion/altered mentality
☐ Nocturia
☐ Sensory Deficit: Sight/hearing/speech impaired
☐ Ambulatory aids/unsteady gait/weakness
  Obtain PT referral from MD if applicable ☐
☐ Postural Hypotension
☐ 24 to 48 hours post-op
☐ Taking high risk medications (hypnotics, psychotropics, diuretics, laxatives, sedatives)
☐ **Fall Prevention Initiated** ☐ **Fall Prevention Not Initiated**

ABUSE ≥ 1 checked Pt. at high risk, immediately notify

Supervisor, *follow with notification of appropriate agency if:*
☐ Verbalizes physical/sexual abuse
☐ Unexplained bruises, abrasions, etc.
☐ Evidence of mistreatment
☐ Evidence of neglect
☐ **Supervisor notified**   ☐ **Supervisor Not Notified**

NUTRITIONAL – send Dietitian Referral if *one or more*

boxes below are checked.
Infants/Pediatrics: number of meals/feedings per day_____
☐ **Infants/Pediatrics/Adolescent Pts.:** At risk if NCHS percentiles over 90th percentile or under 10th percentile.
☐ **Adults:** Weight change (+/- 15 pounds in 2 months)
☐ Chewing/swallowing problems
☐ Diabetes nutrition education
☐ Other nutritional concerns:_____
☐ **Dietitian consult sent**   ☐ **NO CONSULT SENT**

DIABETIC – ≥ 1 checked send referral

☐ Newly diagnosed diabetic
☐ Needs blood glucose monitoring instruction
☐ Needs outpatient diabetic education
☐ **Diabetic Ed referral sent**   ☐ **NO CONSULT SENT**

LEARNING/EDUCATION NEEDS

COMPLETE LEARNING / EDUCATION NEEDS ASSESSMENT SECTION OF MULTIDISCIPLINARY PATIENT TEACHING RECORD.

Date/Time	RN Signature	Init.

Figure 14-4 • *(continues)*

MARQUETTE GENERAL HOSPITAL
Physical Assessment – Patient Data Base

Date:

PATIENT LABEL

Charting By Exception Key:
✓ Findings Within Normal Limits / Pt. tolerated intervention well
✻ Findings Outside of Normal Limits (**Requires entry in Progress Notes**)
→ Status unchanged from previous entry (**Must be updated every 24 hours**)

[Blank] Assessment not indicated according to plan &/or pt. condition
D Intervention Completed

	TITLE		CBE Symbol	NARRATIVE DESCRIPTION—Any abnormal findings, as indicated with an asterisk (*) needs to be documented in the patients progress notes using PIE format.
ASSESSMENT	Skin	Warm, Dry, Intact Color – Patient's Norm. Afebrile		If astericked -- complete skin assessment body outline on reverse side.
	Wound	No redness, hematoma, drainage, swelling.		Document location & reason for presence
	Sutures	Intact, edges approximated.		
	Neuro	A & O for age, equal strength of extremities, Beh. appropriate for situation.		Refer to growth & development charts Infants/Pediatrics/Special Needs Pts
	GI	Abdomen soft; no distention or tenderness; active bowel sounds; no vomiting. Tolerates diet according to developmental age.		Refer to growth & development charts Infants/Pediatrics/Special Needs Pts
	NG/G/Enteral (Circle tube type)	✓Placement by aspirating stomach contents &/or using air bolus; Initials indicate placement verified, tube patient & secured.		
ASSESSMENT	GU	Voids spontaneously; clear yellow urine; output WNL for age; continence appropriate for developmental age.		Refer to growth & development charts Infants/Pediatrics/Special Needs Pts
	Foley	Indicate tube patent & secured (Note; if insertion date unknown may require reinsertion✓with MD		
	CV	Apical pulse regular with no abnormal sounds, Rate and BP WNL for age, peripheral pulses present, no edema.		Refer to growth & development charts Infants/Pediatrics/Special Needs Pts
	Respiratory	Resp regular, rate WNL for age, breath sounds clear & unlabored in all fields, no cyanosis, sputum clear or absent.		Refer to growth & development charts Infants/Pediatrics/Special Needs Pts
	Pain Management Assessment	No pain or pain management acceptable to patient. (Except Cardiac Pain = 0). Use 0-10 scale except as noted. Refer to Policy 100-079.	■	Use appropriate Pain Scale per Pain Policy 100-079. Assessment to be completed on Multidisiplinary Pain Management Flow Sheet.
ASSESSMENT	Psych	Beh normal for age & situation, social support available.		Refer to growth & development charts Infants/Pediatrics/Special Needs Pts
	Family Interaction	Parents interact with child by establishing eye contact & touching child. Child called by name. Parents communicate appropriatly with health care team.		Complete for Infant/Pediatrics/Adolescent/Special Needs Pts.
	Case Manager referral if Pt. readmitted within 30 days of previous discharge for unscheduled admission			
	INITIALS/Signature/Title			

Rev. 1/00, 8/03, 2/04

Figure 14-4 • *(continues)*

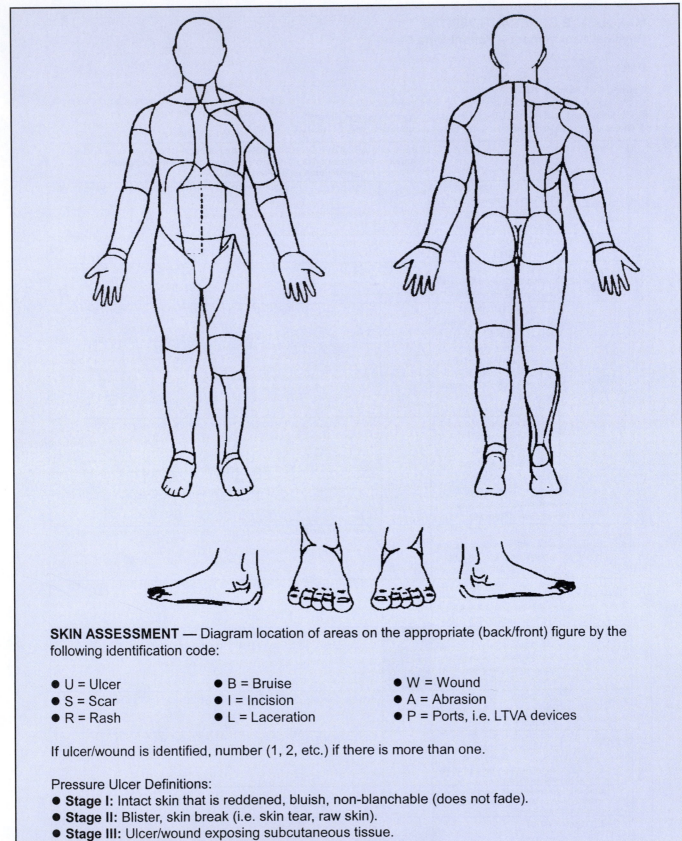

SKIN ASSESSMENT — Diagram location of areas on the appropriate (back/front) figure by the following identification code:

- U = Ulcer
- S = Scar
- R = Rash

- B = Bruise
- I = Incision
- L = Laceration

- W = Wound
- A = Abrasion
- P = Ports, i.e. LTVA devices

If ulcer/wound is identified, number (1, 2, etc.) if there is more than one.

Pressure Ulcer Definitions:
- **Stage I:** Intact skin that is reddened, bluish, non-blanchable (does not fade).
- **Stage II:** Blister, skin break (i.e. skin tear, raw skin).
- **Stage III:** Ulcer/wound exposing subcutaneous tissue.
- **Stage IV:** Ulcer/wound exposing muscle, bone and/or tendon.

Figure 14-4 • *continued*

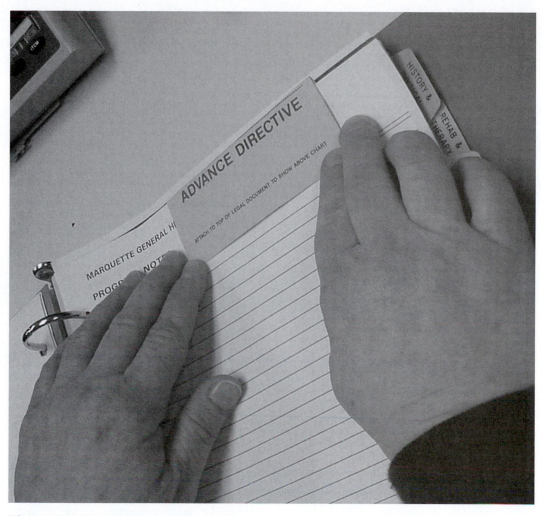

Figure 14-5 • *A copy of the patient's advance directives is filed in the patient chart.*

Patients may be asked if they have completed an advance directive (Figure 14-5). If the patient has an advance directive document, the patient or patient family will be asked to provide it so that the health unit coordinator can make copies of the advance directive to add to the patient's chart. Keeping the advance directive in the patient's chart allows all members of the health care team to be aware of the patient's wishes.

The patient may have come to the health care facility with items of value that need to be put into a safe for safekeeping until the patient is discharged. If that is the case, the health unit coordinator should be certain to carefully follow the health care facility's procedure for the storing of valuables (Figure 14-6).

Patients may bring their current medications to the health care facility. Most health care facilities will store a patient's medications until the patient is discharged. The health unit coordinator may document on the discharge summary if the patient has valuables in the safe or medications in the medication storage area. It is important to document this information so that the patient is not discharged without receiving these items.

MARQUETTE
General Hospital
Regional Medical Center

420 West Magnetic Street
Marquette, MI 49855
Telephone (906) 225-3406

PATIENTS VALUABLE
ENVELOPE No. 1921

CONTENTS OF ENVELOPE
DEPOSITED WITH HOSPITAL

LIST **CREDIT CARDS** DEPOSITED WITH HOSPITAL

- [ ] CASH
- WATCH
- RINGS
- WALLET
- GLASSES
- CHECKBOOK
- [ ] OTHER EXPLAIN
- [ ] OTHER EXPLAIN
- [ ] OTHER EXPLAIN
- [ ] OTHER EXPLAIN

I, the patient or responsible party, assume full responsibility for items which I retain, and certify that items listed above were deposited with the hospital for safe keeping.

PATIENT OR
RESPONSIBLE PARTY _____
(SIGNATURE) ___ (DATE)

OR
HOSPITAL EMPLOYEE
ACCEPTING VALUABLES _____
(SIGNATURE) ___ (TITLE) ___ (DATE)

ADMITTING PERSONNEL
ACCEPTING VALUABLES _____
(SIGNATURE) ___ (TITLE) ___ (DATE)

- -

TO BE COMPLETED UPON RELEASE OF VALUABLES

VALUABLES
RECEIVED BY _____
(SIGNATURE OF PATIENT OR RESPONSIBLE PARTY)

VALUABLES
RELEASED BY _____
(SIGNATURE · ADMITTING PERSONNEL ONLY) ___ (DATE)

PATIENT UNABLE
TO SIGN BECAUSE _____

AUTHORIZATION FOR SOMEONE OTHER THAN PATIENT TO RECEIVE VALUABLES.

PERMISSION IS GRANTED TO _____

TO ACCEPT MY VALUABLES _____
(PATIENT SIGNATURE) ___ (DATE)

WITNESSED BY _____
(DATE)

Figure 14-6 • *The patient's valuables are placed in a valuables envelope and placed in the safe until the patient is discharged or requests that the valuables be returned. (Courtesy of Marquette General Health System, Marquette, MI)*

PATIENT TYPES

The length of stay as well as the guidelines set forth by state and federal agencies define patient types. These guidelines are being defined and redefined as new diagnoses, procedures, and examinations are approved for patient care. As technology and medical treatments improve, a patient type could change from an inpatient to an outpatient. The admission process could be different for each patient type, depending on the health care facility procedures. The common patient types include inpatient, outpatient, same-day patient, and short-stay patient. Some of these types may seem to overlap.

INPATIENT

An individual who resides at the health care facility for a specific amount of time and is receiving treatment is considered an inpatient. These patients are admitted with a diagnosis for health care treatment that requires the patient to be assigned a bed and to stay in the health care facility for a set amount of time. The health unit coordinator will create a patient chart for an inpatient. Examples of criteria for an inpatient stay may include the following:

> **Length of stay (LOS)**, how long the patient can stay in the health care facility, determined by the diagnosis

> Treatment being provided

> Potential side effects from treatment

OUTPATIENT

Outpatients are patients who do not reside at the health care facility in which they are receiving treatment. Outpatients, depending on the type of treatment they require and the time involved, may be assigned a bed in the health care system. Otherwise, they will be provided a bed in the department and assigned to a department. When one is billing charges to an outpatient account, it is very important to charge for only the items that are chargeable outpatient items. The charging of items and services varies for inpatient and outpatients. The health unit coordinator will create a chart for an outpatient; depending on the health care facility, the process for creating an outpatient chart may be different from the process for creating an inpatient chart. Emergency department patients are outpatients, and the charts created in that area of a health care facility may be different from the patient charts on the patient care units.

SAME-DAY PATIENT

Same-day patients are patients who come to the health care facility for tests or procedures that will be performed on the same day. These patients may be assigned a bed, and a chart will be created for them. What the chart contains varies as to the department that is providing the service to the patient. A same-day patient could be a patient attending diabetes education classes, a patient having a procedure done in the endoscopy unit, or a patient having a radiation therapy treatment. A radiation therapy patient could be returning for a period of 5 days per week for an extended time period.

SAME-DAY SURGERY PATIENT

A patient admitted into a health care facility for a surgical procedure that is to be completed with the patient being discharged from the facility after a defined recovery time within that day is called a same-day surgery patient. Same-day surgery patients have continued to increase as the LOS (length of stay) for surgical procedures has decreased. Advances in medical technologies and cost containment initiatives nationwide have affected the increase in same-day surgery. Same-day surgery patients will be assigned a bed on an outpatient surgery unit. The health unit coordinator will create a chart for this same-day surgery patient. The admission process is often shortened for these patients, depending on the health care facility's procedures.

SHORT-STAY PATIENT

Short-stay patients are patients who are admitted to the health care facility for a short amount of time, typically for a period of an hour to a few hours. Each health care facility that uses this patient type would define how long a short stay is and what requirements must to be met for this patient type. These patients could be assigned a bed, and a chart would be created to document the care provided. The health unit coordinator would create the patient chart and assist with processing the patient admission as defined by department procedure. One example of a short-stay patient is a person who comes to the oncology unit for chemotherapy to be infused over a one-hour period. Another example is a patient who comes to a walk-in clinic to be seen by a health care provider for a minor health issue.

TRANSFERS

A **transfer** is the process of moving a patient from one location to another. Transferring a patient can be as simple as moving a patient from one room on a nursing unit to another room on the same unit or as complicated as transferring a patient to a health care facility hundreds of miles away. Patients can be transferred from the patient care unit to another health care facility that is part of the same health care system or to a health care facility that is not part of the same health care system. Health care systems can have many facilities throughout the country. Usually, the physician will write a physician order as to where and when the patient is to be transferred. A physician order is not required if the patient is being transferred within a nursing unit to another room to accommodate the bed needs of the unit. The health unit coordinator processes the order by following the transfer procedure. The procedure is based on where the patient is being transferred.

UNIT TRANSFER

A patient is being transferred within the patient care unit. The need for this transfer arises most often when a bed needs to be available for use by a specific type of patient. The following is an example of a unit transfer. On the patient care unit, all the rooms are semiprivate. There are two females in two separate rooms with no roommates. There are two male patients who require admission to the nursing unit. The health unit coordinator suggests to the health care team that one of the single females in one room be moved into the room occupied by the other single female. This transfer will make a room available for the two male admissions. The nursing staff physically moves the patient and the patient's belongings. The health unit coordinator alerts bed control of the planned move. The health unit coordinator changes the chart forms to reflect the room change, either electronically via the computer or by relabeling the patient paper chart and forms with the new room number.

After the move takes place, the health unit coordinator transfers the patient in the computer system, alerting other departments that the patient is in a different room. It is important that all departments involved in services provided to the patient be alerted as to the patient location. The food trays need to be sent to the correct room, as do the telephone calls from outside callers. A physician's order is not needed for a transfer within the nursing unit, but it is important that the physician be alerted to the fact that the patient has been transferred to a different room.

IN HEALTH CARE FACILITY TRANSFER

When a patient is transferred within a health care facility to a different unit, a physician's order is usually required. An exception could be when a patient bed is needed in a unit for a patient who requires the services provided by the specific unit. For example, a patient is being admitted with a broken leg. The orthopedic unit that provides the services needed by this patient has another patient with asthma who can be transferred to the medical unit. The only reason the patient with asthma is on the orthopedic unit is that, when the patient was admitted to the health care facility, all the beds on the medical unit were occupied. It is in the best interest of both patients to be transferred and admitted to the respective units that are trained to provide the best care for the specific patient types. The physician will be notified of the date and time the transfer is to take place. Whether there is a physician order or not, the health unit coordinator will follow the procedure for transferring patients to another patient care unit. This would include notifying bed control of the request to transfer the patient, either by placing a telephone request or generating a computer request. The health unit coordinator, upon being provided with the room number of where the patient will be transferred, will alert the patient care staff of this information and will prepare the necessary transfer forms. The patient will then be transferred when the nursing care staff physically moves the patient and reports to the receiving unit staff that the patient is now in a room in their unit.

Patients may move to different nursing units during their hospital stay. Some nursing units, such as a rehabilitation unit, are designed to have patients stay for extended periods of time so the patients may be taught skills needed to return to their homes safely. Other patient care units provide acute care. For example, intensive care unit patients spend one or two days on that unit before being transferred to a general nursing unit when they require less intensive patient care. The size and specialties of the health care facility dictate the opportunities for transfer.

OUTSIDE HEALTH CARE FACILITY TRANSFER

A patient's health condition may require transfer to another health care facility that can provide the needed medical care. The health care system may have a facility within its system that meets the patient's needs, or the patient may have to be transferred to a different health care system. There is a transfer procedure that is followed whenever a patient leaves the facility. This type of transfer often requires assistance from other departments within the health care facility. Table 14-1 provides examples of departments and their potential responsibilities in transferring a patient.

When the transporting team removes a patient from the health care facility, the health unit coordinator processes the patient through the system by alerting the necessary departments that the patient is no longer in the facility. The procedure that is followed may be the same procedure or one that is similar to the procedure that is used when a patient is discharged.

TABLE 14-1   Department Responsibilities for Transfer

Department or Service	Responsibility
Admitting	Coordinating with the receiving health care facility admitting department to secure a bed for the patient so that the patient care team can call a verbal report to the receiving team members.
Clinical information department (health information department, medical records)	Preparing the health information releases so that information can be sent to the receiving facility, copying the paper information to be sent to the receiving facility, sending the electronic information, faxing released information. *The health unit coordinator may assist with these tasks.*
Health unit coordinator	Communicating transfer time to all departments so that the required services are coordinated.
Patient care team	Having the patient prepared for transport at the scheduled time. Completing the required transfer form for the receiving health care facility staff (Figure 14-7). Calling in a verbal report to the receiving patient care team members.
Physician	Requesting that the receiving facility and receiving physician are able and willing to accept the patient. *This must be completed before a patient transfer.*
Social work	Contacting the departments to arrange services for the transfer of the patient. Having patient or family sign required release forms. *The health unit coordinator may assist with these tasks.*
Transportation department (EMS department)	Transporting the patient to the health care facility; this could mean air ambulance or ground ambulance.

MARQUETTE GENERAL HOSPITAL

TRANSFER FORM

Facility transferring to:_____

Physician in charge at time of discharge: _____

Health insurance name and claim number: _____

Other facilities from which patient was discharged in past 60 days:
_____

Discharge Summary included with transfer form: _____

ALLERGIES:

MENTAL STATUS
- ☐ ALERT
- ☐ ORIENTATED
- ☐ RESPONSIVE TO ALL STIMULI
- ☐ Disoriented to:
  - ☐ Person ☐ Place ☐ Time
  - ☐ Altered responsiveness
  - ☐ Other

BEHAVIORAL STATUS
- ☐ APPROPRIATE
- ☐ INAPPROPRIATE (specify)
  - ☐ Confused ☐ Non-verbal ☐ Verbally
  - ☐ Withdrawn ☐ Forgetful   abusive
  - ☐ Depressed ☐ Impulsive ☐ Restraints
  - ☐ Noisy ☐ Combative   needed

Comments: _____
_____
_____

NUTRITION ☐ NO PROBLEMS
- ☐ Weight gain/loss problem (specify) _____
- ☐ Dentures
- ☐ Asst. eating _____
- ☐ Problems chewing _____
- ☐ Problems swallowing _____

MOBILITY AND ADL's

	Indep.	Needs Asst.	Comp. Dep.
Daily personal hygiene	☐	☐	☐
Ambulations	☐	☐	☐
Tub or shower	☐	☐	☐
Change positions in bed	☐	☐	☐
Transfers to and from chair	☐	☐	☐
Propel Wheelchair	☐	☐	☐
Toileting: uses commode	☐	☐	☐
Uses bedpan/urinal	☐	☐	☐

Describe transfer: _____

SOCIAL
Previous living arrangement:
- ☐ Alone ☐ Other relative
- ☐ Household help ☐ Non-relative
- ☐ Spouse ☐ Family support

Contact person: _____

SKIN CONDITION ☐ NORMAL
- ☐ Rash (specify) _____
- ☐ Pressure ulcer/decubti (describe/specify location)
_____
_____
_____
- ☐ Incision/wound (location, size, description)
_____
_____
- ☐ Drainage: Color _____ Amount _____
- ☐ Edges Approximated
- ☐ Staples ☐ Sutures ☐ Steri Strips
- ☐ Dressings/cast (specify) _____

BOWEL FUNCTION ☐ NORMAL
Last BM_____
- ☐ Constipation ☐ Diarrhea ☐ Neurogenic
- ☐ Ostomy
- ☐ Incont: Freq. _____
- ☐ Other _____

BLADDER FUNCTION ☐ NORMAL
- ☐ Ostomy ☐ Neurogenic
Catheter: type _____ size _____
Date inserted _____
- ☐ External Device _____ ☐ Incont. freq. _____
- ☐ Other _____

FUNCTIONAL LIMITATIONS ☐ NONE
- ☐ Amputation ☐ Vision ☐ Glasses
- ☐ Contractures ☐ Hearing ☐ Hearing aid
- ☐ Paralysis ☐ Communication
- ☐ Endurance ☐ Cognition/perception
- ☐ Dsypnea with minimal exertion ☐ Developmentally impaired
- ☐ Orthotic device/assistant device ☐ Wheelchair
- ☐ Contractures ☐ Walker
- ☐ High risk for falls ☐ Cane

RN Signature _____ Date _____

REV. 7/95

WHITE: With Patient   YELLOW: Chart   IC# 760268

Figure 14-7 • *Transfer forms must be completed when a patient is being transferred to another health care facility. (Courtesy of Marquette General Health System, Marquette, MI)*

DISCHARGING A PATIENT

Patients are **discharged** or dismissed from the health care facility when their health condition no longer warrants that they remain at the health care facility. Patients can be discharged only with a written physician order, or to a funeral home upon death. Patients may be discharged to home or transferred to another health care facility. A patient also may choose to leave the health care facility without the permission of the physician. This type of discharge is called **AMA**, which is defined as leaving the health care facility **against medical advice**. The patient may ask the physician to discharge him or her but the physician may refuse because the patient's leaving would not be in the best medical interest of the patient. The patient may leave without indicating to anyone that he is leaving. The bed may simply be found empty the next time a member of the health care team enters the patient's room. If the patient indicates a desire to leave AMA, the patient care staff will ask the patient to sign a release form (Figure 14-8) so that the health care facility has documentation that the patient was notified of his or her responsibilities regarding leaving against medical advice. Patients can be forced to stay in the health care facility if they have been ordered by a court to be hospitalized or if they are under the jurisdiction of the police.

DISCHARGE TO HOME

When patients are discharged to home, they are free to go after the necessary paperwork has been completed for the discharge process. Each health care facility has a procedure for discharging patients. After the physician or the physician's designee writes the discharge order, the process for discharge of a patient is followed. The health unit coordinator alerts the nursing care team that the patient is being discharged. Health care facilities may request that physicians discharge patients before a designated time to allow for the admission of scheduled patients. The health unit coordinator may be requested to schedule follow-up appointments for the patient, to schedule tests or procedures for the patient as an outpatient, to order medications from the health care facility pharmacy for the patient to take home, or to arrange for transportation for the patient. The health unit coordinator may need to have releases signed so that the patient records can be sent to the health care providers who will be providing follow-up care (Figure 14-9). If the patient being discharged is on medications, the health unit

---

RELEASE FROM RESPONSIBILITY FOR DISCHARGE

This is to certify that I, _____, a patient in the above Hospital am leaving against the advice of the attending physician and Hospital authorities. I also acknowledge that I have been informed of the risks involved and hereby release the attending physician and the Hospital from all responsibility for any ill effects which may result.

Date: _____

Reason Patient Cannot Sign:

_____

_____

Signed _____
        (Signature of Patient)

or _____
        (Authorized Person)

Witness: _____

Figure 14-8 • *A patient is asked to sign a release before leaving the hospital if the patient's physician has not discharged the patient. (Courtesy of Marquette General Health System, Marquette, MI)*

MARQUETTE GENERAL HEALTH SYSTEM

MARQUETTE, MICHIGAN

Medical Record #:_____
(Office Use Only)

Authorization To Release Protected Health Information

(Required items are in **BOLD** print)

Patient Name:_____ **Birth Date:** _____/_____/_____

Previous Names:_____ **Social Security #:**_____/_____/_____

Address:_____ **City, State & Zip Code:**_____ **Phone #:** _____

I, _____ **authorize** _____
Patient Name   *Name/Organization*

to release information concerning the patient identified above, in accordance with state and federal laws, to the following:

_____   _____
Name/Organization   *Phone Number*

_____   _____
Address   *City, State and Zip Code*

1. **Specific information to be disclosed** *(check all that apply)*

   ☐ Discharge Summary   ☐ Psychological Evaluations   ☐ Progress Notes   ☐ Substance Abuse
   ☐ History & Physical Examination ☐ Lab Reports   ☐ Radiology/X-ray Reports   ☐ Consultation Reports
   ☐ EKG/Stress Test   ☐ Emergency Room Record   ☐ Discharge Instructions   ☐ Operative/Procedure Reports
   ☐ Other _____

   For the following date(s) of treatment or medical conditions: _____

2. **I am requesting this information be released for the following purpose:**

   ☐ Continued Care   ☐ Insurance Claim   ☐ Personal Use   ☐ Attorney Review
   ☐ Other _____

3. With the exception of psychotherapy notes, all records pertaining to psychiatric/mental health, chemical dependency, and/or AIDS/HIV related illness/testing will be released unless otherwise specified here _____.

   Please specify any restrictions: _____.

4. I understand I may revoke this authorization by written request at any time. I understand that the revocation will not apply to information that has already been released in response to this authorization.

5. I understand there may be a fee to process this release of information.

6. This authorization will automatically expire on: _____/_____/_____ or one year from the date of my signature.

7. Marquette General Health System will not condition my continued treatment upon my signing this authorization, except for research-related treatment.

8. I understand that once my health information is used or disclosed pursuant to this authorization, it may be subject to re-disclosure or release by the receiving Party and may no longer be protected by Federal or State law, unless protected by Federal Regulation 42 CFR Part 2 and Public Act 258 in which case it cannot be re-disclosed by the receiving Party without my written authorization.

9. I hereby agree to indemnify and hold Marquette General Health System, their employees and agents free and harmless from any actions against them for alleged invasion of privacy, libel or slander, or defamation arising from or related to disclosure of such information.

_____   _____
Patient or Patient's Legal Representative's Signature   *Date*

_____   _____
Relationship If Other Than Patient   *Witness*

REASON PATIENT IS UNABLE TO SIGN: ☐ Minor   ☐ Deceased   ☐ Other:_____

*☐ **AUTHORITY ATTACHED** (In non-emergency situations documentation of authority must be attached if anyone other than the patient signs this authorization).

☐ Hold for future information request.

C:\PROJECTS\CONSENT\AuthorizeRelPHI.pmd   Rev. 4/03, 3/04   MRURsubApprove: 2/11/04

Figure 14-9 • *Information releases must be signed by the patient or the patient designee before information can be released. (Courtesy of Marquette General Health System, Marquette, MI)*

coordinator will be asked to give the unit nurse information relating to the patient's medications. The nurse will review this information with the patient before discharge.

All patients are provided with discharge instructions. The discharge instructions are individualized to the needs of the patient. The health unit coordinator may write the information on a written discharge summary so that the nurse can verbally review the information with the patient. The patient may have family members or friends present for the nurse's review of the discharge information as well. The health unit coordinator may transcribe on the discharge summary the time and date of the patient's doctor's appointment, medication instructions, and activity limitations, plus any other information the physician has requested in the discharge orders. It is important that the information be transcribed accurately and in a language and readability level that the patient can understand. The health unit coordinator will write the information clearly. The physician order might state the following:

> Discharge patient to home
>
> Make appointment to see me in two weeks
>
> Discharge medications:
>
> > 1. Lanoxin .25 mg po qday
> >
> > 2. Premarin 1.25 mg po qday
> >
> > 3. Motrin 600 mg po Q 6 hours prn for H/A

On the discharge summary, the appointment would be written as:

> Appointment to see Dr. Brown on September 5, 2003, Friday, at 11 A.M. in the Wright Street Clinic. Phone number 801-765-9809

The medications would be written as follows:

> Lanoxin .25 mg to be taken orally once a day in the morning
>
> Premarin 1.25 mg to be taken orally once a day at 8 A.M.
>
> Motrin 600 mg to be taken orally every 6 hours as need for headache

After the nurse reviews the discharge summary with the patient, the patient and the nurse sign the summary. The nurse provides the patient with the written discharge summary and brings a copy of the signed summary to the health unit coordinator to include in the patient's chart (Figure 14-10). The patient is free to go after signing the summary. The health care facility may require that a staff member assist the patient to the health care facility exit, or the patient may request assistance to the exit. When the patient is ready to leave the unit, the health unit coordinator is alerted by the nursing staff or the patient; at that point, the health unit coordinator documents the discharge. This documentation may be done electronically, by paper documentation, or by a combination of the two. The departments that need to be aware of the discharge of a patient include, but are not limited to, the departments listed in Table 14-2.

Once these departments have been notified, the services and all charges to the patient account cease. The time and date of discharge are documented on the patient chart.

MARQUETTE GENERAL HEALTH SYSTEM
580 West College Avenue ● Marquette, MI 49855
(906) 228-9440 ● 1-800-562-9753

PATIENT CARE SUMMARY

Discharge Diagnosis/Major Procedures/Events:

PATIENT LABEL

ALLERGIES:

Discharge Destination and Phone Number: _____

SUMMARY OF PATIENT'S HEALTH STATUS AT DISCHARGE

☐ Patient/S.O. able to manage pain/comfort with appropriate technique(s).
☐ Patient's vital signs stable _____
☐ Patient/S.O. performs activities of daily living within their restrictions: ☐ as tolerated ☐ Other _____

☐ Patient/S.O. is able to tolerate diet: ☐ regular ☐ as prescribed _____
☐ Patient/S.O. is willing/able to follow the plan of care.
☐ Persistent problems (unmet goals) _____

☐ Other _____

SYMPTOMS REQUIRING MEDICAL ATTENTION   ☐ Identify instruction sheet given_____

TRANSFUSION DISCHARGE FORM   ☐ Received   ☐ Not applicable

RESOURCES

☐ Family Doctor/Phone # _____

☐ Lab Location/Phone #   ☐ Home Health Referral/Phone #

☐ Marquette General Hospital
Emergency Department
(906) 225-3560   800-562-9753, ext. 3560

☐ Other: _____

FOLLOW-UP APPOINTMENTS

☐ Call for an appointment   ☐ Physician, date, time: _____

Physician, date, time: _____
Physician, date, time: _____
Post Discharge Labs: _____

EQUIPMENT/SUPPLIES   ☐ None

List: _____   ☐ instructed on use ☐ knowledgeable on use
List: _____   ☐ instructed on use ☐ knowledgeable on use
List: _____   ☐ instructed on use ☐ knowledgeable on use

COMMENTS:

D:/IC MGH/PtCareSumm.pmd 7/95, Rev. 1/04   **WHITE:** CHART   **YELLOW:** PATIENT   **PINK:** PHYSICIAN OFFICE   ITEM # 760437

Figure 14-10 • *The patient discharge summary provides the patient with information needed after discharge. (Courtesy of Marquette General Health System, Marquette, MI)*   *(continues)*

MARQUETTE GENERAL HEALTH SYSTEM
PAGE 2
PATIENT CARE SUMMARY

PATIENT LABEL
HERE

ALLERGIES:

MEDICATION / TREATMENT RECORD

PATIENT / SIGNIFICANT OTHER VERBALIZES KNOWLEDGE OF:
(ONLY TAKE THE MEDICINES LISTED BELOW. DO NOT TAKE OTHER MEDICINES
WITHOUT TALKING WITH YOUR PHYSICIAN. THIS INCLUDES
OVER THE COUNTER MEDICINES AND HERBAL SUPPLEMENTS)

Medication / Treatment / IV	Frequency / Schedule	Last Dose Date / Time

Patient / Significant Other Acknowledges Understanding of Teaching / Instructions and Receipt of Home Meds and Valuables, if any:

_____   _____   _____
Signature   RN Signature   Attending Physician

Discharge Time: _____ Date: _____ Via: _____ With Whom: _____

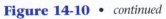

Figure 14-10 • *continued*

TABLE 14-2 Departments to Be Notified of Discharge	
Department	**Reason**
Admitting (bed control)	To be able to assign the bed to an incoming admission
Dietary	To stop sending food trays and nourishments
Housekeeping (unit/bed cleaners)	To prepare the patient room for the next patient (clean the room and furniture)
Medical records	To pick up the discharged patient chart
Pharmacy	To collect the medications from the medication area assigned (charged) to the patient and to not send any more medications
Switchboard	To stop phone calls for the patient being discharged
Therapy	To stop therapy
Transportation department	To discontinue transportation

The health unit coordinator will disassemble the patient chart. Disassembling may mean taking the paper chart apart and making sure all the items are completed. A discharge checklist may be used to document that all items have been completed (Figure 14-11). The discharged chart will be placed in a designated area and will be picked up or sent to the medical records department for processing at a specific time. Each health care facility follows a defined procedure for retrieving discharged patient charts from the patient care units. When the charts arrive in the medical records department, the coding process begins. Once the patient leaves the health care facility and surrounding area, the patient is discharged from the care of the health care facility. The **Emergency Medical Treatment and Active Labor Act (EMTALA)** defines the surrounding area.

Patients may be discharged home and still require nursing care. Private nursing care at home can be provided by private agencies or agencies that are part of the health care system. This type of care is commonly called home health care. The nursing care required by the patient at home will be provided by home health care staff and coordinated by the physician. The home health care staff may see the patient for the first time in the health care facility before the patient's discharge or in the patient's home. The patient must sign a release for the home health care staff to review medical information in the health care facility.

DISCHARGE TO ANOTHER FACILITY

Patients may be discharged to another facility. The facility could be a health care facility from which they were admitted, or it could be to a facility where they reside. Examples are extended-care facilities, assisted-living facilities, prisons and jails, or halfway houses.

MARQUETTE GENERAL HOSPITAL
DISCHARGE CHECKLIST

Discharge Date: _____

Patient Name: _____

RECORD HAS BEEN CHECKED TO VERIFY:

_____ *Old records pulled and in discharge basket*
or
_____ *No old records on Unit.*

_____ Chart thinnings, telemetry strips/alarms removed from file (check for appropriate patient name)
and added to chart.

_____ All pages appropriate to patient and filed accurately (progress notes together, nurses notes, etc.)

_____ Destroy name plate. (Do not send with chart).

_____ Discharge date and time entered on face sheet; face sheet placed underneath the Discharge
Checklist.

_____ Discharge Checklist placed on top of chart.

_____ *Chart rubber-banded, placed inside the front cover of the old record and in discharge basket.*

_____

Verified by:

Figure 14-11 • *Discharge checklists provide a double-check system for the health unit coordinator.
(Courtesy of Marquette General Health System, Marquette, MI)*

When the physician discharges the patient to another facility, the discharge process used is the same as the process for a discharge to home, with the notification of discharge being called to the facility where the patient resides. In other words, the patient will be discharged back to the facility from which he or she was admitted. Usually, the residence facility will arrange for transportation, but the health care facility social worker may assist with this type of discharge by helping with some of the arrangements.

EXPIRATION

Some patients who enter the health care facility die in there. The death may be expected or unexpected. When the patient dies on the patient care unit the health unit coordinator is responsible for preparing the forms that will be required and for alerting the departments within the health care facility that need to know this information. Each health care facility has a specific procedure to follow when a patient dies. It is important that the responsibilities be completed in the correct order according to the procedure. The physician is one of the first health care team members to be alerted to the fact that a patient has died. The physician must examine the patient and pronounce the patient dead before anyone else is told the patient has died. If the patient's death is expected, the family members may have been alerted and may have been at the patient's bedside when the patient died.

If it is an unexpected patient death, most likely the staff member finding the patient will have called for emergency help. If the efforts of the emergency team are unsuccessful at reviving the patient, an unexpected death will have occurred. The emergency team that responds to these requests usually has a physician as a team member. If so, the emergency team physician can examine the patient and certify that the patient is dead. The health unit coordinator may be asked to get the telephone number of the family member from the face sheet and place the telephone call to the patient's family members. The physician, or the patient's nurse, will talk to the family and alert them to the fact that their family member has died and ask them to come to the health care facility if possible to sign the necessary forms and collect the patient's personal belongings. If the family is unable to come to the health care facility, the patient's personal belongings will be sent. Also, if a family member is unable to come to the health care facility to sign the forms, a staff member of the health care facility may sign for the family member with the family member's verbal permission. The verbal permission may be given over the telephone; however, it must be witnessed by two employees of the health care facility.

After the physician has pronounced the patient expired, the health unit coordinator will alert any other departments and staff members that need to know, including nursing supervisors, consulting physicians, departments that have scheduled the patient for procedures, transport staff, and other members of the health care team. The process of notifying departments may be done electronically. Electronic notification decreases the time it takes to notify departments and reduces the chance of omitting a department that needs to know. One department that needs to know is the communication department so that phone calls will no longer be directed to the patient's room nor will visitors be directed to the room. The health unit coordinator will fill out the forms required by the specific health care unit facility's procedure, and the forms will be signed by the necessary persons: members of the staff, the physician, or a family member. The forms include an identification tag, a release of remains form, and, sometimes, an autopsy request.

Identification tags (Figure 14-12) are placed on the body so that the body can be identified by the funeral home. Usually two or more tags are attached to the body. Placement of the tags is defined in the expiration procedure, usually right hand and left ankle.

The release of remains form (Figure 14-13) is a form that the family or next of kin must sign. This form allows the health care facility to release the remains of the patient to a specific funeral home. The family selects the funeral home. The family may ask the health unit coordinator for the names of the funeral homes in the area. The selected funeral home is alerted that the patient has died and the body is to be picked up either in the patient's room on the nursing unit or in the health care system's morgue. A copy of the release of remains form is attached to the remains. The funeral home will usually call the family after the body has been brought to the funeral home.

An autopsy request form (Figure 14-14) is completed when the family requests an autopsy. Not all families request autopsies. If an autopsy is requested, the pathologist is alerted of the request and the request form is sent to the pathologist. A copy of the form is also sent with the remains to the morgue. After the autopsy has been completed, the remains are released to the funeral home. In some deaths, the law requires an autopsy; the legal requirements for autopsy vary by state.

After the remains and the personal belongings of the patient have been removed from the patient room, the health unit coordinator will process the discharge, which alerts all departments that the patient has been discharged and to follow the discharge procedures. Only the health care staff members who have a need to know will be alerted to the fact that a patient has died.

MORGUE RECORD

NAME ______

ADDRESS ______

NEXT OF KIN ______

WARD OR ROOM ______

DATE OF DEATH ______ TIME ______

DIAGNOSIS ______

DOCTOR ______

HOSPITAL ______

INFECTIOUS DISEASE ______

Rev. 5/92

Figure 14-12 • *Identification tags are placed on the patient's body. (Courtesy of Marquette General Health System, Marquette, MI)*

PATIENT LABEL

MARQUETTE GENERAL HEALTH SYSTEM AUTHORIZATION FOR MORTICIAN

Date: _____

NAME OF DECEASED: _____

DECEASED SS#: _____

BIRTH DATE: _____ MEDICAL RECORD #: _____

DATE OF DEATH: _____ TIME OF DEATH: _____

PHYSICIAN WHO PRONOUNCED THE PATIENT'S DEATH: _____

Permission is hereby granted to Marquette General Hospital to release the remains of the above named deceased to _____ Funeral Home.

In addition, the above named Funeral Home is granted permission to embalm the above named deceased.

Date: _____   _____
                                            Signature of Next-of-Kin

Witnesses:

_____   _____
                                            Relationship to Deceased

_____

Received the remains of: _____
                                (Name of Deceased)

on this _____ day of _____, 20____, at _____.

Witness: _____   _____
                                            Signature of Mortician

_____

Figure 14-13 • *A release of remains form must be signed before the funeral home removes the body from the health care facility. (Courtesy of Marquette General Health System, Marquette, MI)*

MARQUETTE GENERAL HEALTH SYSTEM
CONSENT FOR POST-MORTEM

PATIENT LABEL

NAME OF DECEASED: _____

DATE AND TIME OF DEATH: _____

Permission is hereby granted to Marquette General Health System and members of its medical staff to perform a post-mortem examination on the remains of the above named deceased and to retain such portions of the remains as may be necessary for further examination.

The examination is to include: _____
(Specify "trunk only," or "trunk and head", "head only", etc. **DO NOT** use the word "complete.")

This is to certify that the procedure, billing policies, and purpose of the above examination have been fully explained to me.

This is to testify that I am the nearest relative of the deceased.

Date:_____   _____
                                  Signature of Next-of-Kin

Time:_____   _____
                                  Relationship to Deceased

                                  Address:

Witnesses: _____

_____   _____

_____   Phone #:_____

☐ **Bill to Hospital/Clinic**   ☐ **Bill to Patient***

_____   Responsible Party _____

_____   Address _____

                                  Phone #:_____

Acct. No._____   *Insurance will **NOT** cover autopsy charges

NOTE:

1. Consent for post-mortem examination may be given by the following, in order of primary right: spouse, adult son/daughter, parent, adult brother/sister, other next-of-kin, guardian at the time of death.

2. Only one signature is necessary, but if convenient, have more than one signature, each on a separate consent form, dated/timed, and witnessed.

3. If legal permission has already been granted, anyone objecting must submit his objection in writing before the performance of the examination.

4. In the absence of the next-of-kin, a friend or anyone assuming charge of the burial, i.e. public official, may give consent.

5. Telephone permission is acceptable if witnessed by two persons.

WHITE: Patient's Chart   **YELLOW:** Pathologist   **PINK:** Funeral Home

C:\Projects\CONSENT\ConsentPostMortem.pmd 2/85, Rev. 6/03   MRURsubApprove: 5/14/03

Figure 14-14 • *If an autopsy is to be performed, permission must be granted by the next of kin unless the autopsy is required by law. (Courtesy of Marquette General Health System, Marquette, MI)*

SUMMARY

The health unit coordinator plays a key role in the admission, transfer, and discharge processes. Completing the required forms, notifying the appropriate staff members, inputting the correct information, and processing all the information independently and efficiently are all the responsibilities of the health unit coordinator. It is important to remember that the health unit coordinator is often the first person who the patient meets in the health care organization. This first impression is the one that reassures the patient that the choice of this health care system was the right one.

REVIEW QUESTIONS

1. List a form that must be filled out when a patient dies and explain what the form is used for.

2. Describe an inpatient, outpatient, and short-stay patient length of stay in the health care facility. Explain why they differ.

3. Describe an emergency admission.

4. List five items found on the face sheet.

5. List four places patients can be discharged to.

NAHUC CERTIFICATION EXAM

CONTENT AREAS

I. C. 4   Request patient information from external facilities

II. A. 1   Label and assemble patient charts upon admission

II. A. 2   Obtain patient information prior to admission

II. A. 3   Assign beds to patients coming into the unit

II. A. 4   Inform nursing staff of patient admissions, transfers, discharges and returning surgical patients

II. A. 5   Process patient registration

II. C. 1   Assemble necessary forms and perform clerical tasks for patients being transferred to an external facility

II. C. 2   Prepare patient charts and perform clerical tasks for discharge or transfer to other units within the health facility

II. C. 3   Notify appropriate departments and individuals when patients are discharged (i.e., home, expired, AMA, transferred, etc.)

II. C. 4   Disassemble patient charts, put in appropriate order, and send to medical records office upon expiration or discharge.

II. C. 5   Schedule follow-up appointments

II. C. 6   Schedule appointments for diagnostic work at other facilities

II. C. 7   Follow organ procurement procedures

II. C. 8   Schedule ground transportation for patients

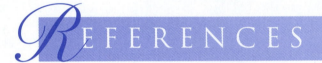

REFERENCES

Kerschner, V. (1992). *Health unit coordinating principles and practices.* Clifton Park, NY: Thomson Delmar Learning.

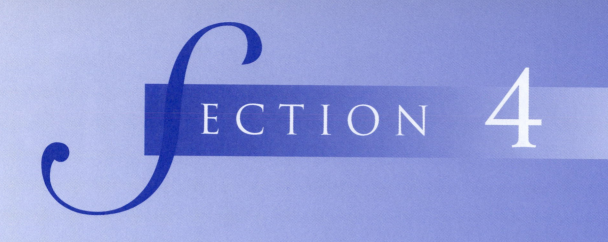

SECTION 4

Communication

Communication Skills

Learning Objectives

Upon completion of this chapter and review questions, the learner should be able to:

1. Explain how communication happens.

2. Describe different types of verbal communication.

3. Discuss nonverbal communication.

4. Explain written communication.

5. Discuss why communication happens.

6. Describe effective communication styles.

7. Discuss effective communication styles in the health care setting.

8. Discuss what affects how communication happens.

Key Terms

communication   The process of sending a message to another person for the purpose of obtaining a response.

communication style   The way or manner used to communicate.

formal communication   Communication that is planned.

informal communication   Communication that is not planned.

nonverbal communication Communicating without using words.

verbal communication Communicating using words; can be spoken or written, but the term usually refers to spoken (oral) communication.

written communication Communicating using written language.

COMMUNICATION

Communication is the process of sending a message to another individual. The person sending the message is called the sender. The sender can send the message using different modes of communication including verbal and nonverbal. The person receiving the message is the receiver. The receiver receives the message, decodes the message sent, and sends back a response to the sender. The sender may encode the message so that only the intended receiver can decode the message.

The communication process can be as simple as the sender's asking the receiver a question and the receiver's answering the question. Communication is a process that is used extensively in the workforce and in health care facilities. Because health care is a business whose purpose is to provide health care to individuals, it is important that the employees be able to communicate effectively with these individuals and their families. Communication skills that are required of health care employees differ according to the situation. Let's look at how we communicate.

HOW COMMUNICATION HAPPENS

When two individuals communicate effectively the results are clear; the message sent by the sender was received and processed by the receiver. That seems like a simple act, but that is not always what happens. It may be that the sender does not speak the language that the receiver understands. In health care, particularly, different terminology is an occurrence. Medical jargon, the language health care professionals speak and write, is not standardized. Terms such as *DTC* may be used to refer to the diagnostic treatment center or to the outpatient treatment department. Health care facilities attempt to standardize medical abbreviations used at their facilities by adopting a standard for all to use. Health care providers come together from all over the world to work at a health care facility and bring different medical jargon and acceptable abbreviations. A good example of different terms and abbreviations is those used for blood cells. Some physicians might ask for PCs, or packed cells; other physicians may ask for CM, or cell mass; still others might ask for RBCs, or red blood cells. All of these terms and abbreviations mean units of blood cells. Also, some health care providers may speak a different language than others, making verbal communication difficult.

In order for communication to happen, the receiver must receive the message sent by the sender. A receiver who is not able to receive the message will not respond. In the health care setting, the channel, or the route through which the message is sent, must be clear for the receiver and the sender to send messages back and forth. Other workers or equipment may block the channel, preventing the message from having a clear path.

Or the channel may be clear but the receiver may misread the message. The receiver reads the message on the basis of knowledge, experience, and what was heard or seen. Most people only hear 35 percent of what is said.

Why is it that people hear and process so little of verbal communication sent to them? Listening to the message sent is difficult in an area where the noise level is high. Health unit coordinators are often at the workstation doing more than one task at a time. When a communication is sent, if they are the intended receiver, the channel may be blocked by the activity at the workstation. Listening is a skill that is learned. It takes practice to be able to hear what messages are sent to you at a busy workstation and block out the messages not intended for you. The health unit coordinator needs to be able to pay attention to the work at hand but still be able to have the workstation under control and running smoothly. The following are some steps you can take to improve your listening skills.

◆ Stop what you are doing and give the person sending the message your attention. Stopping to listen takes time, but the time is well worth it. You will hear the message the first time it is sent so that the sender will not have to repeat the message, and you will be able to provide feedback immediately.

◆ Concentrate on what the sender is saying. This may take practice. We live and work in busy places with lots of stimuli going all the time. Look the person sending the message in the eyes, or focus on an object nearby if your culture dictates that looking someone in the eyes is disrespectful. Listen to the words the sender is sending. Ask questions or nod your head to acknowledge that you are actively listening.

◆ Pay attention to gestures and facial expressions. They may send a message different from the message contained in the words the sender is using.

◆ If you are able to look directly at the sender, don't judge the message sent by what the sender looks like, listen to the message.

◆ Don't interrupt the message sender; let the sender finish the message before you provide feedback. It is easy to jump right in before the sender has completed the message.

◆ Teach yourself to listen to what is being said. Humans speak at between 100 and 200 words per minute.

Health unit coordinators are the senders and receivers of information at the workstation. The information is sent to the health unit coordinator by co-workers, ancillary services, health care professionals, patients, and family members. In turn, the health unit coordinator processes the information received and sends it out to the people who need to know it to complete their responsibilities and tasks. Below is an example of how communication may take place at the unit workstation.

The nurse comes to the unit workstation and asks the health unit coordinator to call for a breakfast tray for the patient in room 657. The health unit coordinator calls the dietary department and requests the tray for the patient. The dietary secretary tells the health unit coordinator the tray will be delivered at 9 A.M. The health unit coordinator then tells the nurse when to expect the tray to arrive in the patient's room.

COMMUNICATION STYLES

Communication styles are the ways or manners used to communicate. There are basically three communication styles. Passive communication is the style used by the communicator who puts the rights of others before his or her own rights. Passive communicators have low self-esteem and often are angry with themselves. Assertive communication is the style in which the communicator believes in himself or herself as having rights and respects the rights of others as well. Assertive communicators are respected by others and, in turn, respect others. Aggressive communication is the style in which the communicator believes in his or her rights but does not respect the rights of others. Aggressive communicators are not liked by others and are seldom welcomed team members.

To see how these three communication styles differ consider the following examples. The health unit coordinator needs to communicate a message to the laundry to have extra laundry delivered.

> The passive communication message sent is: "This is the sixth floor calling and I know you are busy and I am sorry to call you but could you please send up an extra laundry cart at 6 P.M. today."

> The assertive communication message sent is: "This is Roger, the health unit coordinator on the sixth floor, and we would like an extra laundry cart sent up at 6 P.M. today. Thank you."

> The aggressive communication message sent is: "This is Roger on the sixth floor and you need to send an extra laundry cart up at 6 P.M. and don't be late!"

The laundry cart will arrive at 6 P.M. as requested; all three communication styles will get the laundry cart to the department. But which style is the preferred style?

VERBAL COMMUNICATION

Verbal communication is the form of communication used most often in a health care setting. **Verbal communication** is the communication method that uses words to communicate a message to a receiver. The words can be spoken (oral) or written, but the term *verbal communication* is usually used to refer only to oral communication. The receiver and sender must speak the same jargon or at least understand the same jargon in order for the communication process to be effective. Verbal communication is used between co-workers, between health care providers and patient and families, between health care providers and outside vendors, and between health care employees and the community. Verbal communication can be formal or informal. **Formal communication** is communication that has been planned, such as a news conference presentation, a lecture, or a planned education presentation. **Informal communication** is visiting, sharing information, or talking with the patient. The health unit coordinator uses informal verbal communication to communicate with fellow health care providers who are part of the patient care team. When using verbal communication, the health care employees need to pay particular attention to where the communication is occurring. The workstation is often near patient rooms, and the voices of the health care providers can often be overheard in those rooms. It is important to keep voices low when sharing patient information with other health care providers who need to know the information to do their job. Ideally, information regarding patients should be orally communicated only in an area where other people cannot hear.

Verbal communication messages can have different meanings even though the same words may be spoken. Tone, loudness, and pauses can change the meaning of the message. Here are some examples of how they can affect the meaning of messages with the same words.

The pencil is here.

The pencil is *here*.

The pencil *is* here!

Verbal communication styles differ just as people differ. There are different styles used in different situations. Health care facilities provide many different situations for verbal communication styles to be used. Verbal communication is either direct or indirect. Direct verbal communication is communication that is direct between the sender and the receiver. This communication is the method that is used most often. For example, the health unit coordinator calls the dietary department and requests a diet change for a patient from a full liquid diet to a soft diet. The health unit coordinator speaks directly to the diet clerk, whose job responsibilities include answering the phone and recording the diet changes for the dietary department (Figure 15-1).

Indirect verbal communication occurs when the sender sends the message to a receiver other than the person for whom the message is intended. The receiver must

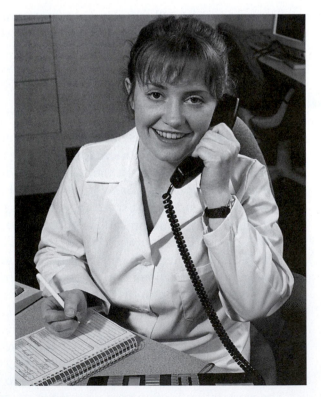

Figure 15-1 • *The health unit coordinator speaks directly to other departments within the health care facility using the telephone.*

then send the message on to the person who is the intended receiver of the message. For example, the health unit coordinator speaks with the respiratory care department secretary, who is handling calls for the respiratory therapist; this call is taped. The secretary must then send the message from the health unit coordinator to the therapist. In some departments, this is an effective communication system as well as a double-check system. The double check system works by the secretary's reviewing the audiotape once on each work shift to make sure that no orders were missed.

Passive verbal communicators talk in a soft voice and can give the impression that they are timid, although in some cultures being soft-spoken is the normal tone. They seem to be apologizing for not doing as well as the other team members. Assertive verbal communicators use a firm voice and usually use "I" statements. Aggressive verbal communicators use a loud voice and use "you" statements.

NONVERBAL COMMUNICATION

Communication without using spoken words is called **nonverbal communication**. Nonverbal communication is 55 percent of all messages received. Included in nonverbal communication are gestures, body language, facial expressions, and eye contact.

Gestures may be used to communicate when verbal communication is not possible or when it is easier and faster than verbal communication (Figure 15-2). Gestures are fast and easy to use, but attention must be paid to the meaning of gestures because most health care facilities have employees from many different parts of the world and many different cultures. The gestures may have the same meaning or totally opposite meanings

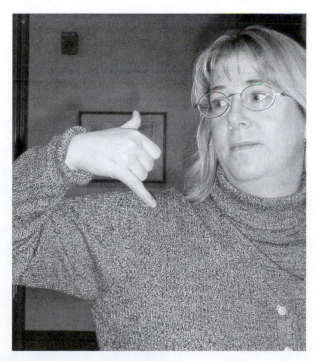

Figure 15-2 • *The health unit coordinator uses gestures to communicate that the nurse is needed for a telephone call when it is not possible to communicate verbally.*
(Courtesy of Marquette General Health System, Marquette, MI)

depending on the culture. If someone approaches the workstation desk and extends his right arm, most often we would assume that was a greeting gesture even without a word being spoken. If someone is on the telephone and extends his hand, we assume he needs paper and a writing instrument to write a note. Often, at the workstation, a member of the health care team may be speaking with one person while using gestures to send a nonverbal request to another team member.

Body language is used to send messages. The message is sent by the sender's using different body positions (Figure 15-3). In the workstation setting, the health unit coordinator may leave the area and return to find other health care workers in her workspace. The message sent by standing and just looking at the staff members says, "Please vacate that space so that I can continue to complete the tasks and responsibilities of my assigned job." A person standing with arms crossed may be sending the message that he or she is not open to other individual's ideas or is not interested in what is going on. A person standing over a health unit coordinator sitting at the workstation might be sending the message that he or she is in charge. In different cultures, being close to another person is disrespectful and invasive of their personal space. At a workstation in a health care facility, the space is limited, and often health care workers are in each other's space.

Facial expressions send nonverbal messages. Smiles, smirks, squints, widening of the eyes, and the like can be used to express approval, dissatisfaction, annoyance, and amazement or surprise. Your eyes are used to send nonverbal messages. The length of time you look at the receiver and how long you hold the eye contact is one way to send a message using your eyes. A long-lasting eye contact sends the message, "I am telling you something important and I am in control." Nonverbal communication sends a clear message and one most all receivers understand.

Passive nonverbal communicators are often seen looking down or not looking directly at the person with whom they are communicating. Assertive nonverbal communicators look directly at the person with whom they are communicating and are in a relaxed posture. Aggressive nonverbal communicators stare at the person with whom they are communicating and often appear tense, even using finger pointing at times.

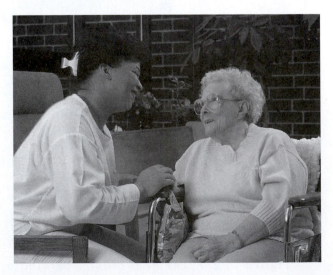

Figure 15-3 • *Body language is used to communicate with people without speaking.*

WRITTEN COMMUNICATION

Written communication is used to communicate information using written words. This type of communication is used when the receiver and sender are not able to communicate orally or when a record of the communication is needed. Written communication may be formal or informal communication. Formal written communication is written information that has been planned, using accepted language, abbreviations, and written using the correct forms and reports. Examples of formal written communication include physician orders, patient reports, and patient documentation by health care providers. Informal written communication may be notes written on notepaper (Figure 15-4). This type of communication is usually short and not in complete sentences but provides the information to the receiver that the sender wanted sent. Health unit coordinators record many informal notes throughout the workshift. These notes could be patient lab values that the lab called to the workstation; they could be messages for health care workers from other health care facility departments; they could be messages from physicians for the nurses caring for the patients; or they could be messages from ancillary departments regarding test times. The written notes must be accurate, and they must be able to be read by the receiver. It is important that the health unit coordinator know the acceptable medical language so that the written message is correct. A notepad form for informal written communications may be used by the health unit coordinator (Figure 15-5).

The manner is which messages are given to the intended recipient is defined by the unit or department. Often the health unit coordinator will define the process of communicating written messages to other employees. One of the responsibilities of the health unit coordinator is to answer the telephone and communicate the information to the people who need to know the information to do their jobs. For example, the health unit coordinator answers the telephone, and the caller asks her to ask Sally to call the

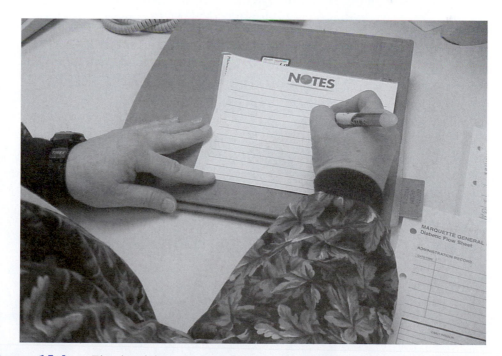

Figure 15-4 • *The health unit coordinator takes notes to provide information to others. (Courtesy of Marquette General Health System, Marquette, MI)*

To   J. Sampson   ☐ URGENT
Date___4-29-XX_____Time____6:10____ Ⓐ.Ⓜ.
                                              P.M.
WHILE YOU WERE OUT
From_____Dr. Olegna_____
Of_____Hillside Medical Center_____
Phone____123____555____1212_____
          Area Code   Number   Ext.

Telephoned	X	Please call	
Came to see you		Wants to see you	
Returned your call		Will call again	

Message ___Call before noon-re:_____
          _____laboratory tests for_____
          _____Donelda Dirickson_____
          _____
          _____
          _____
          _____

Signed _L. Winslow, CHUC_____

Figure 15-5 • *This type of notepad is used by a health unit coordinator on a patient care unit.*

pharmacy at extension 4563. Sally doesn't work until the next day, so a written message is posted on the message board (Figure 15-6) in the report room. The health unit coordinator tells the caller that Sally is not working until tomorrow but a written message will be posted for Sally. In this particular unit, the health care coordinators always post messages on the report board, and one of the first things other team members do upon starting their workshift is to check the report board for messages.

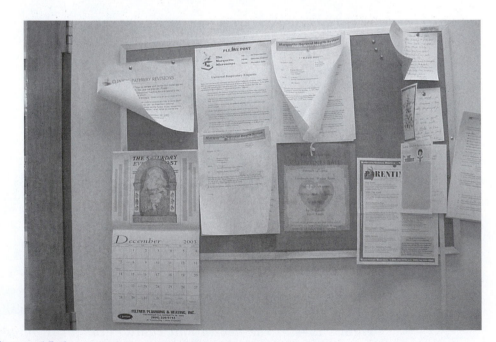

Figure 15-6 • *Messages for the staff are left on this message board.* (Courtesy of Marquette General Health System, Marquette, MI)

WHY COMMUNICATE?

Communication allows us to share information with one another. That information can be shared verbally, nonverbally, or in writing. We communicate to provide information. In a health care facility, we communicate information continuously. We communicate to process the orders and requests of the clinical health care providers to take care of the patients. We communicate in person, both verbally and nonverbally. We communicate using communication devices. Communication is powerful, and it is important to communicate so that the receiver can correctly interpret or decode the message sent. Health unit coordinators communicate to fulfill the tasks and responsibilities of the position. Competencies are the skills required to complete the functions and responsibilities of the position. The position of health unit coordinator requires the ability to communicate effectively in a variety of situations.

An example of a competency that may reflect the reason we communicate is stated as:

1. Communicates effectively to process the tasks and responsibilities of the position
   a. Demonstrates verbal communication skills
   b. Demonstrates written communication skills
      - Phone messages
      - Memos
   c. Demonstrates use of communication equipment
      - Telephone
      - Fax
      - Beeper system
      - Electronic mail

EFFECTIVE COMMUNICATION

Effective communication means the sender sends the message to the receiver and the receiver receives the message and sends feedback to the sender. What is effective differs in each situation and with the people involved in the sending and receiving. In a health care facility, communication must be accurate. The message received must be the message sent. All health care facilities must have a standard language that is used throughout the facility. It is important for the surgeon in the operating room to be communicating to the operating room staff in the language that they understand; and the operating room staff must communicate effectively to the recovery room staff.

We adjust how we communicate on the basis of our perception of the receiver. In the health care facility, the health unit coordinator communicates with co-workers, patients, family members, outside vendors, and the community. The number of people with whom the health unit coordinator interacts varies with the department population, the size of the health care facility, and the department scope of service. In a unit that provides services to geriatric patients, the communication skills you use would be different from the skills you would use if you were employed on a pediatric unit. If you spend time communicating with different age groups, you must be competent in communicating with that group. Table 15-1 presents communication skills for different age groups.

TABLE 15-1 Communication Skills for Different Age Groups

Name of Group	Age (Years)	Skill Level of Group	Example Message
Infant	Birth to 1 year	May understand many words and be able to follow simple directions	Would you like the Teddy Bear?
Toddler	1–4	Play and simple instruction	Would you like some milk?
Preschooler	4–6	Able to answer questions in sentences	What would you like to eat?
School-age	6–12	Able to recall events past and have a feel for the future	Can you tell me what you had to eat yesterday?
Adolescent	13–18	Able to process information and create a plan	Let's plan your menus for the next week.
Early adulthood	18–29	Able to use experiences to understand	Provide me with examples of balanced menus.
Young adulthood	30–44	Experience-based learning	On the basis of your previous experiences, what kinds of meal planning will work for you?
Middle adulthood	44–65	Same as young adulthood but increased experience	In the past, you were eating . . . and . . . happened. What if we try . . .
Geriatric	65 and older	May have difficulty hearing	(Look directly at the person and speak clearly.) What would you like to eat today?

WHAT AFFECTS COMMUNICATION

It is possible to communicate in different ways not only on the basis of the age of the person with whom you are communicating but also on the basis of how you feel toward the person and how you feel physically and mentally. Other factors that affect communication are education, noise, culture, and location.

The education level of the person you are communicating with affects communication. In a health care facility, communication happens between people of varying education levels. Remember, as a health unit coordinator you will be a member of the patient care team. The members of the team will have different levels of education. If you do not understand something—for example, "this patient will be going for a cholecystec-tomy"—ask the person requesting the service to explain what is needed because you are unfamiliar with the term. The opportunity to expand your knowledge is within your reach.

Noise and activity affect communication. The message is difficult to hear or see if the level of noise or activity interferes with the receiver or sender of the message. Communication devices can be difficult to use if noise or activity interferes. It is hard to hear on the telephone if people are talking close by.

Cultures affect communication. You must be knowledgeable about the cultures that use your health care facility and how they communicate. In some cultures, people nod in agreement to be polite not to agree or acknowledge what has been said. It is important for health unit coordinators to be aware of such cultural aspects of communication as they provide information for follow-up appointments and directions on how to get to those appointments.

The receiver affects how communication happens. If the receiver has a hearing problem, make sure that you carefully pronounce your words and that you have the person's attention before sending a message. If the receiver is quiet, you would most likely use a quiet tone when sharing information.

The location and time of day can dictate how we communicate. If it is a busy and loud area with lots of conversation happening at once, so then will the conversation be busy and loud. If it is quiet, you will find employees speaking in quiet voices. There are usually more people around, all conversing, during the day, whereas at night fewer people are around, and it is much quieter.

An important point to remember is that communication can, in turn, affect location. In a health care facility, patient confidentiality is protected. This means that patient information cannot be shared with people who do not have a need to know it to do their job. In the hallways, where many people can hear information, you would not communicate diagnosis information or medication information. This information would be communicated or shared in a room where only the health care providers caring for the patient could hear it. We guard the manner and place in which information is shared so that it is not broadcast indiscriminately.

People can also create barriers to communicate by choosing not to receive the message sent because:

- They do not believe the sender because of past experiences

- They do not like the sender

- The sender is the boss

- They are not interested in what the sender is sending

- They are preoccupied

SUMMARY

Communication is powerful. It happens both verbally and nonverbally in the health care facility. Written communication is an accurate way to communicate and is a record of what was communicated. The sender and the receiver of the message affect communication. Noise, cultural differences, co-workers, education, location of communication, and activity can affect communication. There are three common communication styles: passive, assertive, and aggressive. Communication styles vary not only on the basis of who is communicating with whom but also because of the physical and mental health of the communicator and receiver and the environment in which communication is taking place. Health unit coordinators must have excellent communication skills that can be demonstrated for all age levels that they communicate with.

REVIEW QUESTIONS

1. What term is used for communication that is planned?

2. What is the term for communicating using words?

3. What is the term for communicating without using words?

4. What is the person sending the message called?

5. What is the person receiving the message called?

6. What term is used for communication that is not planned?

7. What is the term for the process of sending a message to another person?

8. Name three common communication styles.

NAHUC CERTIFICATION EXAM

CONTENT AREAS

II. B. 1   Receive diagnostic test results

II. B. 3   Report diagnostic test results to nursing staff

II. F. 6   Greet patients, physicians, visitors, and facility staff who arrive on the unit

II. F. 7   Respond to patient, physician, visitor, and facility staff requests and complaints

III. A. 4   Answer and process unit telephone calls

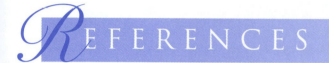

THROUGH THE EYES

OF A HEALTH CARE PROFESSIONAL

In discussions of what qualities are needed to be a successful health unit coordinator, one that is stated over and over again is that a health unit coordinator must have good communication skills. The person must be able to send a message that can be received and decoded by the receiver as it was sent. The workstation is the targeted area for information, with many people coming to that area—patients, upset families, lost visitors, busy co-workers, ancillary department staff, and physicians. The health unit coordinator needs to communicate with each person who approaches the workstation, and they all require a response. It is quite a feat to keep the unit running smoothly by sharing the correct information with the correct people. It is important that the customers at the unit workstation have their concerns and questions addressed with effective communication.

REFERENCES

Kerschner, V. (1992). *Health unit coordinating principles and practice*. Clifton Park, NY: Thomson Delmar Learning.

LaFleur-Brooks, M. (2004). *Health unit coordinating* (5th ed.). Philadelphia: Saunders.

C HAPTER 16

Communication Devices

Learning Objectives

Upon completion of this chapter and review questions, the learner should be able to:

1. Define the purpose of communication devices.

2. Discuss appropriate use of the telephone.

3. Describe telephone etiquette in the health care setting.

4. Explain how the computer is used as a communication device.

5. Describe the function of the pneumatic tube system.

6. Identify four frequently used communication devices in the health care setting.

Key Terms

communication board   A board used to communicate information to others.

communication device   A device used to assist with communication.

computer   A device used to process, store, send, receive, and retrieve information.

copiers   A machine used to make copies of written material.

emergency call light system A system that turns on a warning light that goes on at the workstation, or at an overhead location, when an emergency is happening in a patient room or area.

fax machine A machine used to send and receive written materials from one place to another place.

pneumatic tube A system using containers placed in a "tube" that uses air pressure to move the container from one station to another.

room call system A system used to notify the staff that the patient or family is requesting assistance in the patient's room.

telephone A device used to send speech from one person to another person.

Abbreviations

PDA Personal Digital Assistant

COMMUNICATION TOOLS

Communication devices are tools used to assist the sender in efficiently and effectively sending a message to the intended receiver. Communication devices allow the sender to communicate with a receiver who may be miles away. These devices have allowed information to be communicated across the world as well as across a room. Health care workers use various communication devices to communicate information and requests. The use of these devices assists in providing quality patient care. In this chapter, you will be introduced to communication devices that are used frequently in the health care setting.

TELEPHONE USAGE

The **telephone** is one of the most widely used communication devices. The telephone allows health care workers to communicate verbally with anyone who has access to a telephone. Health unit coordinators use the telephone to communicate information to people who need the information in providing care to patients and to receive information that they need to do their job.

In the past, in order to communicate using the telephone, the users had to have the telephone connected to a telephone line. As technology has continued to develop, people can now use telephones that are able to connect without the "line." Users are no longer forced to stay in one place to communicate using the telephone. With a portable telephone, the user can travel within a defined range while using a telephone and is not restricted to a space that is limited to only as far as the cord will reach. With the addition of the cell phone to the types of telephone available, people can be connected no matter where they are. The cell phone is free of connecting lines. Their primary limitation is the need to recharge as the battery light indicates.

TELEPHONE SKILLS FOR THE RECEIVER

Using the telephone to communicate requires that you develop some basic skills. These skills seem simple on the surface, but they are important because, even on the telephone, the message sent could be more than just the words spoken. When using the telephone to answer calls, use these basic skills:

1. Answer the telephone by identifying:

   ◆ Your name. This allows callers to know to whom they are speaking.

   ◆ Where you are located. This allows callers to know to which department or nursing unit they are connected.

   ◆ What you do in the department, your title. This allows the caller to ask the correct question or request of the person.

   This identifying information provides the caller with the basic information as to where the call was answered. Here are two examples of how to answer an incoming call.

   "Good morning. This is Linda, health unit coordinator on the surgical unit. How may I help you?"

   "Surgical unit. Linda, health unit coordinator. How may I help you?"

2. Use simple courtesies.

   Customers appreciate the telephone courtesies provided to them by the telephone answerer. These courtesies include the following:

   ◆ Be cheerful.

   ◆ Be friendly. Often people are calling a strange place, and a friendly voice builds an atmosphere in which the caller feels comfortable asking questions. Do not make callers feel they are a bother or that you do not have time for them. Remember, in a health care facility a variety of people will call: health care professionals, co-workers, patients, concerned families, and customers.

   ◆ Be helpful. The health unit coordinator is the communication expert in the patient care department; share the information that you are able to share with the caller without breaching patient or employee confidentiality.

   ◆ Be polite. Everyone responds to phrases that are labeled "good manners" "Please," "thank you," and "you're welcome" usually put a smile on everyone's face.

   ◆ Be a person who does what you commit to do. Callers expect you to do what you say you are going to do. If you say you will search for the patient care provider, page and locate the provider and then return to the caller and let the caller know that the provider will come to the phone momentarily.

3. Speak clearly.

It is important that the caller can understand and hear what you are saying. Do not have food in your mouth when you answer the telephone, and do not put food in your mouth while you are talking. It is difficult to understand someone who is attempting to talk and eat at the same time. Do not chew gum or suck on candies because they make it difficult to speak clearly and produce smacking mouth sounds and distracting background noises. Remember, those noises are louder over phone lines. Speak into the receiver so that your voice will travel clearly to the caller. Speak at a normal rate. Keep in mind that callers are unable to read your body language to interrupt the message you are sending. They must rely entirely on what they hear.

4. Put a smile in your voice.

Even though callers cannot see the person answering the telephone, they still form a mental picture of the receiver. Smile, and the caller will hear it through the conversation. The tone, pitch, and pauses send that smile through the phone lines. If this is difficult to do try the following exercise: Place a mirror next to the telephone, and when you answer the phone look into the mirror and smile. That is the mental picture the caller will see.

5. If possible, answer the telephone call before the third ring.

It is important to answer the incoming call as quickly as possible. Health care facilities use the telephone as a main communication device. Often incoming calls can be processed in less than one minute communicating information quickly and effectively.

6. Place a caller on hold only after you have asked for the caller's permission.

If you must put a caller on hold, ask for permission and wait for an answer. All callers should be placed on hold if information to respond to their questions requires leaving the phone. If the caller agrees to be placed on hold, check back every minute to make sure he or she wishes to continue to be on hold. Also inform of the caller of the progress being made to respond to the request. Some callers may not have the time to be placed on hold and would rather leave a message.

7. Process phone messages accurately.

If the caller wishes to leave a message, follow the message procedure established in the health care facility. The health unit coordinator can take messages and process them in conformance with the message procedures in place.

- ◆ Written messages
- ◆ E-mail
- ◆ Voice mail
- ◆ Pagers

Written messages may be processed using paper and pencil and placed in a designated area, or they may be processed using communication devices such as computers or pagers. When the caller requests that a message be taken, the following should be done:

◆ Repeat the message you will write to the caller.

◆ Write the message clearly.

◆ Address the message to the intended receiver.

◆ Record the date and time when the message was received.

◆ Sign the message so that the receiver can identify who took the message.

TELEPHONE SKILLS FOR THE SENDER

Using the telephone as a communication device to request a service or supplies requires that the sender of the message use telephone skills to communicate effectively. When calling another person or department, the caller should be prepared to do the following:

◆ Identify who you are.

◆ Indicate from where you are calling.

◆ State what you are requesting.

This gives the receiver the information needed to quickly process the call.

Before placing a call, following these simple rules will save time:

1. Have all the information you need to complete the call. State the reason you are calling and proceed with business. Small talk encourages conversations to be lengthy. Here is an example: Mr. Smith is going home and needs a follow-up appointment with Dr. Jones on Monday. To make this appointment, you will need to have Mr. Smith's address and phone number, his diagnosis, and his discharge date. All this information is stored on different screens in the computer system. To prepare for this call, you will need to have all three screens open.

2. Have the telephone number you need to call in front of you. Some phone systems allow frequently called numbers to be placed in a speed dial system. This is fast and convenient for callers. There may be telephone directories that list often-called numbers. These directories may be created by the health system, or the health unit coordinator may create one unique to the unit.

3. Place one phone call for multiple requests. If there are five patients being discharged by Dr. Jones, call Dr. Jones's office once and make the follow-up appointments for all five patients. Making all the appointments in just one call saves time not only for the health unit coordinator but also for Dr. Jones's office staff. It also reduces the number of outgoing phone calls.

4. Place calls when the receiver is available. If possible, call when you know that the intended receiver is able to take the call. The following example illustrates this point: Dr. Jones's office hours are from 9 A.M. to 4 P.M. The

health unit coordinator needs to know not to call Dr. Jones's office after 4 P.M. to make appointments.

5. Always end telephone calls with a thank you. This indicates an end to the phone conversation and that you, the caller, have received the information requested.

IMPORTANCE OF THE TELEPHONE

You will most likely find the telephone to be one of your most frequently used communication devices. Remember that even though you cannot physically see the person on the other end of the line, you can still feel an attitude on the telephone. To project a positive attitude to others keep your:

1. Body language positive. Your body language will be reflected in your message.

2. Voice tone appropriate. It should be soft yet assertive.

3. Vocabulary appropriate. Use terms you think the caller will understand.

4. Often, a first impression is made during a telephone conversation. These first impressions are based on voice volume, voice tone, and interest level. First impressions are powerful. and there is never a second chance to make a first impression. Use positive telephone techniques to make positive first impressions.

TELEPHONE SYSTEMS

Telephone systems in health care facilities are as varied as the health care facilities. There is usually a published phone number that the community can call to access the health care facility. A switchboard operator answers this phone number. The switchboard operator is employed in a department in the health care facility called the switchboard or communications. The main function of this department is to answer all incoming calls and direct the calls to the correct departments in the health care facility. The communications department is responsible for educating personnel on the use and function of the telephone system within the health care facility. They may also be responsible for the repair of the system and equipment as well.

The telephone device used in the health care facility will have a receiver and a dial pad. The receiver may or may not be directly connected to the dial pad. The telephone may have a headset that replaces the traditional receiver. A telephone headset allows the health unit coordinator to have both hands free and to move about the workstation. A remotely connected headset will have a limited use range. The health unit coordinator should be aware of headset's range as not to inadvertently exceed it. Health system staff members may carry wireless telephones. These devices allow the staff to answer and send calls from defined range areas. Wireless telephones allow staff members to complete tasks throughout the patient care department but still be able to send and receive calls. The telephone pad will often have a hold button, or, if no hold button is on the keypad, there is a simple procedure for placing the caller on hold

(Figure 16-1). It is important to never put the telephone headset or telephone receiver down without putting the call on hold. If the call is not put on hold, the caller may hear the conversations that are being conducted in the immediate area. This practice is especially important at a workstation where patient information is exchanged and may be heard by the caller.

Each workstation at the health care facility may have more than one telephone extension or line. Usually one telephone device can access all the telephone lines coming into the workstation. This type of system is efficient for the health unit coordinator because she can access all the calls coming into the unit from one telephone device. These devices allow the health unit coordinators to not only answer the call but to also transfer calls to another extension if the need arises. Transferring calls within the health care facility is accomplished by depressing a button or following a simple procedure. Most phone systems also allow additional people to listen to or participate in a call. This feature is especially useful when two people must witness verbal permission from a third person for a procedure. For calls placed outside the health care facility, there may be a number that must to used to access an outside line. For example, Dr. Smith has his office outside the health care facility and is not an employee of the health care facility, so to call Dr. Smith's office, it is necessary to dial 8-225-4657. It may be that an office is off-site but still part of the health care facility phone system so that only a short extension number need be dialed. There is usually an additional charge to place phone calls outside the health care facility's telephone system.

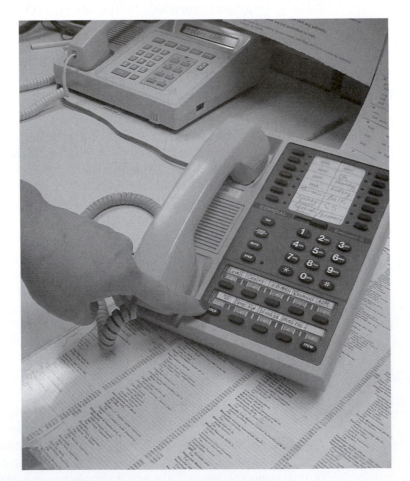

Figure 16-1 • *It is important to use the hold function on the telephone correctly. (Courtesy of Marquette General Health System, Marquette, MI)*

PAGING SYSTEMS

A beeper system is one type of paging system. The communications department is the department that coordinates the beeper system at the health care system. Beepers allow people who are not readily accessible to the telephone system to be contacted if needed. Beepers can provide a message in voice or typed text format. When a message is sent, it is announced to the recipient by an alert. The alert can be a sound, a movement (vibrating), or a flash. The user can customize the type of alert to his or her personal needs. Some health care facilities' paging systems require all health care team members to carry beepers. In others, only certain designated staff members carry beepers. The use of beepers saves time by allowing the health unit coordinator to beep the needed individual and go on with other duties until the needed party returns the call. The following examples illustrate different situations.

The patient in room 206A has family coming from out of town who would like to speak with the physician regarding the condition of the patient. The patient does not know when the family will arrive, and the physician has a full office schedule and also has to make rounds at the health care facility across town. Dr. Wong asks the health unit coordinator to beep him when the family arrives. The pager allows Dr. Wong to continue with his schedule and be alerted when the family arrives.

The lab provided Mr. Stein's lab values by telephone to the health unit coordinator in the patient care unit. Because the lab values were in the panic range, the health unit coordinator immediately beeped the doctor. By beeping the doctor, the health unit coordinator could give the doctor the lab values right away so that the patient treatment could be quickly adjusted.

FAX MACHINE

The **fax machine** is a telecommunication device used to transmit written information. The written information is sent through the phone lines to a receiving fax machine. This communication device can transmit written information to another fax machine in the health care facility or anywhere in the world. The fax machine has become a communication tool that is used to communicate information that at one time could be communicated only in person or by paper mail. The fax machine copies the written information that is fed into the machine and transmits the information. Some advantages of having access to a fax machine are:

1. Reduces errors. For the health unit coordinator, this transmission reduces errors by transmitting the written material directly to the receiving site. No longer is it necessary for the health unit coordinator to hand write reports that can be sent via fax.

2. Reduces time. The fax machine reduces the time it takes to retrieve information from other facilities. Information can be faxed within minutes.

3. Confidential information is secure. Information is sent directly to the person requesting the information or to the person having a need to know. The information bypasses many sets of hands of people who do not have a need to know.

It is important to adhere to fax etiquette when using the fax machine. The fax machine should be in an area where the users are able to easily access the machine and still protect the information from being assessable to people who do not need to know the information. Here are some ways to protect health information faxed and reduce the risk of the faxed information ending up in the wrong place.

1. Fax only information that must be sent right away. Send other information using the paper mail system.

2. Double-check with the receiver that the fax number you have is correct. Fax numbers, like telephone numbers, change.

3. Always double-check that the fax number that you have entered or dialed into the fax machine is the correct number. It is easy to press an incorrect number on the keypad.

4. If the fax machine is equipped with a password system, use the system. This helps ensure that the receiver will be the intended receiver.

5. If you are expecting a fax, make sure that you are listening for the cue that indicates a fax is being sent and prepare to retrieve the fax.

6. Make sure that your fax includes a cover sheet that includes a disclaimer (Figure 16-2). This protects the sender and provides an unintended receiver with instructions as to what to do with the fax.

In the health care facility, the fax machine is used to send information to departments from the patient care units. The health unit coordinator can fax reports to physicians' offices, physician orders to the pharmacy, patient information to social workers, and lab reports to the operating room. Faxing these types of documents provides important patient information in a timely and ongoing manner for the health care providers who make decisions for patient care and support. The health unit coordinator may be responsible for faxing information to extended-care facilities concerning a patient being transported to the facility, or for faxing patient reports to a large health care facility so that the patient will not need to have a procedure or test repeated at the facility. This faxing of information saves the patient time and money.

COMPUTERS

Computers, which process, store, send, receive, and retrieve information, have become a workplace assistant at the workstation. Most health care facilities have computers installed in each department. Some facilities have stand-alone computers. These are computers that are not connected to other computers. They work independently. Usually, individuals responsible for functions that are unique to that individual use these stations. Most health care facilities have a network interconnecting all the workstation and department computers within the facility so that the computer users can communicate with each other and share information.

COMPUTER STATIONS

Health unit coordinators may either have their own computer at their workstation or they may share a computer with other health care team members. The computer is

MARQUETTE GENERAL
HEALTH SYSTEM

CONFIDENTIAL INFORMATION ENCLOSED

❑ **Urgent**
❑ Return Phone Call
❑ Fax Back Reply
❑ Informational

Recipient Information

Name: _____

Organization: _____

Phone number: _____

Fax number: _____

# of pages: _____ (including cover sheet)

**MGHS
Education
Department**

580 W.College Ave.
Marquette, MI 49855
906-225-3470

Sender Information

Name: __Education Department__

Phone number: __906-225-3470__

Fax number: __906-225-3037__

Message:

Fax Back Reply:

CONFIDENTIALITY NOTICE

This facsimile transmittal is intended only for the use of the individual or entity to which it is addressed. It may contain Protected Health Information, which is privileged and confidential. Protected Health Information may only be used or disclosed in accordance with law and you may be subject to penalties under law for improper use or further disclosure of the Protected Health Information in this transmittal. If you are not the intended recipient of this transmission, you may not read, copy, distribute or otherwise use or disclose the information contained in this transmission. If you received this transmission in error, please notify the sender immediately and request instructions on return or destruction of the information in this transmission.

Figure 16-2 • *A fax cover sheet with a disclaimer (Courtesy of Marquette General Health System, Marquette, MI)*

placed at the workstation so that it is easily accessible for the users. The computer monitor, also called the computer screen, should be positioned so that information on the screen is visible only to the authorized staff. Some organizations may use screen protectors to further protect the visibility of the information.

The keyboard is placed at the correct height for the users. There are many types of keyboards to choose from, but they all have a keypad resembling a typewriter keypad (Figure 16-3). It is not necessary to have typing skills to be proficient at using a computer.

The third component of the computer system is the computer itself. This is the component that is the "brains" of the system. It is a cabinet that houses the power supply, devices in which programs and files are stored, and other components required for the computer to function. When this cabinet is narrow and tall, it is commonly called a "tower." This is in contrast to older desktop models, in which these computer components are housed in a more compact horizontally oriented box.

The computers store programs and files. Some of the programs are well known and readily available, such as word processing, data base, or spreadsheet programs that may be purchased and used on home computers. Other programs that are in the workstation computer have been created specifically for that patient care unit. For example, a unit might have a program that tracks the number of supplies used for each patient according to the patient's identification number assigned by the health care facility.

Not all programs or applications used in the health care system must reside in the individual workstation computer towers. Health care facilities typically link many individual

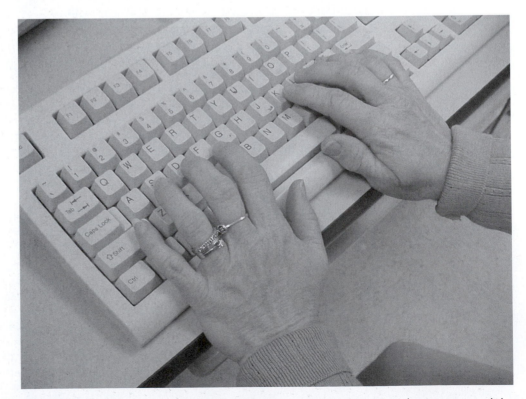

Figure 16-3 • *All computer keyboards have letter keys in the same positions. (Courtesy of Marquette General Health System, Marquette, MI)*

computers together in a network. Then programs and files may reside in the health care network. Networks are computer systems that allow more than one workstation access or use of the same computer programs. Networks can be in the same building, same town, or same health care system. Network programs allow authorized users to access information from different workstations and departments.

Each health care system purchases or develops computer program applications that are best suited to its overall needs. Because of the health care facility's security needs, especially those regarding protecting the confidentiality of patient records, user access is limited to a need-to-know basis. For example, people who do not have a need to know about patient billings or health histories are denied access to those records in the computer network. This limited access, or security access as it is usually called, is accomplished by issuing a user identification code and a password to each authorized computer network user. In order to use the computer programs, each person must log into the network by using an assigned user identification code and password. The combination of the identification code and password will give that person access to only the information, records, and programs needed to do his or her job; the person will not be able to access any other records, information, or programs. Below is an example of a process that may be used.

> A newly hired employee is sent a user identification code and a password through the interoffice mail system in a sealed envelope labeled confidential. The user identification code and the password will permit the employee to access certain records and programs in the computer network or system. The degree of access the employee is permitted is determined by the employee's need to know, based on the employees' position within the health care system and the department where she will be employed. Before the user identification code and password are provided by the security department, the newly hired employee is given a copy of the health care facility's computer policies. The employee is required to sign a release, which states that the employee has read, understands, and agrees to adhere to the policies. This document is retained as a permanent record in the employee's personnel file.

One function computer programs may be used for is to communicate information. The information communicated can generate orders, schedule procedures, bill insurance companies, and provide test and procedure results. The communication possibilities are defined by the health care system through their policies and procedures.

ELECTRONIC MAIL

One type of electronic communications commonly used in health care facilities is called electronic mail, or e-mail. It is the transmission of messages over communication networks. Some e-mail systems are confined to the health care system's single computer network. This means users can communicate electronically only with people who have e-mail accounts within the computer network. There are many programs that can be purchased and used to provide an e-mail system within a network. Lotus Notes and Microsoft Outlook are examples of electronic mail programs that are often used to set up an e-mail system within a health care system.

Some organizations have an electronic mail system that can connect to the Internet, which then opens electronic communication with the world. Not all organizations allow all computer users access to all options. The use of the computer programs is based on the responsibilities of the position. Health unit coordinators communicate information to the health care team members and receive information from health care team members and departments both within and outside the unit and facility. They use all the communication equipment that allows the completion of their tasks in an efficient and timely manner. Electronic communication allows communication to take place, for the most part, instantaneously. The following are often cited advantages of communicating electronically:

1. It reduces time in transporting information.

2. Information is written, therefore it is not likely to be misunderstood.

3. The information can be read at the convenience of the receiver and thus does not interrupt current activities.

4. The sender may keep a written copy of the communication.

5. Communication with people regardless of where they are located is possible providing they have e-mail technology.

PERSONAL DIGITAL ASSISTANT (PDA)

As technology continues to advance the role of the personal digital assistant (PDA) device will continue to grow and expand. The PDA is a handheld computer. In the future, health unit coordinators may likely use a personal digital assistant. It is envisioned that this device will be used to receive messages, provide telephone numbers, medical coding information, and updated drug information. The possibilities are endless. The uses are limited only by the health care system. The following example illustrates the use of a PDA at the point of care—the patient bedside.

> Dr. Lopez is writing discharge orders for Mr. Brown. Mr. Brown's daughter, who is visiting her father in his hospital room, asks the physician how much a 10-day supply of the new medication Dr. Lopez is prescribing for her father will cost. Dr. Lopez accesses that information on her PDA and is able to give Mr. Brown's daughter the amount Mr. Brown's pharmacy will charge for it.

PNEUMATIC TUBE

A **pneumatic tube system** is a means of rapid communication and transportation of small sized items that is used within health care facilities. It is an air-operated system in which a cylindrical carrier is inserted into a pneumatic tube where air pressure conveys it to its destination. The sender, before engaging the operating control that sends the carrier on its way, selects the destination. This system can carry almost any item that will fit inside the carrier. Typically, these items include paper reports, supplies, lab specimens, and medications. The health unit coordinator is a frequent user of the pneumatic tube system, using it to transport information to other departments and receive information from other departments. The pneumatic tube station is located in the patient care unit, and it is usually at the workstation so that the health unit coordinator is able to quickly and easily retrieve the sent item.

An example is a health unit coordinator removing a unit of blood that has been sent by the blood bank in the laboratory. The health unit coordinator received a phone call from the blood bank that they were sending the blood, and she knows that when it arrives in the pneumatic tube it must be brought to the nurse in the patient room so that it can be given to the patient. Sending it through the pneumatic tube system enables the patient to get it as soon as it is prepared.

The pneumatic tube system can also be used as a communication device when it is used to deliver written messages throughout the health care system. This device is a useful timesaver, decreasing the amount of time that was physically spent walking items and written information from one department to another. Some facilities that do not have pneumatic tube systems must physically walk the needed supplies and information from one area to another. Health unit coordinators may be responsible to transport information and supplies from one area to another.

ROOM CALL SYSTEMS

Health care facilities often have a **room call system** that enables a patient to communicate directly with the workstation via a two-way voice system. The room call system allows the patient (or members of the patient's family) to verbally request service from the bedside. The health unit coordinator, who may be at the workstation, might be the health care team member who responds to the patient call (Figure 16-4). If the patient's request is something the health unit coordinator can process she or he would

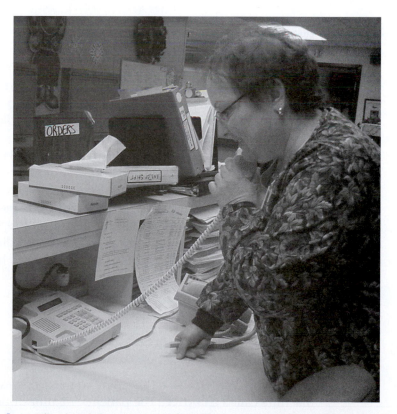

Figure 16-4 • *The health unit coordinator answers the patient call.*
(Courtesy of Marquette General Health System, Marquette, MI)

do so. Otherwise the appropriate health care team member would be "beeped" or otherwise notified to respond to the patient's request.

Patient call systems vary by health systems, as does the responsibility of answering the call system. These systems allow patients and health care team members to communicate quickly and conveniently with the responsible health care team members who respond to the patients' calls. It is an effective communication system, saving time and providing rapid response to patient requests.

EMERGENCY CALL LIGHT SYSTEMS

An **emergency call light system** turns on a warning, or alert light of some type, that is usually located either at the workstation or at a highly visible overhead location. The emergency call light system may be included in the patient's room call system or it may be a separate stand-alone system. All facilities inform patients and families how to get someone to come right away if an emergency arises. As the health unit coordinator, you must be aware of your role in an emergency situation and respond accordingly. If you are at the workstation and someone in a patient's room actuates an emergency call, you may be the health care team member who beeps the other team members or you may be the one who goes to the room to assist. Whatever your role is in an emergency situation, you should be prepared by knowing what to do and how to do what is expected and needed.

COMMUNICATION BOARDS

Communication boards are tools used to communicate information to other members of the nursing care team. The board could be simply a white board indicating nursing team members' assignments by patients so any member of the health team can look to see which team members are responsible for which patients (Figure 16-5). The communication board could also be a patient census kept at the unit workstation by the health unit coordinator. The patient census board would contain the information that the health unit coordinator needs in order to communicate with the responsible patient care provider the correct information regarding a specific patient. Figure 16-6 is an example of a communication board used by a health unit coordinator. Health unit coordinators use communication boards for shift reports, sharing both oral and written information with the next shift's health unit coordinator. Communication boards come in different sizes and shapes, dictated by the health care facility and its staff needs.

COPIERS

Health care facilities have the ability to make copies of written materials using a machine called a **copier**. The patient care unit or department may or may not have a copier, but regardless of whether a copier is located within the unit or department, the health unit coordinator will have access to a copier in the facility. Copies of patient

September 20 Friday

Blue Side

Team Leader Sally–1

Team Members
Andy, NA–2
Peggy, LPN–1
Ruth, RN–2
Greg, UC

Green Side

Team Leader June–2

Team Members
Sue, LPN–1
Robin, NA–2
Bill, RN–1
Bonnie, UC

Medical Unit South Tower

Figure 16-5 • *Patient care assignments are written on the communication board so that the health unit coordinator can quickly look at the board to find out who is responsible for which patients on the shift.*

Neuro Unit   September 10, 2004   05:00

601-D	Callie Smith	76	White	w/c	IV, CXR
601-W	Tina Brown	72	Green	cart	OR today
602-D					
602-W	Tom Bess	45	White	w/c	IV
603-D	Greg Like	34	Kosin	w/c	Plan D/C today
603-W	Bob Lord	39	Kosin	BED	NO CODE
604-D	Lily Wentla	47	Lyon	cart	IV
604-W	Tammy Bleau	53	White	w/c	Bae

Total beds 8
Beds available 1

Figure 16-6 • *The health unit coordinator has a census board that is kept at the workstation within easy reach for information.*

medical records may not be made without written permission of the patient and health care facility. The health unit coordinator may have the patient sign the copy request before actually copying patient medical records. Copying is done according to the policies and procedures of the health care facility.

BULLETIN BOARDS

Posting information on bulletin boards is an effective way of sharing information with staff members who work a variety of shifts on the same unit. The health unit coordinator will find this form of communication to be an efficient and effective way of sharing information with members of the nursing care team. The information posted is information of interest to the staff. It would typically include staff schedules, policy updates, procedure changes, and health system changes and updates, as well as information specific to that unit or department.

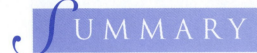

SUMMARY

Communication devices are devices that allow the health unit coordinator to provide members of the health care team with the information they need in order to provide the best possible patient care to each individual patient. They can range from devices as simple as a bulletin board, where written information can be posted for a set amount of time, to as technologically innovative devices as a handheld computer that communicates lab values to health care providers when tests are completed. The telephone is the most frequently used communication device, but computer systems, capable of providing information at the touch of a fingertip from anywhere in the world, are running a close second. Communication devices will continue to be developed to make sharing of information faster, more reliable, and more secure. Health unit coordinators will be the users of these communication devices, communicating information to health care team members who have a need to know the information so as to provide quality care to patients in the most efficient time.

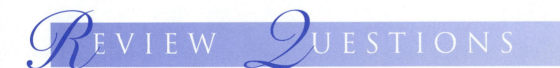

REVIEW QUESTIONS

1. Explain the value of communication devices in a health care setting in a paragraph of 10 sentences. Include all the key terms for communication devices.

2. List four communication devices that may be on a patient care unit and describe what they are used for communicating.

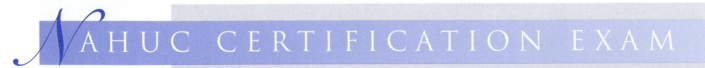

NAHUC CERTIFICATION EXAM

CONTENT AREAS

II. B. 1   Receive diagnostic test results

II. B. 3   Report diagnostic test results to nursing staff

II. D. 6   Maintain unit bulletin board

II. E. 6   Maintain patient census boards

II. E. 8   Maintain patient assignment board

II. F. 7   Respond to patient, physician, visitor, and facility staff requests and complaints

III. A. 1   Communicate with patients and staff via intercom

III. A. 2   Send and receive documents via fax machine

III. A. 3   Contact personnel via telecommunications systems (e.g., pagers, cell phones)

III. A. 4   Answer and process unit telephone calls

III. B. 1   Maintain computer census (i.e., ADT functions)

III. B. 4   Enter orders via computers

III. B. 5   Schedule appointments via computers

III. B. 6   Prepare documents using computer software

III. B. 7   Generate reports using computers

III. B. 8   Operate computers safely and correctly

III. B. 9   Troubleshoot problems with computers

III. D. 1   Duplicate documents using a copy machine

III. D. 2   Transport patient specimens, supplies, and medication using pneumatic tubes

THROUGH THE EYES

OF A HEALTH CARE PROFESSIONAL

Communication devices are the tools of the health unit coordinator profession. The telephone and computer are communication devices that are used throughout the shift. The phone never seems to stop ringing. It is constantly bringing information and answers to questions. The computer system allows the health unit coordinator access to people, places, and results at the touch of a few keystrokes. Communication devices have allowed communication to happen at an accurate and faster rate than ever thought possible.

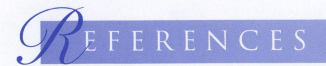

REFERENCES

LaFleur-Brooks, M. (2004). *Health unit coordinating* (5th ed.). Philadelphia: Saunders.

Simmers, L. (2004). *Diversified health occupations essentials* (6th ed.). Clifton Park, NY: Thomson Delmar Learning.

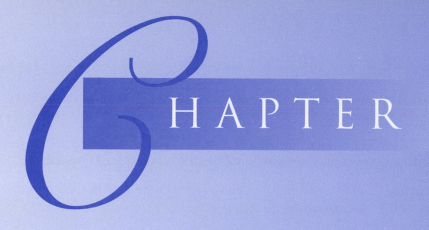

C HAPTER 17

Orientating and Training Personnel

Learning Objectives

Upon completion of this chapter and review questions, the learner should be able to:

1. Define key terms.

2. List four situations in which health unit coordinators may train or be trained.

3. List the three primary roles of the preceptor, or trainer.

4. Describe the four phases of reality shock.

5. Explain how to apply adult learning principles to orientation and training.

6. List three methods to identify learning needs.

7. List three learning activities to meet learning needs.

8. Demonstrate how to give constructive feedback.

Key Terms

advocate One who supports or helps another by defending or comforting.

educator One who teaches or shares knowledge with another.

internship A form of on-the-job training that usually combines job training with classroom instructions in trade schools, high schools, colleges, or universities.

mission statement   A written statement of purpose that defines the essence of the health care system.

organizational culture   A pattern of shared values and beliefs giving members of an organization meaning and providing them with rules for behavior.

orientation   The planned introduction of new employees to their jobs, their co-workers, and the organization.

preceptor   An employee assigned to act as a role model, advocate, and educator for someone learning a new task or job responsibility.

role model   One who serves as an example worthy of imitation.

rounds   A term given to the practice of health care team members or students and their instructor reviewing patient cases, usually involving a face-to-face visit with the patients.

social norms   The customs or culture of the department.

vision statement   A written statement defining the health care system's future and the direction that will be pursued in achieving it.

TEACHING IS A FUNCTION OF HEALTH CARE

Teaching and training are primary functions in the health care field. In order to provide the best care possible, health care facilities have to grow and change to keep pace with rapidly expanding technology and patient care delivery systems. Learning and training are ongoing activities within health care facilities. Training takes place in a variety of settings within the health care field.

HEALTH CARE FACILITIES TEACH THEIR EMPLOYEES

Health care facilities provide training for their own employees. Examples of training for employees include training for newly hired employees to teach them about the facility; training to meet the safety requirements of regulatory agencies (see Chapter 10); training to become proficient in the use of job-related equipment such as computers, nursing equipment, and x-ray machines; and training to learn procedures for the job such as administering medication or transferring a patient to another unit (Figure 17-1).

HEALTH CARE FACILITIES TEACH STUDENTS

Many health care facilities develop partnerships with schools. For example, a hospital may have a partnership with a university that teaches student physicians, more commonly referred to as medical students. The hospital may provide **internships** for the medical students. Mathis and Jackson (1994) define an internship as "a form of on-the-job training that usually combines job training with classroom instructions in trade schools, high schools, colleges, or universities." The university benefits because the medical students are able to learn from exposure to real patients. The hospital benefits by having the prestige of being associated with an institution of higher learning and from the diversity and skills offered to the patients from the students and their instructors. The hospitals, by being able to directly observe the work habits, knowledge,

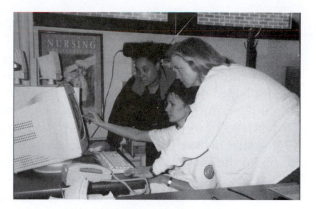

Figure 17-1 • *Training is needed to become proficient in the use of the hospital information system.*

and attitudes of the students are able to better select job candidates who will both meet the job requirements and have good compatibility with the health care facility and its other employees. Besides partnerships with medical schools involving internships for medical students, health care facilities often enter into partnerships with extended-care facilities to provide training programs for nurse's aides, or with community colleges that offer health unit coordinator training programs.

TRAINING AND THE HEALTH UNIT COORDINATOR

A health unit coordinator will have the opportunity to be trained and to train. A health unit coordinator will receive initial training when newly hired and ongoing training as the need arises. In turn, a health unit coordinator will train students and employees. Because a health unit coordinator will play the role of both the learner and the teacher, this chapter addresses orientation and training from both perspectives. Training situations for health unit coordinators include:

◆ Training a newly hired health unit coordinator who has formal job-specific education

◆ Training a newly hired health unit coordinator who does not have formal job-specific training

◆ Training a newly hired health unit coordinator who has experience

◆ Training a newly hired health unit coordinator who does not have experience

◆ Training the health care facility staff to use the hospital information system

◆ Orienting the new nursing staff to the nonclinical operations of the department

◆ Orienting the medical staff to the nonclinical operations of the department

◆ Training internship students

◆ Training volunteers

ORIENTATION

Orientation is defined by Mathis and Jackson (1994) as "the planned introduction of new employees to their jobs, their co-workers, and the organization." Orientation may be divided into two phases: orientation to the employer and orientation to specific job duties. In most health care facilities, orientation to the employer occurs within the first few days of employment. New employees from all departments are assigned to meet together to have the opportunity to learn about their employer (Figure 17-2). Information about the employer's mission statement, vision statement, and organizational culture is given to the new employee. Both the mission statement and vision statements were discussed in Chapter 8. The **mission statement** is a written statement of purpose that defines the essence of the health care system. Mission statements often outline the organization's purpose and goals as well as the services it aspires to provide. A **vision statement** is a written statement defining the health care system's future and the direction that will be pursued in achieving it. Both the mission statement and vision statement can help the new employee become familiar with the company. Mathis and Jackson (1994) define **organizational culture** as "a pattern of shared values and beliefs giving members of an organization meaning and providing them with rules for behavior."

The orientation of newly hired employees to the health care facility often includes presentations and information from senior management of the organization as well as from key members of such departments as administration, human resources, employee health, education, and security (Table 17-1). The format for orientation will vary from one health care facility to another. Individual health care facilities design an orientation program to meet their specific situation, to be compatible with their culture, and to help in meeting their mission and vision.

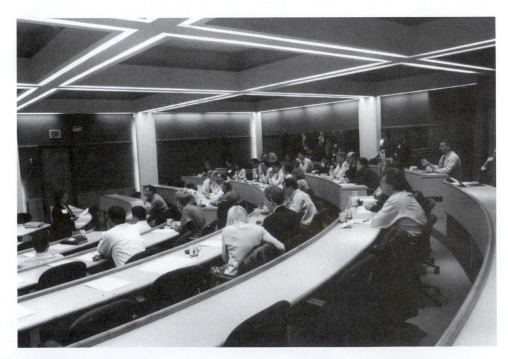

Figure 17-2 • *Orientation of employees in a health care facility (Courtesy of Aurora Health Care, Milwaukee, WI)*

TABLE 17-1   Sample Orientation Schedule

DAY	TIME	TOPIC	PRESENTED BY
Day 1	8:00 A.M.	Welcome and Mission Statement	Chief Executive Officer
	8:15 A.M.	Forms and Benefits	Human Resources
	9:30 A.M.	Employee Wellness and Immunizations	Employee Health
	10:30 A.M.	Break	
	10:45 A.M.	Safety	Environmental Services
	11:45 A.M.	Security/Parking	Security Department
	12:15 P.M.	Lunch	
	1:15 P.M.	Infection Control	Epidemiology
	2:15 P.M.	Employee Assistance Program	EAP
	2:30 P.M.	Tour and Scavenger Hunt	Human Resources
	3:45 P.M.	Preview of Day Two	Human Resources
Day 2	8:00 A.M.	Confidentiality/HIPAA	Risk Management
	10:00 A.M.	Break	
	10:15 A.M.	Customer Service	Guest Relations
	12:15 P.M.	Questions and Answers	Human Resources

PRECEPTOR/TRAINER

A health unit coordinator will also be oriented to the specific work area and trained to the specific job responsibilities. Training may take place in a classroom or within the department. Many health care facilities utilize **preceptors** in the training process. Following are some of the definitions that apply to a preceptor:

◆ An experienced employee selected according to specific criteria to serve as a resource person to new employees.

◆ Someone who provides role support and learning experiences while continuing to perform some or all of the other responsibilities of his or her position.

◆ Someone who assists and supports a staff member through a planned orientation.

◆ One who teaches health professional students.

◆ An experienced and competent staff member who has received formal training to function in this capacity and serves as a role model and resource person to new staff members.

The common themes in the above definitions are experienced employee, support, and teacher or resource person. For the purposes of this chapter, the definition of *preceptor*, from the Primedia *Ensuring Success* video is used and written as "an employee assigned to act as a role model, advocate, and educator for someone learning a new task or job responsibility." The proportion of the three roles (role model, advocate, and educator) of the preceptor, or trainer, is determined by the training situation. In some training situations, such as having a health unit coordinator student observe the department activities, the role model role will be emphasized. When an experienced health unit coordinator who has transferred in from another department within the same facility is being introduced to the staff, the advocate role will be emphasized. When a registered nurse is being trained in the use of the computerized order entry system, the educator role will be emphasized. An understanding of all three roles—role model, advocate, and educator—can be beneficial when training and also when being trained.

ROLE MODEL

A **role model** is one who serves as an example worthy of imitation. A health unit coordinator role model's key responsibility is to perform all of the duties and responsibilities of a health unit coordinator as they are defined in the job description. The role of the health unit coordinator in modeling is that of a competent health unit coordinator. In the many definitions of the term *preceptor*, the words *experience* and *competence* are often used. The first step in being a preceptor is being able to perform the job one is teaching.

In Chapter 2, health unit coordinator responsibilities were shown in a variety of job descriptions. In most health unit coordinator job descriptions, there are statements about fulfilling duties as described; demonstrating safety; utilizing resources effectively; communicating effectively with patients, families, and staff; and maintaining effective working relationships.

The first step in fulfilling the responsibility of role model as a preceptor is to make sure one does the job one is hired to do and that one is fulfilling the described duties. Preceptors aspiring to be role models may first want to examine their own job descriptions and compare their performance against the written job description to determine if they are fulfilling the duties as described. Preceptors could also compare their behavior with the National Association of Health Unit Coordinators (NAHUC) Code of Ethics and their performance with the NAHUC Standards of Practice.

As a role model, a preceptor should demonstrate safety according to the policies of the health care facility. A role model uses resources efficiently and effectively. Last, and definitely not least, a role model has effective communication skills and positive customer relations. The first three points—fulfilling duties, demonstrating safety, and utilizing resources effectively—are extremely important in modeling the role of a competent health unit coordinator, but without effective communication skills, the role model is incomplete. The person who is being trained looks not only at what is done but also at how it is done.

ADVOCATE

An **advocate** is one who supports or helps another by defending or comforting. The preceptor responsibility as advocate is how the preceptor facilitates the social integration of the trainee into the work group. As an advocate, the preceptor is responsible for helping the trainee fit in and feel welcome. Things the preceptor can do to assist the trainee in becoming part of the health care work team include:

- ◆ Introduce the trainee to the staff, including the physicians

- ◆ Make sure the staff knows the new employee is in training

- ◆ Explain the department's routine schedule, such as hours of operations, start and stop times for shifts, and break times

- ◆ Explain how time off is requested and awarded

- ◆ Include the trainee in breaks and meals

- ◆ Provide a tour of the department

- ◆ Explain the social norms to the employee

Social norms are the customs or culture of the department. Examples of social norms are outside activities in which the staff participates, birthdays or holidays that are observed, how money is collected for gifts, what gifts are purchased, and what is done for bereavement. Knowledge of the social norms is beneficial. Being familiar with the social norms allows one to fit in, to be accepted by other employees, and to be comfortable in the work environment.

Reality Shock

An understanding of the four stages of reality shock and biculturalism can assist the preceptor in understanding the needs of the trainee. Most trainees have completed some classroom training before their arrival to the new workstation. For some trainees, the new job may be their first job or their first job in health care. For others, the new job may be the same role within a new department or facility. Whatever the training or work background may be, the trainee brings expectations to the new work environment. The term *reality shock* is sometimes used to describe the reaction of trainees when they discover that the new work environment does not always match the values and ideals that they had anticipated. According to the Health Sciences/Columbia Web page, there are four stages, or phases, of adaptation to reality shock: "the honeymoon, the shock, the recovery, and the resolution" (Figure 17-3).

The honeymoon stage is one of excitement and exhilaration. Often, the trainee sees only the good about the new job or employer. The trainee may have the impression that everything is great. During the honeymoon stage, the trainee usually performs well. The trainee may master new skills easily and appear to be fitting in well in the

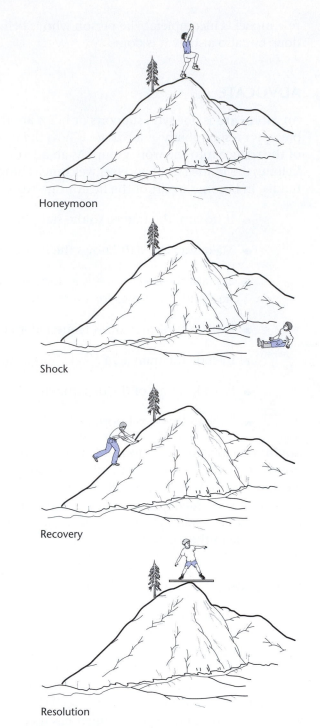

Honeymoon

Shock

Recovery

Resolution

Figure 17-3 • *The four stages of reality shock: honeymoon, shock, recovery, and resolution.*

new environment. During the honeymoon stage, the preceptor can share the trainee's enthusiasm and show the trainee new tasks and ideas.

The shock stage follows. During the shock stage, the trainee realizes that the new job is not exactly what was expected or prepared for. The trainee may experience conflict, including conflict about expectations and reality, between school and work. The trainee may also be disappointed with her own performance, feeling she is not learning the skills as quickly as she had expected. During the shock phase, the trainee may display anger, fatigue, and confusion. During this stage the preceptor can listen and provide the trainee an opportunity to vent. The preceptor can encourage the trainee to write down her feelings and negative observations and her recommendations for change, encouraging her to reevaluate her observations at a later date. Trainees may benefit by being able to spend time with other trainees to share coping techniques. During the shock phase, the preceptor can make sure that the trainee has a chance to perform the skills that she does well to encourage her.

Recovery is the third stage of reality shock. During this stage, the trainee is able to view the situation with a balanced perspective. The trainee realizes that not everything about the new job is bad when compared with the original expectations or beliefs about the job. The trainee's performance may improve, and a returned sense of humor may lift the negative feelings of the shock phase. The preceptor can continue the advocate role, encouraging the trainee to recognize the positives of previous and current situations. The preceptor can also explain the facility's channels for change and quality improvement.

The fourth and last stage of reality shock is resolution. During this stage, the trainee is able to combine past and present beliefs or expectations, thereby keeping the best of both worlds. This combination or blending of beliefs may be referred to as biculturalism and it is the desired outcome or end of reality shock. There may be outcomes or resolutions other than biculturalism. The trainee may resolve the reality shock conflict by rejecting previous values or expectations and may change careers. The trainee may reject the new values and change employers. Some trainees continue to battle conflict between their previous values and expectations and their current job throughout their career. These trainees may stay with the new job but continue to complain and be unhappy. If the trainee continues to experience conflict, the preceptor may need to refer the trainee for help with transition. The following is an example of how the preceptor can be an advocate and role model for the trainee.

> A preceptor has been assigned to work with a new health unit coordinator student during his internship. The trainee is a recent high school graduate and is attending a training program at the local vocational school. The trainee tells the preceptor that he admires her and the work she does. The trainee often quotes the preceptor and tries to mimic the preceptor's behavior. The trainee is displaying behaviors in the honeymoon stage of reality shock. As the trainee's advocate, the preceptor can use this upbeat period to introduce the student to new people and tasks. The preceptor recognizes that she is being observed closely at this time and strives to be a positive role model.

EDUCATOR

The third primary role of the preceptor is that of educator. An **educator** is one who teaches or shares knowledge with another. In the educator role, the preceptor has three responsibilities:

1. Identify learning needs.

2. Plan learning experiences.

3. Evaluate learning experiences.

Principles of Adult Learning

It is important for a preceptor to know basic principles of adult learning. There are many adult learning models. The Malcolm Knowles model is summarized below. When a person is training or being trained, it is helpful to apply the principles of adult learning. In 1970, in *The Modern Practice of Adult Education*, Knowles defined *andragogy* as an emerging technology for adult learning. He proposed that andragogy, a learner-focused approach for adults, be considered an alternative to pedagogy (the art of teaching children). His four andragogical assumptions are that adults:

1. Move from dependency to self-directedness.

2. Draw upon their reservoir of experience for learning.

3. Are ready to learn when they assume new roles.

4. Want to solve problems and apply new knowledge immediately.

Accordingly, Knowles suggested that adult educators should:

- Set a cooperative learning climate

- Create mechanisms for mutual planning

- Arrange for a diagnosis of learner needs and interests

- Enable the formulation of learning objectives based on the diagnosed needs and interests

- Design sequential activities for achieving the objectives

- Execute the design by selecting methods, materials, and resources

- Evaluate the quality of the learning experience while rediagnosing needs for further learning

Identify Learning Needs

Before learning needs can be identified, expectations have to be identified. The expectations are what the trainee needs to know. Expectations will vary according to various learning situations. Often, the very first part of identifying learning needs, identifying expectations, is overlooked. The tools that can be used to identify expectations are:

- Orientation assessments

- Orientation checklists

- Job descriptions and competencies required

- Policies and procedures

- Practice standards

- Job duty checklists

Once the expectations or what the trainee needs to know have been identified, learning needs are identified. The learning needs are the gaps between the expectations and what the trainee is currently able to do.

According to the adult learning model, each trainee will have a unique background and experience. As an educator, the preceptor should not assume what the trainee does or does not know. As Knowles wrote, the educator can arrange a diagnosis of learner needs and interests. To identify learning needs, the preceptor can:

◆ Ask the trainee questions about work experience

◆ Review the trainee's application and résumé

◆ Observe the trainee

◆ Listen to the trainee

◆ Administer a pretest

◆ Ask the trainee to do a self-assessment of a list of skills and indicate which items he or she is not able to perform, is able to perform with assistance, or is able to perform independently

Plan Learning Experiences

After identifying learning needs, the preceptor and trainee can set objectives for learning. These objectives are based on the identified needs and, to be valid, should be written in clear, observable, measurable terms. The preceptor should write expectations in terms of behaviors that can be observed. For example, how does one observe and measure whether someone is remembering something or understanding something? However, one can observe someone doing something. For example, one can observe someone stating something, describing something, or demonstrating, writing, listing, or reciting.

Learning objectives should include an action, an object or skill, a standard of performance, conditions, and a target date. For example:

Action: Demonstrate

Object: Patient admission

Standard of performance: According to steps listed in HUC Entry Level Education Competencies

Conditions: Without assistance

Target date: Friday Aug 16

Once the objectives have been decided, according to Knowles's principles, educators should design activities for achieving the objectives and then select methods, materials, and other resources for executing the designed activities. It is important to involve the trainee in choosing the instructional method or learning activity. Some educators will choose what they think is the easiest way to teach something without determining the trainee's situation. The hazard in this approach is that everyone learns differently. As an educator, the preceptor can try to determine the easiest way for the trainee to learn something. Most people can identify the way they learn best. The preceptor can ask the trainee the preferred learning methods and use this information for a successful learning experience. The preceptor can observe if the trainee prefers to read, hear, see, or do.

In most training situations, observing and practicing are key ways of learning. But having the trainees observe and practice may make the preceptors feel they have a permanent shadow and may make the trainees feel they are underfoot and in the way. Using a variety of learning experiences and activities can prevent those feelings (Figures 17-4 and 17-5). There are many instructional methods or experiences the preceptor can use:

◆ Hospital procedures manuals

◆ Books

◆ Self-learning modules

◆ Audiotapes and videotapes

◆ CD-ROMs

◆ **Rounds** (reviewing patient cases and, usually, visiting the patients)

◆ Tours

◆ Computer simulations

◆ Computer-assisted instruction

◆ Observation and practice

◆ Search-and-find exercises

◆ Skills labs

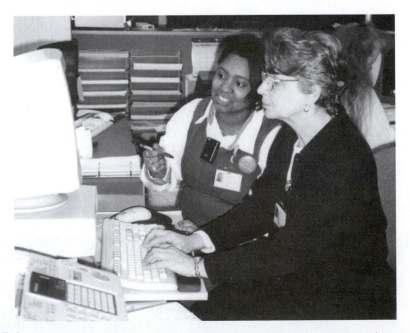

Figure 17-4 • *The preceptor arranges time for the trainee to observe and practice. (Courtesy of All Saints Health Care, Racine, WI)*

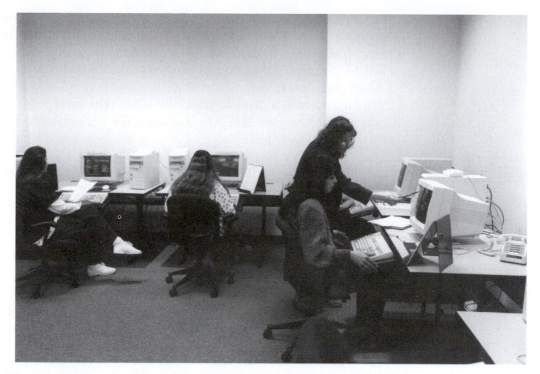

Figure 17-5 • *Participating in simulated computer training is a learning experience. (Courtesy of Aurora Health Care, Milwaukee, WI)*

Evaluate Learning

The third responsibility of the preceptor, as an educator, is to evaluate the quality of the learning. According to Knowles, both the educator and the trainee should evaluate the training on an ongoing basis. There are various methods of evaluation:

- Post-tests

- Written exercises

- Simulation exercises

- Discussion

- Feedback from other staff

- Attendance at in-services

- Attendance at department meetings

- Attendance at classes

- Observation

The majority of the evaluation process will involve the preceptor's observing the trainee. The preceptor and trainee will spend a fair amount of time exchanging information. This information exchange, or feedback, can provide information about performance and how to improve performance and can build confidence for the trainee.

It is important for the preceptor to give positive feedback and praise when the trainee is performing well. Although praise can be given in public for other health care team members to hear, criticism should be offered in private. Feedback should be offered as close to the time of the observation as possible. In addition to on-the-spot feedback, allow some quiet time for reviewing the learning needs and activities (Figure 17-6). Evaluation should include feedback from both the preceptor and the trainee. Let trainees evaluate themselves. To encourage the trainees to do this self-evaluation, ask them to share their perceptions of what is going well and what could be improved.

A nonthreatening way for the preceptor to share observations is to use "I" statements. An "I" statement is phrased to guard against putting someone on the defensive. Use the following five steps and examples for creating "I" statements.

1. Describe the behavior that has been observed. What actions need to be reinforced or corrected? Describe behavior, not a personality trait. Be specific about the behavior, include the who, what, when, and where of the behavior.

   Preceptor: "I see charts piling up on the desk and phones are not being answered before the third ring."

2. Describe reactions, the consequences, and how the behavior made you feel.

   Preceptor: "I worry that we are not carrying through with the physicians' orders and meeting our patients and families needs."

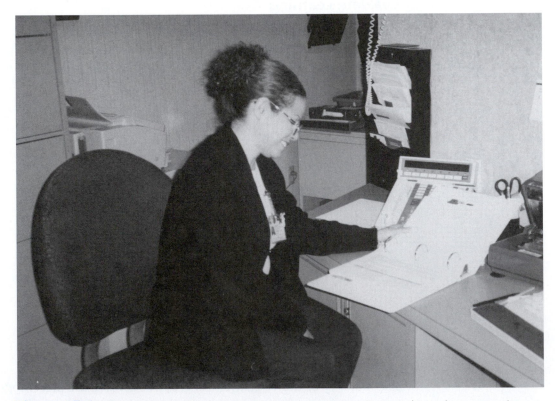

Figure 17-6 • *Reading policy and procedure manuals is a learning experience. (Courtesy of All Saints Health Care, Racine, WI)*

3. Give the trainee an opportunity to respond.

Trainee: "I know. It seems like as soon as I start to transcribe information into a patient's chart the phone rings. Then I answer the phone and it seems to take me forever to locate whatever information the person on the phone wants. When I finally get back to the charts I have forgotten where I was at or which chart I was working on. Meanwhile, two more charts have mysteriously been added to my desk. I just don't know where the time goes."

4. Suggest alternative behaviors and share ideas.

Preceptor: "Yes, I agree. One nice thing about this job, there is seldom time to worry about having too much time on your hands. I suggest that together we can make up a little procedure for you to follow until you become more familiar with the job. It will help you identify what has to been done right away and what can be postponed for a while. What do you think?"

Trainee: "That would be neat. I haven't been able to figure out what to do first. I was beginning to think I should just take the phone off the hook until I get caught up."

Preceptor: "Well, I'm happy you haven't lost your sense of humor—I know you are just joking. We have to find a way you can keep up with the charts and still answer the phone before the third ring. For a start, I suggest you consider making it a habit to read through the physician's orders as they are written, prioritize charts, and begin transcribing orders when they are received."

Continue discussing how prioritizing and other techniques will help.

5. Summarize and express support.

Preceptor: "OK here is what I believe we are going to do. I'll stop by every hour and we can discuss any problems that come up or anything you do not understand. I'm sure in very little time you will have no problem in handling the phone traffic and in keeping the charts current."

ORIENTATION AND TRAINING RECORD

Documentation is a huge component of health care. Physicians' orders, nursing observations, and patient information are documented. Staff information is also documented. Job applications, immunization records, and evaluations are examples of employee information that is documented. Most health care employers document the orientation or training process. Most health care training programs document the internship process as well. An orientation tool, or form, may be used for documentation. The orientation form may include a list of job competencies, a self-assessment key, learning activities or requirements, and evaluation comments (Table 17-2). A structured tool such as an orientation record can assist both the preceptor and trainee in understanding expectations.

TABLE 17-2 Orientation Tool					
Performance Expectations	**Self-Assessment**	**Learning Options**	**Evaluation Mechanisms**	**Date Met/ Signature**	**Comments**

ORIENTATION AND TRAINING BENEFITS AND CHALLENGES

A training experience has important benefits and challenges. Consideration of the benefits and challenges is part of preparation. The value of providing a training experience is dependent on preparation. Benefits of being a trainer include:

◆ Joy of watching a student develop

◆ Opportunity to share one's knowledge and experience

◆ Feeling useful

◆ Chance to reenergize

◆ Regaining fun of job

◆ Reminder of why chose profession

◆ Revitalized interest in work

◆ Enhanced self-esteem and confidence

◆ Supporting and strengthening the profession

◆ Helping shape the next generation of professionals

◆ Learning about precepting through preceptor development and training programs

◆ Fulfillment of own developmental needs

◆ Exposure to new and different thinking styles, knowledge, and perspectives

◆ Recognition

Challenges of training include:

◆ Burn-out

◆ Lack of confidence in an educator role

◆ Workload too heavy or lack of time

◆ Difficulty balancing needs of unit and needs of preceptee

◆ Unsupportive colleagues

◆ Personality conflicts

◆ Lack of clarity of expectations

ORIENTATION AND TRAINING RESOURCES

One approach to training challenges is to look at the challenges as needs. One may state the needs to one's supervisor or manager, education department, or instructor. Present at least one option for a solution when stating the challenge or need. For example, if one does not feel confident in the educator role, state this need to the supervisor and ask for additional training. If one is having difficulty training and keeping up with the workload, this problem can be brought to the supervisor's attention along with a request to be relieved from the desk periodically to teach and answer questions away from the pressing needs of the workstation. If there is a lack of training expectations, one can ask to work with someone in the education or staff development department to clearly define what is expected. A department manager or supervisor can be a resource for a preceptor when the preceptor identifies a need. The human resources and education departments may have preceptor learning resources such as staff development and training journals, books, and videotapes for both the preceptor and the trainee. Successful preceptors have access to resources and support. Ask for them.

SUMMARY

Training is an important function in the health care environment. The three primary roles of a preceptor are role model, advocate, and educator. As a role model, remember that the trainee is watching what is done and how it is done. As an advocate, make the trainee feel welcome and be aware of the stages of reality shock. As an educator, identify learning needs by comparing the role expectations with the trainee's current capabilities. Plan activities to address the needs. Follow up with constructive feedback, and allow trainees to evaluate themselves and the training experience.

REVIEW QUESTIONS

1. List four health unit coordinator training situations.

2. List three primary roles of a preceptor.

Match the scenarios in the right column with the reality shock stage that best describes it in the left column.

3. Honeymoon   a. Angry and frustrated with new job

4. Shock   b. Able to see more than one side or perspective

5. Recovery   c. Absolutely loves new job

6. Resolution   d. Biculturalism

7. "Although an adult may be new to a job, she brings her own previous experiences to the job." Is this statement true or false?

8. "Adult learners are eager to apply knowledge to the new job." Is this statement true or false?

9. List three examples of learning activities.

10. Give an example of constructive feedback using an "I" statement.

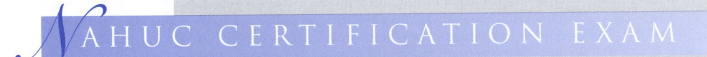

NAHUC CERTIFICATION EXAM

CONTENT AREAS

II. F. 1   Orient new staff members to the unit

II. F. 2   Precept new or student unit coordinators

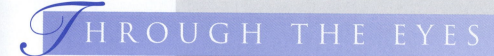

THROUGH THE EYES

OF A HEALTH CARE PROFESSIONAL

A health unit coordinator who successfully completed her orientation and training shares survival tips for the new health unit coordinator:

Take notes when you ask questions to avoid having to ask the same thing over and over.

Ask for time with your preceptor during breaks or downtime to review your notes and your progress.

Accept corrections with an open mind. Learn from your mistakes.

Be friendly, but do not involve yourself in personal conversations that do not pertain the work.

Find positive ways to cope with stress.

Congratulate yourself on a job well done. Write down your successes and remind yourself that you are making progress.

Keep a daily log to show yourself how far you have come.

Remember, you can't learn everything at once.

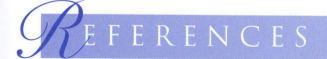

REFERENCES

Knowles, M. S. (1970). *The modern practice of adult education: Andragogy versus pedagogy.* New York: Association Press.

Mathis, R. L., & Jackson, J. J. (1994). *Human resource management* (7th ed.). Saint Paul, MN: West Publishing.

Primedia/HSTN (Producer). (2001). EDA 314-0103 *Ensuring success: Health unit coordinator preceptor roles presented by Sandy Ayres.* [Video program]. Carrollton, TX: Primedia/HSTN.

Reality shock, or from novice to expert. *http://www.healthsciences.columbia.edu/dept/nursing/preceptors/realityshock.html* Accessed December 2003.

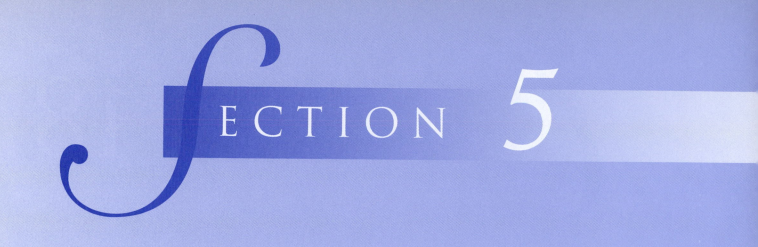

SECTION 5

Critical Thinking and Cultural Diversity

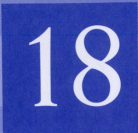

CHAPTER 18

Critical Thinking

Learning Objectives

Upon completion of this chapter and review questions, the learner should be able to:

1. Define key terms.

2. Explain why critical thinking is important in the workplace.

3. Explain how to prioritize.

4. Describe how to use a "to-do" list to manage time.

5. Give two examples of each of the three group interaction roles.

6. Describe problem-solving techniques.

Key Terms

critical thinking The ability to solve problems by making sense of information using creative, intuitive, logical, and analytical mental processes.

prioritization Organizing tasks in order of importance.

quality circle A small group of employees who monitor specific practices or trends and suggest solutions for improvement.

to-do list A form that can be used to plan and organize the tasks that need to be completed.

Abbreviations

SCANS Secretary's Commission on Achieving Necessary Skills

STAT Immediately or urgent

CRITICAL THINKING IN A CHANGING WORK WORLD

A health unit coordinator is a member of the health care team and works within an environment of change. Health unit coordinators face the same challenges as other members of the health care team. Those challenges include working with rapidly expanding technology, working with smaller budgets, facing more competition for health care revenue, being asked to do more with less, being asked to be self-directed, and working well with diverse team members. In the broader picture, these are challenges faced by all members of the work world.

These challenges demand that employees be clear thinkers. Employees must know how to manage their time. They need to know how to use resources. They need to know how to make decisions and solve problems. The term to describe these skills in health care is **critical thinking**. Snyder (1993) describes critical thinking as "the ability to solve problems by making sense of information using creative, intuitive, logical, and analytical mental processes. . . . and the process is continual." Jo Ann Klein identified skills that are required in critical thinking such as "the ability to set priorities by weighing risks and benefits, identification of appropriate interventions, decision making, and exceptional communication skills." To be a high-performance employee, one needs to quickly think through a situation and determine the best course of action for the desired outcome, whether it be mastering a new computer application or assisting a disgruntled family member.

THE SECRETARY'S COMMISSION ON ACHIEVING NECESSARY SKILLS

As stated in the U.S. Department of Labor Web site: "The Secretary's Commission on Achieving Necessary Skills (SCANS) was appointed by the U.S. Secretary of Labor to determine the skills that people need to succeed in the world of work. The Commission's fundamental purpose is to encourage a high-performance economy characterized by high-skill, high-wage employment. As outlined in the SCANS report, a high-performance workplace requires workers who have a solid foundation in basic literacy and computational skills, in the thinking skills necessary to put knowledge to work, and in the personal qualities that make workers dedicated and trustworthy. But a solid foundation is not enough. High-performance workplaces also require competencies: the ability to manage resources, to work amicably and productively with others, to acquire and use information, to master complex systems, and to work with a variety of technologies. This combination of foundation skills and workplace competencies is what is needed in the world of work."

The workplace know-how identified by SCANS is made up of five competencies and three foundation skills and personal qualities that are needed for solid job performance. These are listed in Table 18-1.

TABLE 18-1 Workplace Know-How	
Workplace competencies: Effective workers can productively use:	◆ Resources. They know how to allocate time, money, materials, space, and staff.
	◆ Interpersonal skills. They can work on teams, teach others, serve customers, lead, negotiate, and work well with people from culturally diverse backgrounds.
	◆ Information. They can acquire and evaluate data, organize and maintain files, interpret and communicate, and use computers to process information.
	◆ Systems. They understand social, organizational, and technological systems; they can monitor and correct performance; and they can design or improve systems.
	◆ Technology. They can select equipment and tools, apply technology to specific tasks, and maintain and troubleshoot equipment.
Foundation skills: Competent workers in the high-performance workplace need:	◆ Basic skills. Reading, writing, arithmetic and mathematics, speaking, and listening
	◆ Thinking skills. The ability to learn, to reason, to think creatively, to make decisions, and to solve problems
	◆ Personal qualities. Individual responsibility, self-esteem and self-management, sociability, and integrity

TIME MANAGEMENT

The SCANS report states that a successful worker knows how to allocate time. The report states, "A successful worker selects relevant, goal-related activities; ranks them in order of importance; allocates time to activities; and understands, prepares, and follows schedules." Health unit coordinators work in an environment requiring multitasking and prioritizing. It is not uncommon to have a visitor asking directions, a physician asking where a patient is, ambulance drivers awaiting paperwork, the phone ringing, and at least eight charts with orders to be transcribed all within the same time. A health unit coordinator is expected to manage time and tasks. A key aspect of time management is being able to prioritize.

PRIORITIZATION

Prioritization can be defined as organizing tasks in order of importance. In health care, the term *stat* is used to mean immediately. All of the health care team members know that a stat request must be taken care of immediately. The problem arises when more than one stat request is made at a time and when other requests are pending too. For example, a health unit coordinator encounters a physician writing stat orders to be transcribed, a nurse asking for a respiratory treatment to be performed stat, and a patient care technician bringing a specimen that has to be delivered to the lab stat. The health unit coordinator must determine which stat task has to be performed first. This determination of what needs to be done first is prioritization. In determining what needs to be done first, patient safety is the main factor. One must tend to the stat requests that pertain to patient safety before all others. Another factor in prioritization is the length of time that will be required to complete the task. In other words, a health unit coordinator may determine that he or she will perform several of the quickest tasks first to allow time for the longer tasks. For example, the health unit coordinator may page the respiratory therapist to request a stat breathing treatment, return a phone call to surgery letting them know the patient is ready, fax a lab result to the physician's office and then focus on the new set of admission orders that need to be transcribed. Another factor in prioritization is grouping tasks that can be performed together. For example, the health unit coordinator may determine that it will save time to make phone calls and print chart forms from the computer at the same time. The ability to successfully perform more than one task at a time is called multitasking. With experience, a health unit coordinator will be able to multitask. Prioritization is a skill that is developed with experience over time. Inexperienced health unit coordinators may have to ask for assistance in prioritizing until they become familiar with the type of tasks they will be encountering.

ORGANIZING TASKS

A health unit coordinator must manage time well. Usually, the health unit coordinator is responsible for completing the work without having someone give him or her a schedule. Health unit coordinators' workload is determined by factors and events over which they have no control. For example, the health unit coordinator has no control over what time the physicians will make rounds and write orders. The health unit coordinator has no control over the emergencies that bring the patient to the health care facility for services. Because the health unit coordinator has no control over these events, it is important to manage time well so that all the tasks will be completed in a timely fashion.

There will be routine tasks that the health unit coordinator has to do every workday or work shift. Routine tasks include entering patient charges, stuffing and thinning charts, ordering patient and clerical supplies, and entering daily lab tests. The efficient health unit coordinator will manage those tasks and allow time for the nonroutine tasks. One way to manage the workday is to develop a "**to-do list**." A to-do list is a form that can be used to plan and organize the tasks that need to be completed. Other terms for a to-do list are activity sheet, memory board, and brainboard. At the beginning of the work shift, the health unit coordinator can determine the routine and scheduled activities that must be done and create a to-do list (Table 18-2). For example, the health unit coordinator may pull the department census and scheduled activities from the hospital information system or from listening to the staff report at the beginning of the work shift. In addition to the patient activities, the health unit coordinator can also list routine tasks that need to be completed. The list can also be used to track and record phone calls.

The to-do list is just a tool. The health unit coordinator has to use the tool for it to be effective. Sometimes the to-do list fails to keep one on track. Table 18-3 lists common problems and suggestions for the to-do list.

TABLE 18-2   Health Unit Coordinator To-Do List

Room	Name	Labs	Diagnostics	Diet	Other
401					
402					
403-A					
403-B					
404					
406-A					
406-B					

Today's Tasks	Deadline	Completed
Chart maintenance	Beginning of shift	
Chart maintenance	End of shift	
Patient charges	Noon	
Update bulletin board with new policies	End of shift	
Set up charts for evening admissions	2:00 P.M.	

Long-Term Tasks		
Complete patient satisfaction committee assignment	June 4	
Complete mandatory safety self-study packet	June 18	

Date/Time	Phone Calls (Name/Purpose)

TABLE 18-3 To-Do List Suggestions	
Problem	**Suggestions**
The list gets longer each day and is never finished.	Be realistic; record what is actually accomplished each day for a week to give a realistic picture of what can be done in an average workday.
A crisis interferes with plans on the list.	A health unit coordinator will always have unexpected requests and situations. Allow time each day for the unexpected.
Someone else wants to prioritize for the health unit coordinator.	Establish better communication with the supervisor and work team. Consider using one of the problem-solving techniques mentioned later in this chapter.

TEAM PLAYER

The SCAN report states, "High-performance workers can work on teams and work well with people from culturally diverse backgrounds." A health unit coordinator does not work in isolation. The health unit coordinator is a member of a health care team. Health unit coordinators attend staff meetings and are included in work groups to improve performance. Many issues will be discussed as a team or group. As a team player, the health unit coordinator should understand group interaction roles.

GROUP INTERACTION ROLES

Stewart L. Tubbs (1995) explains that people play a variety of roles in a variety of settings. One can learn and assume different roles or functions to help the work group function. Tubbs (1995, p. 215) reports, "Group interaction roles consist of:

◆ Task roles—goal- or objective-oriented roles such as contributing, elaborating, seeking and giving information, evaluating, recording, seeking and giving opinions, orientating, gate-keeping or keeping on track

◆ Building and maintenance roles—interpersonal roles such as encouraging, harmonizing, and observing, praising, listening empathetically

◆ Individual roles—self-centered roles such as dominating, withdrawing, blocking, and seeking recognition, aggressing, pleading special interest"

GROUP INTERACTION ROLES IN PROGRESS

The following conversation in a typical health care team staff meeting already in progress demonstrates group interaction roles.

Ed: Okay, before we close the meeting, does anyone have any concerns they'd like to discuss with the group?

Thanh (whispering to next person): Go ahead, you've been talking about this all week. Now's your chance to get it out into the open.

Maria (whispering back): No, I'll be misunderstood.

Ed: Maria, please let us know if you have a concern. You may learn that others share your concern, also.

Maria: Well, I know the census has been extremely high and we've all been really busy, but it seems like I'm the only one who ever answers the phone around here. And the one in a million time someone answers the phone, they can never take a complete message. I'm just sick and tired of it, that's all.

Aiesha: Hey, I've answered that phone plenty of times when you're not around. Seems like I even take more than my fair share of personal messages for you.

Maria: Oh, don't get me started on personal phone calls. Believe me, you don't want to go there.

Ed: Okay, we're all feeling overworked and a little defensive right now. Maria, can you describe the problem as you see it, without pointing any fingers?

Maria: Okay, the way I see the problem is that the phones have been so busy that I don't have time to do anything else.

Thanh: Exactly what are the phones preventing you from doing?

Maria: Normally, I check inventory and order supplies the first thing in the morning. Lately, the phones have been busier in the morning and it takes me too long to order supplies because I keep getting interrupted.

Aiesha: You said something about incomplete phone messages, too.

Maria: That's right. When someone does answer the phone for me, it seems the message is never complete and then I have to spend more time clarifying the information.

Ed: Thank you, Maria, for sharing that with the group. It seems like we have two issues: the tasks of ordering supplies and answering calls are conflicting with each other, and then there's the issue with the messages. Any ideas on what our next step should be?

Thanh: Personally, I shy away from the phone because I'm unfamiliar with the questions people ask.

Maria: I've never thought about that.

Aiesha: There have been times when I've answered the phone and can't find anything to write on.

Ed: Our meeting is scheduled to end in five minutes. We better think of our next step.

Maria: If you all think it would help with messages, I can create a phone log to keep at the phone so we all can record date, time, caller, number, and request.

Thanh: Make sure you put a pen next to the phone log.

Aiesha (laughing): Make sure it's attached with a string so it can't walk away.

Ed: The phone log can be our immediate solution. We may also want to attach a list of frequently asked questions and answers to help those who aren't used to the calls we receive.

Aiesha: Let's all think of common questions we receive and bring them to the next staff meeting.

Ed: Thank you all for your ideas. We'll add this issue to the next meeting agenda and monitor our progress. We can also address the issue of the supplies inventory task being interrupted by the phones. Meeting adjourned.

Aiesha (finishing writing): Okay, it's in the minutes.

This meeting demonstrates examples of all three group interaction roles: task roles, building and maintenance roles, and individual roles. The staff meeting conversation has examples of each of the roles:

Thanh demonstrates a building role when he encourages Maria to talk. Ed echoes the encouragement.

Maria demonstrates an individual role when she initially withdraws.

Maria also demonstrates an individual role when she states her problem in blaming or attacking terms.

Maria and Aiesha then take on individual roles when they defensively bicker among themselves.

Ed demonstrates a building role of harmonizing when he states they are all overworked. He then moves to the task role of information-seeker when he asks for the facts of the problem.

Thanh demonstrates a task role when asking for clarification.

Ed demonstrates the building role of praise-giver when he thanks the group for their contributions.

Thanh and Aiesha demonstrate the task role of opinion-giver when they share why they don't like to answer the phone.

Ed plays the task role of gatekeeper when he reminds the participants the meeting ends soon.

Aiesha plays the building role of tension-reliever when she interjects a little humor about the pen being attached to the phone log.

Aiesha also demonstrates the task role of direction-giver when giving an assignment for the next meeting.

Ed closes the meeting in the task role of summarizer.

Aiesha demonstrates the task role of recorder throughout the meeting.

It's important for all work team members to take an objective look at the roles they play in meetings. Each member can identify the task and building roles he or she plays well and use those strengths to support the work team. One can develop the task and building roles where they are weak and eliminate the individual roles that can hinder the work team. As demonstrated in the meeting script, fulfilling a role such as opinion-giver or harmonizer can move the team forward.

DECISION MAKING AND PROBLEM-SOLVING TECHNIQUES

The SCANS report states, "The successful worker:

◆ Recognizes that a problem exists (i.e., that there is a discrepancy between what is and what should be)

◆ Identifies possible reasons for the discrepancy

◆ Devises and implements a plan of action to resolve it

◆ Evaluates and monitors progress

◆ Revises the plan as indicated by findings"

The first step in problem solving is to identify the problem. The nature of the problem should be defined, along with possible causes of the problem. Once the problem has been identified, possible solutions can be generated. Once the best solution has been determined, a plan of action can be developed. The plan of action should be evaluated and adjusted as necessary once the plan has been implemented.

Health care work teams are often called upon to make decisions. Making decisions holds the organization together. Health unit coordinators may also participate in **quality circles**. A quality circle is a small group of employees who monitor specific practices or trends and suggest solutions for improvement. Structured communication can improve work group performance. An international technology company, the 3M Company, states, "structured techniques support work team effectiveness and efficiency and amplify feelings of fairness and satisfaction among members." Three decision-making techniques are brainstorming, force field analysis, and the Kepner-Tregoe approach.

BRAINSTORMING

Brainstorming can be used in many phases of problem solving such as the generation of ideas and to boost creativity. Brainstorming can be used to think of possible solutions for a problem. To use brainstorming as a technique to get the creativity flowing, one can display a common object to the group and ask them to think of as many uses for that object as possible. Another example of brainstorming could be to ask for ideas to increase participation in meetings.

It is a good idea to review some guidelines before brainstorming. Brainstorming works best in a relaxed environment so everyone feels comfortable sharing.

1. State the issue or problem. Make sure everyone understands the problem. An example of an issue would be to ask the members to brainstorm ideas to increase participation in meetings.

2. Instruct the team members to generate as many ideas as they can. Assign a time limit. Appoint one member to write down the ideas as they are generated.

3. Review the ground rules for brainstorming:

   ◆ No criticism, evaluation, or discussion of ideas is allowed during the idea-generating phase

   ◆ Go for quantity

   ◆ Strive for creativity—wild and crazy ideas are accepted

   ◆ Build on the ideas suggested by others

4. Evaluate the ideas. Select a small number of ideas that are agreed upon to be the best solutions. The best ideas can be judged or examined. Criteria for judging the ideas can be determined. The Kepner-Tregoe table described later in the chapter can be used to evaluate the ideas.

FORCE FIELD ANALYSIS

Wherever there is change, there will be opposing sides. Paul Hersey and Kenneth Blanchard describe Kurt Lewin's development of a tool for constructively analyzing the forces for and against the change. The team can use this tool to determine the probability of success of a proposed change. The team can then concentrate on strategies to increase the driving forces and decrease the restraining forces. The process for the force field analysis follows:

1. Identify the desired change and situation.

2. Make a list of the forces working against the change (the restraining forces) and a list of the forces in favor of the change (the driving forces). The forces can be people, finances, attitudes, cultures, and internal or external factors—anything that is either inhibiting (restraining) or enhancing (driving) the ability to make a change.

For example, the work team members have identified that low attendance in training sessions is having a negative impact on work performance. The work team feels it is important to increase attendance at meetings. The group is considering a policy change to enforce attendance at training. The force field analysis can be used to assess the current situation. Then the group can work on ideas and tactics to increase the driving forces and decrease the restraining forces.

Restraining Forces

- Coverage not available to allow attendance

- Workload does not allow time for training

- Lack of encouragement from supervisor to attend training

- Training not relevant to real-life job issues

- Training scheduled before or after shift interferes with family

- Training scheduled before of after shift interferes with transportation

Driving Forces

- Training can improve quality of patient care

- Content of training is good

- Training can result in better performance appraisals

- Training can help meet professional goals

- Training can help meet personal goals

- More time spent in classroom training could decrease preceptor's time commitment

- Training offered in-house is free to employee

Once the group assesses the current situation, they can focus on strategies to improve the chances of success of increasing attendance. The chances of success will improve if they can increase the driving forces and decrease the restraining forces. The group can list factors that could increase each driving force, thereby bringing about a positive change.

KEPNER-TREGOE APPROACH

The Kepner-Tregoe approach proposes a variation on the criteria phase of problem solving. Musts and wants can be used to evaluate solutions that are proposed to solve the problem. Criteria are then ranked in order of importance.

For example, the Kepner-Tregoe approach can be used to decide upon the location for a new computer workstation. A work team has been informed that they will be receiving a much-needed additional computer workstation. Their task is to determine where to place the computer in their already crowded department. In using the Kepner-Tregoe approach, the team members will first determine their needs, their musts, and their wants. In the following example, the team members decide that the workstation should be conducive to confidentiality, accessible to staff, quiet, and comfortable. These factors, the musts and wants, are then ranked in order of importance and listed on the left of a table. Then the team members list the possible locations for a new computer workstation. The team decides on four possible locations: the staff office, the office lobby, the conference room, and the photocopy machine cubicle. The locations are listed at the top of the table columns. The members then rank each location on

	Staff Office	Office Lobby	Conference Room	Photocopy Machine Cubicle
TABLE 18-4 **Kepner-Tregoe Table Sample**				
Conducive to confidentiality	Satisfactory	Poor	Outstanding	Satisfactory
Accessible to staff	Poor	Outstanding	Good	Satisfactory
Quiet work area	Good	Poor	Outstanding	Poor
Comfortable work area	Good	Satisfactory	Outstanding	Poor

how well it meets the established needs of accessibility, confidentiality, noise level, and comfort. The group uses the ranking of poor, fair, satisfactory, good, and outstanding. The location with the highest marks in the most important factors appears to be the best solution. In this example, the conference room appears to be the best choice for the location of the computer workstation (Table 18-4).

SUMMARY

The U.S. Department of Labor has identified the skills that a high-performance worker needs. These skills include managing one's time, working in teams, and identifying and solving problems. People can work on developing those skills to ensure they are an invaluable employee whatever their profession. Critical-thinking skills develop over time. A health unit coordinator needs to learn the basic tasks and gain experience in the new role before developing critical-thinking skills specific to the job. Keeping this idea in mind can help one set realistic expectations for critical-thinking ability.

REVIEW QUESTIONS

1. What is the most important factor to consider when prioritizing?

2. What is a tool that can be used to assist in time management?

Indicate what type of group interaction role is represented: task (T), building (B), or individual (I):

3. _____ Withdrawing from the team

4. _____ Explaining an idea to the team

5. ____ Having a side conversation at a team meeting

6. ____ Asking questions for clarification

7. ____ Thanking the team members for participating

8. ____ Telling a joke to lighten the mood

9. ____ Blaming a team member for a problem

10. ____ Encouraging a quiet team member to participate

11. ____ Bringing the team members back to an agenda item

12. "Brainstorming is a technique that can be used to generate solutions to a problem." Is this statement true or false?

13. "Wild ideas should be discouraged when brainstorming." Is this statement true or false?

14. "A force field analysis can help the team assess the powers for and against a desired change." Is this statement true or false?

15. "A Kepner-Tregoe table can be used to evaluate several possible solutions to a problem." Is this statement true or false?

NAHUC CERTIFICATION EXAM

CONTENT AREAS

I. A. 4   Prioritize orders and tasks

I. A. 5   Process orders according to priority

I. A. 19 Recognize order categories (i.e. standing, one-time, prn, and stat)

THROUGH THE EYES

OF A HEALTH CARE PROFESSIONAL

A health unit coordinator supervisor shares her thoughts: Critical thinking can be described as being able to solve problems by making sense of data and information. To me, developing my critical-thinking skills is important to my own and my staff's professional growth. It is important to continually evaluate one's work practices and find ways to be more effective. When one of my staff members comes to me with a problem, I ask him to be part of the solution. I think that person has to be part of the process for the solution to be effective. And maybe next time, that person will be able to successfully solve the problem on his own. Generally, we try to look at the whole problem and how it affects all the team members, not just the health unit coordinators. To become more skilled at looking at the big picture, I encourage my staff to participate on committees outside of their own department. Working with members of other work teams and departments broadens their perspective and improves their problem-solving skills.

REFERENCES

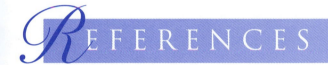

3M Meeting Network. Processes to move groups ahead. *http://www.3m.com/meetingnetwork/readingroom/meetingguide* Accessed December 2003.

Klein, J. Critical Thinking in Nursing. *http://www.nursingnetwork.com/critthink1.htm*

http://www.kepner-tregoe.com Accessed December 2003.

Hersey, P., & Blanchard, K. H. (1993). *Management of organizational behavior: Utilizing human resources.* (6th ed.). Englewood Cliffs, NJ: Prentice Hall.

Snyder M. (1993). Critical thinking: A foundation for consumer-focused care. *Journal of Continued Education Nurse, 24*(5), 206–210.

Tubbs, R. L. (1995). *A systems approach to small group interaction* (5th ed.). New York: McGraw-Hill.

U.S. Department of Labor. Learning a living: A blueprint for high performance: A SCANS report for 2000. *http://www.wdr.doleta.gov/SCANS/lal/LAL.HTM*

CHAPTER 19

Cultural Diversity and Ethics

Learning Objectives

Upon completion of this chapter and review questions, the learner should be able to:

1. Discuss how culture affects the health care environment.

2. Describe the health care practices of the major cultural groups.

3. Describe how the generations affect health care.

4. Discuss the impact the education of health care providers can have on health care delivery.

Key Terms

advocacy Providing support to others in the decision-making process.

autonomy Independent decision making by an individual in his or her best interest.

beneficence The duty to act in the best interest of the person involved in the issue.

boomers The group of people born between 1943 and 1960.

cultural competence Sensitivity to and knowledge of different cultures.

cultural diversity How one culture or group is different from another.

culture Patterned behavioral response that develops over time as a result of imprinting the mind through social and religious structures and intellectual and artistic manifestations.

ethics Practices that are conscious reflections expressing our values or moral beliefs.

fidelity Being faithful to the promises made.

generation Grouping of people based on age or birth date.

generation X The group of people born between 1961 and 1979.

justice A just distribution of resources.

millennial generation The group of people born after 1980.

nonmalfeasance The duty to do no harm.

veracity Telling the truth.

veterans The group of people who were born before 1943.

CULTURE

Culture is defined as a "patterned behavioral response that develops over time as a result of imprinting the mind through social and religious structures and intellectual and artistic manifestations" (Gigner, 2004). Culture, in part, forms who we are. It affects the decisions that we make in our life as well as how, when, and why we interact as we do. Our culture is a part of each of us. It develops and changes throughout our life. Our heritage, our community, our generation, our families, and our education affect us. Culture influences our decision-making process, our work ethics, and our values. Culture affects how we interact with others in the workplace as well as our expectations of others. In the health care environment, staff from many different cultures work together to provide health care to patients from many different cultures.

Health care facilities provide care to people from different countries and cultures. Those patients may have beliefs and health care practices that are different from those of their health care providers. It is important for health unit coordinators to be aware of the cultural practices of the people for whom they provide care as well as the cultural practices of staff with whom they work. This sensitivity to and knowledge of other cultures is called **cultural competence**. In order to better understand different cultures, one needs to examine some key factors and how they affect each culture. Some of these key factors include communication, space, time, social organization, environment, and biological differences.

COMMUNICATION

Communication includes the primary language spoken, voice quality, how words are pronounced, the use of silence, and nonverbal communication. People whose native language is not English may often have a more limited understanding of spoken English than is apparent. While seeming to speak somewhat fluently, often they have a limited vocabulary and either may not understand what is being said or may misinterpret the meaning. A number of cultures believe it is impolite to disagree, so often instead of asking a question or saying no they will nod or otherwise agree.

It is often useful to find multiple ways of imparting a message. Some people understand the written word better than the spoken word. One might write the key words, if not the entire message, in addition to the spoken words. Reinforce the spoken words with gestures. For example, hold up two fingers when saying "two." When saying, "one glass" pick up a glass. Remember, some cultures regard disagreement as not being polite, and it is common for many people, regardless of culture, to not want to reveal their lack of understanding; consequently, just because a person agrees does not mean he understands and will carry out the instructions. Stress the importance of compliance with the instructions. Whenever possible follow up to ensure instructions are being correctly followed.

Eye Contact

A number of cultures believe that direct eye contact should be avoided because it is not respectful, or it is aggressive, or for other reasons. Still other cultures value direct eye contact. It is regarded as an indication of veracity and of being straightforward. Do not assume when talking to a person who does not make direct eye contact that the person is "shifty" or is being evasive. On the other hand, do not assume that a person who maintains direct eye contact with you during a conversation is being disrespectful or aggressive. In some cultures, direct eye contact between members of the opposite sex is regarded as improper.

Voice Tone

The tone of voice, that is loudness or softness, may have more meaning in some cultures than it does in one's own culture. A loud voice may mean aggression, or it may indicate a perception that the speaker's message is not being understood ("If he can't understand what I am saying in a normal conversational tone, I will speak louder.") Avoid speaking in a loud voice. Do not assume people speaking in a low tone are submissive.

SPACE

Space addresses how comfortable the person is with others, how physically close the person is to another person, and body movement. Personal space is the distance between two people engaged in normal conversation. People tend to be uncomfortable when this distance is less than that to which they are accustomed. Generally, people living in densely populated areas tolerate proximity with others better than do people from more sparsely populated areas. Americans, for example, tend to require more personal space than do Europeans. People also tolerate proximity with people they know very well. A person whose personal space is invaded will feel uncomfortable and move away. In this case, the other person should not try to close up the gap. It is better to be at a little greater conversational distance than too close. Avoid physical contact while engaged in a conversation. For example, putting an arm on someone's shoulder, nudging, and touching the person's hand, all may be too intimate and cause the other person to be uncomfortable.

TIME

Time addresses the use, definition, and measurement of time: for example, whether there is a difference between work and social time and whether the orientation is to future, past, or present. People of different cultures regard time in different ways. In some cultures time is approximate. A two o'clock appointment this afternoon may mean simply "sometime this afternoon." Patients with this concept of time may arrive at almost anytime in the afternoon other than promptly at two o'clock. People with this concept of time do not perceive themselves as being late if not arriving at the scheduled time. Because health care facilities are typically run in a highly time-specific manner, conflicts can occur.

In other cultures, time is thought of in present terms. Only what happens today is important. Tomorrow's event will take care of itself. This time concept may cause problems with patients who are required to take preventive medications or need follow-up procedures. Special care will have to be taken to explain the importance and the need for the patient to continue to take the medication, or the ongoing procedure, even when the patient may no longer have any outward symptoms.

SOCIAL ORGANIZATION

Social organization addresses the family unit and how is it organized, the roles of family, work, church, friends, and religion. The extended family is important in a number of cultures, especially in times of illness. The patient gains comfort from having family nearby, and the family in turn finds comfort in being near the patient. Whenever it is feasible, involve designated family members in decisions by keeping them informed.

In some cultures, the eldest male acts as the family spokesperson; in others it is an older female; and in still others the patient will act as his or her own spokesman. A patient who seems reluctant to make a decision concerning his or her own health care may want to first consult with the family spokesperson.

In some cultures, at times, the family spokesperson will be very insistent and repetitious, making demands in a loud tone of voice and with a demanding demeanor. The family spokesperson may behave in this manner to indicate authority and as a means of demonstrating he or she wants the best of care for the ill relative.

ENVIRONMENT

Environment addresses the climate, the community, the job availability, the land, and the values that are associated with the environment.

BIOLOGICAL VARIATIONS

Biological differences have to do with appearance. This includes body structure, eye color and shape, hair color, skin color, and nutritional needs and illnesses people may have.

CULTURAL DIVERSITY

Cultural diversity is how each person's culture is different from others. There are no right or wrong cultural beliefs or customs. They are just different. No one culture is better than another culture. It is important to be aware of the nature and magnitude of the diversity of the people in the region in which one works. In the United States, we have a population that continues to grow in its diversity. The United States was called the Melting Pot of the world as it opened its doors to all who chose to come. Many people came from many different parts of the world to become Americans. They brought with them the different cultures and passed these traditions to their descendants. The United States continues to welcome people from throughout the world even today, and these people, as did the people of the past, bring their own culture, adding to the diversity of our nation. It is an interesting and diverse group of people health care providers care for today.

Patients and co-workers may also come from families that have blended cultures. They may practice some customs that are part of one culture and other customs that are part of the other culture. Some of the different cultures and the diversity of cultures that we may encounter in the health care setting are addressed in the following paragraphs. The following information is generalized and does not hold true for all individuals of the described culture. The following descriptions are some generalizations about cultural behavior. Generalizations can be dangerous because people are individuals and do not necessarily conform to the generalization. With that caveat in mind, the following aspects of culture may be helpful in understanding the behavior of others.

NATIVE AMERICANS

Native Americans may have a distrust of a white-dominated health care system. This distrust may be identified as a problem dating back to the time the white man came to North America. At that time, the white man brought diseases that proved to be a disaster for the Native Americans because many European diseases such as smallpox, measles, and mumps were unknown in America. The Native Americans had not built up natural immunities for them. Hence, many lives were lost when the Native Americans contracted these unfamiliar diseases.

◆ Native Americans in general speak in a low tone of voice. It is expected that the health care provider will pay close attention to what the Native American patient has to say. Native Americans may not look directly at you when you speak to them. Just because they are not looking at you does not mean they are not listening.

◆ Time is not clock time; it is governed by need not by the hour.

◆ Families are extended.

The medicine man plays an important role in healing using traditional medicine. This medicine can include natural remedies and rituals. Ideally, these natural remedies and rituals can be included in modern health care facilities as patient health care needs dictate and allow. Health unit coordinators need to know whom to contact and what can be brought into their facility to meet the needs of this patient population.

MEXICAN AMERICANS

Mexican Americans are usually of mixed Spanish and Indian ancestors. They are individuals who have a Mexican cultural heritage. The language spoken by Mexicans is Spanish. English may be a second language for some Mexican Americans. It is important to remember that even though people can speak English, they do not always understand all the English words that are used. Spanish is the second most common language spoken in the United States. Many forms used in health care, including consent forms, are available in Spanish. People of Mexican descent may engage in small talk before addressing the business at hand (Gigner & Davidhizar, 2004). They may appear to be agreeable on the surface because of their value of courtesy but not always carry through on the previous agreement (Gigner & Davidhizer, 2004). A health unit coordinator may schedule a Mexican American patient for a follow-up appointment and ask the person to arrive 30 minutes early. The patient may agree to do this but may not understand the request with the language barrier. It is important to get an interpreter if needed to explain the importance of the appointment. It may be a requirement for the interpreter to be a medically competent interpreter.

The Mexican culture places great value on family. Therefore, people of Mexican descent are very likely to bring family members with them when they arrive for an appointment. Mexican families are often large and extended. They believe that when someone dies it is the will of God. They are a very faith-based culture. Time in the present is the focus of this culture—what is happening at present, not what will happen in the future.

Roman Catholicism is the primary religion practiced by Mexicans. If a patient of Mexican descent is hospitalized, the health unit coordinator may be asked to call a Catholic priest for the patient and family.

The health unit coordinator may also be asked to call a traditional healer. Traditional healers are important members of the community to the Mexican Americans who use traditional medicine.

Mexican American may also request special food to maintain their health such as eggs, bread, and tea. Requests of this nature would be communicated to the dietary department by the health unit coordinator.

ARAB AMERICANS

The Arab populations immigrating to the United States after 1970 are generally professionals, married, and well educated (Lipson, 1996). They speak English well, but their understanding may be limited. They generally are very respectful to elders and professionals. When a loud voice is used, it is usually an indication that what is being said is important.

The Arab population, as a group, believes in, and honors, oral contracts and agreements. They are a modest population and may tend to appear shy and expressionless. When a family member is very ill, they may prefer to protect the ill person from receiving this information at first, and then gradually give the information to the patient.

Their belief is that the patient should rest to get well. It is the nursing staff and the family who should provide nursing care and support to the patient. To illustrate, a patient who is capable of walking and being ambulatory may be reluctant to walk on her own. The health care staff is responsible for explaining the importance of self care to both the patient and the family.

Food preferences should be addressed. Many Arabs are Muslims, and most Muslims do not eat pork or food cooked in alcohol. They prefer to not have ice as well. The health unit coordinator would make a referral for the dietitian to see the Arab patient and family for the food preferences.

CHINESE AMERICANS

Chinese people have a history of being strong users of traditional medicine. This includes acupuncture, herbal medicine, massage, skin scraping, and cupping. Cupping is placing a cup with burnt special materials inside it over the affected area. This cup creates a vacuum over the area it covers, and it is kept there until it is easy to remove. This might cause a burn on the skin. The health unit coordinator may be transcribing orders for these therapies that can be performed in the health care facility. The people of this culture generally feel that excessive eye contact or touching is not welcome. They bow when they greet each other rather than undergo the touching of a handshake. They value silence, avoid disagreement, and do not like raised voices. They use many nonverbal communication tools, including facial expression, speed of speaking, and movements. The location where the conversation is taking place is important. It could be viewed as inappropriate to ask a patient of Chinese descent about health care issues in the emergency department interview area, where strangers may be able to overhear the conversation.

Family and family loyalty are very important to the Chinese. Family members take care of family. It not only is expected but also is regarded as an honor to do so.

The Chinese culture places importance on the role of diet in one's health. Yin is associated with cold food, and yang with hot food. Food is considered to be the reason the illness exists as well as the treatment for the illness. The health unit coordinator may be requested to order certain hot and cold foods as part of the traditional treatment process for Chinese patients.

AFRICAN AMERICANS

African Americans are affectionate; they hug, touch, and sit close to each other (Lipson, 1996). Religion may be very important to many African Americans. Usually, a minister will be requested to visit a patient either by the patient or the patient's family. The health unit coordinator may be asked to notify the clergy of a request for a visit. Time may be considered flexible, and life issues may take priority over keeping appointments (Lipson, 1996). In a clinic setting, the health unit coordinator may schedule appointments for the morning or afternoon, taking people as they arrive instead of giving a specific time. This time frame would allow the flexibility needed for the patients and also for the health care providers.

HMONG AMERICANS

The Hmong group began immigrating to the United States after 1975. Originally from Laos and of Asian descent, there are now large groups of Hmong in cities throughout the United States. Most of the older members have no formal education. They speak

Hmong but have no written language of their own. They may be unable to read and write English. They may want family members to serve as their interpreter, not someone at the health care facility. They may be concerned that a health system interpreter may not be truthful and would instead do what is good for the health system. The Hmong are very polite and consider it disrespectful to not be so. They may have a large family. They tend to not want to be alone. They may want another member of the family to stay with them in the hospital. The health unit coordinator then could be involved in making sure that a bed is put in the room so that a family member can stay with the patient.

Calling a married woman by her first name is regarded as disrespectful to the woman's husband. It is not welcomed. Handshakes and smiling are often used in greetings. When a Hmong is ill, it is expected that the female members of the family will provide the care, not the patient care staff. Elders of the family make the decisions. They meet and decide what needs to be done. When someone is near death, the Hmong dress the dying family member in his or her finest clothing so that the family member will enter the next world properly dressed.

EUROPEAN AMERICANS

Europeans are a group of people who are reserved and distant, with a time orientation of future over present (Gigner & Davidhizar, 2004). They tend to not get too close to other individuals, and they like noncontact, nontouching. They use the modern health care system but may also use some folk or traditional medicine. They believe in what is called traditional health care and do participate in preventive medicine. They expect to be provided with health care by health care providers. They are the group that provides the majority of health care providers to the health care systems. They speak English as the primary language and practice Christian religions. They like to be part of social groups, sharing information and beliefs. The majority of patient care staff in a health care facility belong to this cultural group. The level of education among European Americans is varied, as it is among other cultures, and this variation may or may not affect their understanding of health care practices. It is important to be aware of all patients' education levels so that the correct information can be provided at the correct reading and understanding level.

SENSITIVITY TO DISCRIMINATION AND PREJUDICE

The people of almost any ethnic or cultural background, when in a different ethnic or cultural environment, may be unusually sensitive to perceived discrimination and prejudice. For example, an Anglo in a Hispanic population or conversely a Hispanic in an Anglo population may suffer a feeling of discrimination when none was intended. To avoid any inference of discrimination or prejudice, always be courteous. Avoid being too familiar. Do not call patients or their family members by their first name, unless requested to do so. Call them by their title and surname: Mr. Smith, Ms. Jones, Miss Jones, Reverend Smith, or Dr. Smith. Never use terms of address such as "boy," "girl," "gal," "chief," "man," "brother," or "sister."

Health care providers are members of different cultural groups as well. They, too, come to the health care facility interacting with the health care team members from different cultural backgrounds. It is important to be knowledgeable about the different cultures that are part of the health care community. Many requests for services that the health unit coordinator coordinates and processes are unique to the culture the patient is associated with. Consider this example of a situation that could happen in a facility where residents practice.

Doctor Ling is a new resident from China. In China, the nursing staff does not question a physician order because doing so would be considered rude. When the health unit coordinator questions a duplicate order he has written, he may not respond to the question. In his country, only another physician would question an order written by a physician. The health unit coordinator asks the chief resident to explain to Dr. Ling that the health unit coordinator is not being disrespectful or rude but protecting the patient from a potential error, and that is part of the health unit coordinator's job responsibilities.

COMMUNITY DIVERSITY

Health care is affected by the size and customs of the community just as it is affected by the different cultures that use the health care system. Large communities and small communities offer and provide different advantages and expectations for health care facilities. Small communities tend to provide services on a limited scale, not offering all the specialized services that larger communities can provide. Health care providers who provide services in small communities tend to be someone everyone knows. They are the neighbors and friends. They are often from the same cultures. They frequently are members of the local churches. Small communities often are involved in activities that are unique to the area, such as church fairs, volunteer fund raising, school programs where students visit and entertain patients. In small communities, health care support activities are often financed by small donations from many individuals. Volunteers usually run the gift shop in the health care facility of small communities (Figure 19-1).

Large communities can support large health care facilities. Large health care facilities can provide specialized services. In a large facility, there are many health care workers from many different cultures. Usually, patients do not know any members of the facility before admission. In larger communities, foundations support activities through large monetary donations not requiring as much involvement by community members. Paid staff members are in charge of the gift shops.

Communities celebrate and recognize different events during a year. The health care facilities are a focal point in a community and contribute to the community at large. They are a gathering place for events for communities and provide the health care for the communities. They provide health education and resources for communities. The diversity of the community is reflected in the health care facility just as it is in the local school systems.

GENERATIONAL DIVERSITY

In health care facilities, patients range in age from newborn babies to older adults. A **generation** is a grouping based on age or birth date, and employees range in age through many generations, from young people just entering the workforce to older people of retirement age (Figure 19-2). Young people born after 1980 are called the

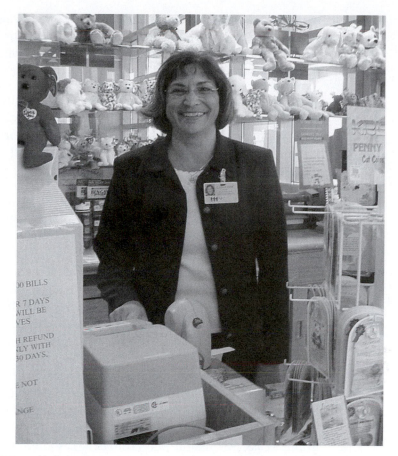

Figure 19-1 • *Volunteers are important members of the health care facility, assisting with the operations of the gift shop.* (Courtesy of Marquette General Health System, Marquette, MI)

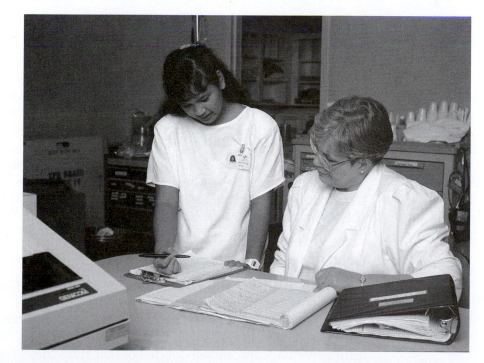

Figure 19-2 • *Employees of different age groups often work together as health care team members.*

millennial generation or the Nexters. The baby boomer generation, **boomers**, are people who were born between 1943 and 1960. This is the group that is closest to retirement age. As a health unit coordinator, you will interact with co-workers throughout these ranges.

Most health care facilities limit the ages of the family members who are allowed to visit patients. The age of the visitors are limited because children at certain ages could be disruptive to the other patients as well as the workflow of the health care facility. It is also difficult to be responsible for children in the facility; there are many things happening that could be frightening to children.

The health unit coordinator should be aware of some basic traits of the different generations to be prepared to provide services at an acceptable and expected level. The following are some generalized characteristics often associated with specific generations.

VETERANS

The **veteran** group is described as the generation born before 1943. They are, for the most part, the group most likely to be using the health care services and are insured through Medicare. They are often described as looking forward to retirement if they are not already retired. They are not thrilled with all the technology and would like the environment to be quiet. They like to see health care employees dressed in uniform so it is easy to identify who is a nurse. They like to be addressed as Mr., Mrs. or Miss. When they are provided with written materials, the type should be large enough to read because often their vision has diminished. Be respectful of the veteran generation and ask permission to do things. It is sometimes difficult for them to be given information by someone who is from the younger generations. Here is an example: "Mr. Smith, I am the health unit coordinator who can make your follow-up appointment to see Dr. Jones. Would you like me to make the appointment? I can make it for Monday in the morning or in the afternoon. Thank you Mr. Smith."

BOOMERS

The boomers are the generation consisting of people born between 1943 and 1960. They have a strong work ethic and have been in the workforce since graduating from high school. They tend to be driven to succeed. They are very dedicated to their profession. They enjoy people relationships and work well in groups or teams. They like to be comfortable and enjoy interactive activities. They are the workers in the health care facilities. They like to be called by their first name, and technology is used in the workplace to do what needs to be done. Here is an example of a good approach to use when making an appointment for a boomer: "Hi Jennifer. I am the health unit coordinator, and I will be making your appointment to see Dr. Jones on Monday afternoon. Will that interfere with your work schedule?"

GENERATION X

Generation X refers to people who were born between 1961 and 1980. Gen Xs have a different orientation to time and space. They tend to believe as long as the job gets done it is not always important when and how. Gen Xs value personal time and would take a day off to enjoy life, even without pay. They are highly motivated to learn new things and are self-directed in that area. They love to have fun. They move from job to job seeking what fits their lifestyle. Here is an example of a possible exchange with a gen X: "Hi Sally, I am the health unit coordinator and was wondering if you would like me to make an appointment for you to see Dr. Jones?" "Oh no, I will make my own appointment because I am not sure what I will be doing so I want to be flexible with the date and time."

MILLENNIAL GENERATION

People of the millennial generation are just beginning to enter the workforce. They are the generation born from 1980 to the present. They have been introduced to technology as students and they use it. They love new technology and always want the newest item to use. They like to be doing and are easily bored if thing are not moving. They work in teams and do not like difficult people. This generation likes to read and learn new things. Here is an example of making appointments in this group: "Hi Richard. I am the health unit coordinator. Dr. Jones would like to see you in two weeks. If you give me your e-mail address I will send the appointment date and time to your electronic calendar and have your calendar alert you two days before your appointment through your cell phone."

UNDERSTANDING GENERATIONAL DIVERSITY

It is important to know why people respond to other people as they do. People often expect the same response as they would give, but as you can see, each person responds differently depending on what generation he or she represents.

The members of the patient care team can be members of different generations all working together to provide the patient with the best possible outcome. Being aware of the generational differences enables the health care team members to work together efficiently and effectively to provide quality patient care.

EDUCATIONAL DIVERSITY

The level of education that has been completed is diverse in the United States. Health care providers should provide information to patients and co-workers at their level of understanding. Whether you are telling a patient how to get to the radiology department or providing drug information handouts, it is important to recognize that not everyone has attained the same level of learning. In a blue-collar community, the health care facility may provide services to patients who are high school graduates. In a white-collar community, the majority of the patients may be college graduates. The patient education handouts that the health unit coordinator provides to the nursing care staff to give to the patients and families should be available at different reading levels to meet the educational diversity of the patient population.

ETHICS

Ethics is the conscious practices and reflections expressing our values and morals. Values are actions or ideas people believe are desirable. Morals are actions or ideas people believe are right. Values and morals are based on beliefs, attitudes, and behaviors.

Ethics enters into how people make decisions. The focus of ethics is the evaluation of behavior as well as the desire or search for quality, value, and meaning. Issues that are included in the scope of practice of the health unit coordinator position are professional ethics regarding patient rights. These include:

- ◆ Health

- ◆ Confidentiality

- ◆ Autonomy

- ◆ Informed consent

Societal issues or obligations may be ethical issues. Society dictates that the health unit coordinator, as a clerical health care provider:

Act in patients' best interest

Ensure that there is a just allocation of resources

Ensure that all people have access to health care

Some health care professional responsibilities are ethical issues. Professionals adhere to a written code of ethics. The Code of Ethics of health unit coordinators includes:

- ◆ Respect and confidence

- ◆ Protect rights (privacy)

- ◆ High level of competency

- ◆ Keep current

- ◆ Report unethical, illegal professional practices

The health unit coordinator Code of Ethics is found in Chapter 2. The National Association of Health Unit Coordinators as a profession promotes and adheres to the Code of Ethics.

Health unit coordinators are accountable for the correct use of funds and resources in health care. Funds used by health unit coordinators may include correct charging and use of supplies and services. Accountability is an ethical issue.

Health unit coordinators make ethical decisions. Those decisions may be based on any of the following beliefs:

- ◆ What is right is what the *sacred* text tells me to do.

- ◆ Conscience tells me what is right or wrong. Follow your conscience.

- ◆ The only person to look out for is yourself.

- ◆ Doing your duty is the right thing to do.

- ◆ Respect others, even if they have different beliefs.

- ◆ All people are created with certain rights.

◆ We can make the world a better place.

◆ Be fair.

◆ Be a good person; good people make good choices.

◆ What happens is out of my control.

The basic principles of ethical decision making can provide the framework to be used in the health unit coordinator role when making decisions. It is important to understand that health unit coordinators are involved in ethical decision making. The extent of involvement does depend on the situation at hand. The following basic principles will assist in the process:

◆ **Autonomy** is independent decision making by an individual in his or her best interest.

◆ **Nonmalfeasance** is the duty to do no harm.

◆ **Beneficence** is the duty to act in the best interest of the person involved in the issue.

◆ **Justice** is a just distribution of resources.

◆ **Veracity** is telling the truth.

◆ **Advocacy** is providing support to others in the decision-making process.

◆ **Fidelity** is being faithful to the promises made.

When an ethical issue arises, it is important to get the facts, not what you think or what someone else thinks are the facts. Determine what is at risk, what values are at risk. Look for the conflict between values and the professional norms. Make a list of all the possible actions and look for the alternatives. Be open. Consider the following ethical issues:

You are the clerical support person for a large nursing unit. Recently, because of a shortage of available licensed support professionals, administration combined four units into the one you are now working on. Recently, your hospital has been very successful in recruiting four new physician specialists who admit to your unit. Your community marketing department has aggressively promoted these physicians' practices, and as a result your department is severely understaffed. The clerical staff was having difficulty processing all the patients that you had before this expansion. Admitted patients have to wait for beds, and the nurses are not able to discharge patients in a timely manner. You notice the clerical workers are taking much longer than ever to process patient information. However, this is still faster than the nurses can attend to your finished orders. You observe that critical problems are attended to but that routine care is not being done. You are very worried about the quality of care patients are receiving. You believe that there are some ethical considerations involved in assuming more work than your department can handle. What are some ethical issues or principals involved in this case?

A part of your clerical duties includes taking a daily inventory of equipment and supplies in each patient room. You know that the patient in the room you are in is a 28-year-old woman who was involved in a car accident last evening. She suffered a concussion, severely fractured ankle, and facial lacerations. She underwent emergency surgery early this morning and is now becoming alert enough to begin postoperative treatments. Her 4-year old daughter was killed in the accident, but authorities have not been able to inform the rest of the family. The nurses have told you this to ensure that the staff does not inform anyone until the family is informed. You have also been informed that the patient's physician has decided not to tell her about her daughter's death until she is more medically stable. As you begin your inventory, the patient looks you in they eye and asks you directly to tell her how her daughter is doing. What should you say or do? What are the possible alternatives?

You have been a health care clerical worker for 8 years and have worked in a small rural hospital your entire career. Two months ago you moved, and the only position you could find was in a large metropolitan hospital. There are too many hospitals in this city, so the emphasis is on competition and on high productivity. Last week, one of the health care clerical workers on this unit was fired for not being able to keep up with the pace. You are worried about the daily equipment quality assurance checks that you forgot to do 10 days ago. The unit manager, who returned from a 3-week vacation last week, has not yet discovered your oversight. You really need this job because you recently got divorced and are raising two children alone. You do not have enough money to move to another city, and there are no other jobs available in this area. You feel certain that you will be fired if your mistake is discovered. What should you do? How will your actions be related to the principles of autonomy, beneficence, and nonmalfeasance?

SUMMARY

Diversity affects each and every one of us. In a diverse health care facility, not only do the patients have diverse cultural backgrounds but so do the employees and staff. It is important to be aware of the different cultures in the health care facility. Heritage, community, education, and generations affect culture.

Ethics affects how we make decisions. It is what we believe to be right based on our culture and diversity. Who we are, how we respond, what our decisions are based on, and how we interact with others are all affected by our unique cultures.

REVIEW QUESTIONS

Fill in the blanks.

1. _____ is the duty to act in the best interest of the person involved in the issue.

2. _____ is a just distribution of resources.

3. _____ is telling the truth.

4. _____ is providing support to others in the decision-making process.

5. _____ is being faithful to the promises made.

6. _____ is shared, learned, and passed on to others through community, education, generations, and families.

7. _____ are groupings of people based on age or birth date.

8. _____ is the practices that are conscious reflections expressing our values or moral beliefs.

9. _____ _____ is how one culture or group is different or diverse from another.

10. _____ _____ is being sensitive to and knowledgeable about different cultures.

11. The group of people who were born prior to 1943 are _____.

12. The group of people born between 1943 and 1960 are _____.

13. _____ are the group of people born between 1961 and 1979.

14. The group of people born after 1980 is _____.

15. _____ is independent decision making by an individual in his or her best interest.

16. _____ is the duty to do no harm.

THROUGH THE EYES

OF A HEALTH CARE PROFESSIONAL

As a health unit coordinator I am working daily with diverse people. These people are my co-workers as well as the customers of the health care facility. I must be aware of different cultures and practices, as well as have a keen awareness of my beliefs and culture. I must be able to access individuals who can assist with the health care needs of our patients whether it is an individual who is able to communicate with the patient and family in the preferred language or a medicine man who can assist with the rituals of health care. I must be able to work well with my co-workers who are older and younger and have different religious beliefs and different levels of education. We are a diverse group coming together to provide for the needs of our entire patient population and their families.

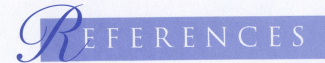

REFERENCES

http://www.youth.co.za/bushrgenstr.htm Accessed March 2003.

Gigner, J. (2004). *Transcultural nursing assessment and intervention* (4th ed.). St Louis: Mosby.

Hecox, C., Jr. (2003). Ethics: How your beliefs influence your decisions. Healthcare Clerical Conference. Marquette General Hospital, Marquette, MI.

Lipson, J. G. (1996). *Culture and nursing care: A pocket guide.* San Francisco: UCSF Nursing Press.

Spector, R. (1996). *Cultural diversity in health and illness* (4th ed.). Stamford, CT: Prentice Hall Health.

Spector, R. (2000). *Cultural diversity in health and illness* (5th ed.). Stamford, CT: Prentice Hall Health.

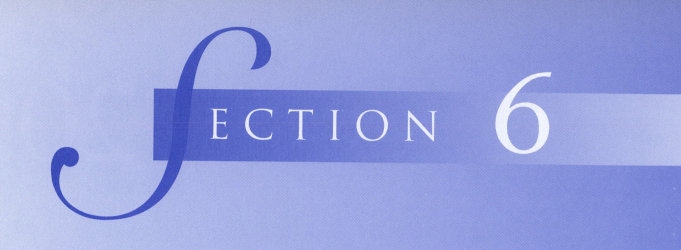

Medical Terminology

Introduction to Medical Terminology

Learning Objectives

Upon completion of this chapter and review questions, the learner should be able to:

1. Define common prefixes, word roots, and suffixes used in medical terminology.

2. Explain two functions of a prefix.

3. Explain two functions of word roots.

4. Explain two functions of a suffix.

5. Name the most common combining vowel.

6. List pronunciation rules.

Key Terms

combining vowel Used to join a word root to a suffix and to join two word roots together.

prefix A word part that is attached to the front of a word to produce a new word with a new meaning.

suffix A word part that is attached at the end of a base word to form a new word with a new meaning.

word root refers to the origin of the word

MEDICAL TERMINOLOGY INTRODUCTION

This chapter is an introduction to basic medical terminology. Health unit coordinators in a true sense do not use much medical terminology throughout the workday. Instead, they use terminology and approved medical abbreviations pertaining to different tests and treatments regarding patients with a variety of ailments. To have an understanding of what and why various exams and treatments are required health unit coordinators need a basic understanding of the body systems and medical terminology.

The origin of most medical terms is Greek or Latin. Other medical terms are derived from the inventor or discoverer, such as pasteurization, discovered by Louis Pasteur. There are thousands of medical terms used in the health care field. This chapter includes explanations on the different parts of word structure. An understanding of various prefixes, word roots, and suffixes is necessary in order to form the many different medical terms. Lists of the most commonly used prefixes, word roots, and suffixes are included in this chapter.

One of the many challenges faced by a new health unit coordinator is reading the written physician orders. However, what the health unit coordinator needs to keep in mind is that physicians use many medical abbreviations when writing orders, and therefore a good knowledge of medical abbreviations as well as medical terminology is essential. Medical abbreviations will be addressed in a separate chapter later in this unit.

WORD STRUCTURE

The best way to learn medical terminology is to learn the parts of a word: prefixes, suffixes, wood roots, and combining vowels. A **prefix** is a word part that is attached to the front of a word to produce a new word with a new meaning. For example when the prefix *mis*, which means "wrong," is attached to the base word *spell*, a new word, *misspell*, is formed. A **suffix** is a word part that is attached at the end of a base word to form a new word with a new meaning. When the suffix *ize*, which means "to make," is attached to the base word *social*, a new word, *socialize*, is formed. The term *word root* refers to the origin of the word.

Putting together the various word parts will form thousands of words. Not all words have prefixes, and not all words will have suffixes. Some words include prefixes, word roots, and suffixes. A **combining vowel** is used to join a word root to a suffix and to join two word roots together. A combining vowel is not necessary to join a prefix and a word root. A root word is the main component of a word. The word root usually describes a part of the body. Some word roots describe medical conditions. The medical term *hematology* can be used as an illustration. Broken into medical terms *hemat*, the root word, means "blood," *logy*, the suffix, means "study of," and "*o*" is the combining vowel. Hence, *hematology* means "blood study." However, in English it would not be referred to as blood study but "study of the blood." When translating medical words into English, remember to read the suffix first.

PRONUNCIATION

In addition to word building, the health unit coordinator must enunciate medical terms correctly and with confidence. Many of the rules for pronouncing medical terms are the same as pronunciation rules for English. Phonetic spelling of terms is found in most medical dictionaries. A guide to the various symbols used in the phonetic spelling is found in the front of the dictionaries. Examples in this chapter are listed with a phonetic spelling. Below is a guide to the phonetic spelling of vowels used in this chapter.

ă	apple
ā	fate
ä	father
ĕ	bet
ē	she
e	(a neutral vowel, always unstressed) *ago, focus*
er	air
ĭ	hit
ī	ice
ŏ	proper
ō	go
ŭ	cup, love
ū	you
ü	loot

PREFIXES

Prefixes are found at the beginning of a word. Prefixes modify a word root and often give a clue to the location or amount. Not all words will have a prefix.

Prefix	Refers to or Means	Example with Pronunciation and Definition
a-	not, without	**a**caudal \ā-kŏd-l\ having no tail
ab-	from, away, off	**ab**normal \ăb-nōr-mel\ off of the norm
ambi-	both	**ambi**dextrous \ăm-bī-dĕk-str*e*s\ using both hands with equal ease
ante-	anterior, forward, in front of, prior to	**ante**partum \ăntī-pärt-*e*m\ relating to the period before childbirth

Prefix	Refers to or Means	Example with Pronunciation and Definition
anti-; ant-; anth-	opposing in effect or activity; inhibiting; serving to prevent, cure, alleviate	**anti**biotic \ănt-*e*-bī-ät-ĭk\ prevent, inhibit, or destroy life
auto-	self	**auto**logous \ŏ-täl-ō-g*es*\ one individual as both donor and recipient of blood
bi-	two, into two parts, twice	**bi**lateral \bī-lăt-*er*-el\ both sides
brady-	slow	**brady**cardia \brăd-ĭ-kärd-ē-ä\ slow heartbeat
con-	with, together	**con**fluent \kän-flü-*ent*\ running together
de-	down, lack of	**de**colorize \dē-kŏl-*e*-rīz\ lack of color
dys-	abnormal, difficult, bad, painful	**dys**pnea \dĭs(p)-nē-*e*\ difficult breathing
e-	missing, absent	**e**dentulous \ē-dĕn-ch*e*-l*es*\ toothless
ec-	out of, outside	**ec**topic pregnancy *e*k-täp-ĭk\ pregnancy outside of the uterus
epi-	upon, beside, attached to	**epi**cranial \ĕp-ĭ-krā-nē-äl\ situated on the cranium
ex-	out, away from	**ex**tubation *e*k-stü-bā-sh*en*\ removal of a tube
extra-	outside, beyond	**extra**pulmonary *e*k-stre-pŭl-m*e*-ner-ē\ situated or occurring outside the lungs
hyper-	excessive	**hyper**tension \hī-p*er*-ten-ch*en*\ abnormally high blood pressure
hypo-	under, beneath, less than normal	**hypo**glycemia \hī-pō-glī-sē-mē-*e*\ low blood sugar
infra-	below, within	**infra**umbilical \ĭn-fr*e*-em-bĭl-ĭ-k*el*\ situated below the navel
inter-	between	**inter**cellular \ĭnt-*er*-s*e*l-ye-l*er*\ occurring between cells
intra-	into, within	**intra**venous \ĭn-tr*e*-vē-n*es*\ into the vein
macro-	large, thick	**macro**cranial \măk-rō-krā-nē-*el*\ having a large or long skull
mal-	bad	**mal**aise \m*e*-lāz\ bad feeling
meta-; met-	change, after	**meta**biosis \m*e*t-*e*-bī-ō-s*es*\ a medical change
neo-	new	**neo**natal \nē-*e*-nāt-ăl\ new birth

Prefix	Refers to or Means	Example with Pronunciation and Definition
non-	not, reverse of, absence of	**non**ambulatory \nän-ăm-bye-le-tōr-ē\ not able to walk
para-; par-	beside, abnormal, closely resembling, almost	**para**kinetic \păr-e-ke-net-ĭk\ relating to a disorder of motor function resulting in abnormal movements
peri-	around, surrounding	**peri**renal \per-e-rēn-ăl\ the tissue surrounding the kidney
poly-	many, much	**poly**uria \păl-ē-yūr-ē-e\ excessive secretion of urine
post-	after, behind	**post**operative \pōst-ŏp-ră-tĭv\ the period following a surgical operation
pre-	earlier than, prior to, in front of, before	**pre**term \prē-term\ born by premature birth
pro-	immature, being a precursor to, forward	**pro**tract \prō-trăkt\ to extend forward or outward
pseudo-	false	**pseudo**pregnancy \süd-ō-preg-nen-sē\ false pregnancy
re-	back, again	**re**mission \rē-mĭsh-en\ a state or period during which the symptoms of a disease are abated
retro-	behind, backward	**retro**grade \re-tre-grād\ occurring in a direction opposite the normal
sub-	under, beneath, below	**sub**cutaneous \sŭb-kyū-tā-nē-es\ under the skin
supra-; super-	super, transcending	**super**spinal \sü-per-spī-nel\ situated or occurring above the spine
syn-; sym-	with, along with, at the same time	**syn**drome \sĭn-drōm\ to run together
trans-	through, such as, to change or transfer	**trans**plant \trăns-plănt\ to transfer from one place to another
ultra-	beyond in space, on the other side, transcending	**ultra**structure \ŭl-tre-strŭk-cher\ an especially fine structure not visible through a light microscope

WORD ROOTS

A **word root** is the main component of the medical term. Examples of word roots listed here are used with only suffixes to allow more concentration on the word root. This is not a complete list of all word roots; only the most commonly used word roots are listed. Notice that some word roots are spelled similarly yet have different meanings. For example, the *ileum* is a part of the small intestine, and the *ilium* is a part of the pelvis.

Word Root	Refers to or Means	Example with Pronunciation and Definition
abdomin	abdomen	**abdomin**al \ăb-däm-*e*n-l\ pertaining to the stomach
acr	extremities, top, peak	**acr**omegaly \ăk-rō-m*e*g-*e*-lē\ enlarged extremities
acu	performed with a needle	**acu**puncture \ăk-y*e*-pŭk-chŭr\ Chinese practice of puncturing the body (with needles) at specific points to cure or relieve disease or pain
aden	gland	**aden**itis \ăd-ĭn-īt-*e*s\ inflammation of a gland
adren	adrenal gland	**adren**alectomy *e*-drēn-ăl-*e*k-t*e*-mē\ removal of adrenal gland
angi	blood or lymph vessels	**angi**oplasty \an-jē-*e*-plăs-tē\ surgical repair of a blood vessel
anter	front	**anter**ior \an-tēr-ē-*e*r\ pertaining to the front
arteri	artery	**arteri**al \är-tēr-ē-*e*l\ relating to an artery
arthr	joint	**arthr**oscopy \är-thräs-k*e*-pē\ surgical examination of the interior of a joint
audio	hearing, sound	**audio**logy *o*d-ē-äl-*e*-jē\ study of hearing, and hearing impaired
bar	weight, pressure	**bar**ometer \b*e*-rŏm-*e*-t*e*r\ an instrument for measuring atmospheric pressure
bi, bio	life, living organism	**bio**logy \bī-äl-ō-jē\ study of life
bili	bile, gall	**bili**ary tract \bĭl-ē-*e*r-ē\ includes the liver, gallbladder and ducts that excrete bile into the duodenum
carcin	tumor, cancer	**carcin**oma \kär-cĭn-ō-m*e*\ cancerous tumor
cardi	heart	**cardi**ology \kärd-ē-äl-*e*-jē\ study of the heart
cele	tumor, hernia	encepholo**cele** \ĭn-s*e*f-*e*-lō-sēl\ hernia of the brain
cephal	head	**cephal**ic \s*e*-făl-ĭk\ pertaining to the head
cerebr	brain	**cerebr**al \s*e*-rē-br*e*l\ relating to the brain
cervic	neck, cervix of an organ	**cervic**al \s*e*r-vĭ-k*e*l\ pertaining to the neck of the uterus
chol-, chole	bile, gall	**chole**cystectomy \kō-l*e*-sĭs-t*e*k-t*e*-mē\ removal of the gallbladder
chondr	cartilage	**chondr**otomy \kän-drăt-*e*-mē\ cutting or dissection of cartilage
cost-, costo	rib	**cost**ophrenic \käs-tō-fr*e*n-ĭk\ relating to the ribs and the diaphragm

Word Root	Refers to or Means	Example with Pronunciation and Definition
crani	cranium	**crani**al \krā-nē-*e*l\ relating to the skull or cranuim
cry	cold, freezing	**cry**ostat \krī-*e*-stăt\ a device for maintaining low temperature
crypt	hidden, covered	**cypt**ococcus \krĭp-te-käk-*es*\ fungus that causes lung, brain, and blood infections
cyan	blue	**cyan**osis \sī-*e*-nō-s*es*\ a bluish or purplish discoloration
cyst	bladder	**cyst**oscopy \sĭs-täs-k*e*-pē\ use of a cystoscope to examine the bladder
cyt	cell	**cyt**ology \sī-täl-*e*-jē\ study of cells
dent, denti	tooth, dental	**dent**al arch \dēn-tal\ the curve of the row of teeth in each jaw
derm	skin	**derm**al \d*e*r-m*e*l\ pertaining to the skin
dextr	right, on or toward the right	**dextr**ad \d*e*k-străd\ toward the right side
duoden	duodenum	**duoden**um \dü-äd-ĭn-*em*\ first part of small intestine
encepal	relating to, affecting the brain	**encephal**ogram \ĭn-s*e*f-*e*-le-gram\ an x-ray of the brain
erg	work	**erg**onomics *e*r-ge-näm-iks\ designing things that people will interact and work with effectively and safely
erythr	red	**erythr**ocyte \ĭ-rĭth-r*e*-sīt\ red blood cell
fibr, fibro	fiber, fibrous tissue	**fibr**oma \fī-brō-m*e*\ benign tumor consisting mainly of fibrous tissue
gastr, gastro	belly, stomach	**gastr**itis \gă-strī-t*es*\ inflammation of the stomach
gloss	tongue	**gloss**opathy \glä-sä-pă-thē\ a disease of the tongue
gynec	woman	**gynec**ic \jī-nē-sĭk\ relating to or treating women
hepat	liver	**hepat**itis \h*e*p-*e*-tīt-*es*\ inflammation of the liver
hydr, hydro	water, liquid, fluid	**hydr**othorax \hī-dr*e*-thō-raks\ fluid in the pleural cavity, thorax
hyster	womb	**hyster**ectomy \hĭs-t*e*-r*e*k-t*e*-mē\ surgical removal of uterus

Word Root	Refers to or Means	Example with Pronunciation and Definition
ileum	part of the small intestine	**ile**itis \ĭl-ē-īt-*es*\ inflammation of the small intestine
ilium	part of the pelvis	**ili**ac crest \ĭl-ē-ăk\ the thick curved upper portion of the pelvis
leuk, leuko	white, colorless	**leuk**ocyte \lü-k*e*-sīt\ white blood cell
lip, lipo	fat, fatty tissue	**lip**oblast \lĭp-*e*-blăst\ a connective tissue cell destined to become a fat cell
lith	calculus	**lith**otripsy \lĭth-*e*-trĭp-sē\ breaking of calculus, often by shock waves or surgical instrument
mal	bad, abnormal	**mal**acia \m*e*-lāsh-ē-*e*\ abnormal softening of a tissue
mast	breast, nipple	**mast**ectomy \mă-st*ek*-t*e*-mē\ surgical removal of the breast
mono	one, single	**mono**phobia \män-*e*-fō-bē-*e*\ a morbid dread of being alone
morph	form, shape	**morph**ometrics \mōr-f*e*-m*e*-triks\ the measurement of forms
multi	many, multiple	**multi**rooted \mŭl-tē-rüt-*e*d\ referring to a tooth with several roots
my	muscle	**my**algia \mī-ăl-jē-*e*\ muscle pain
myc, myco	fungus	**myc**osis \mī-kō-s*es*\ disease or infection caused by fungus
myel, myelo	marrow or spinal cord	**myel**ogram \mī-*e*-l*e*-grăm\ picture or x-ray of the spinal cord after a contrast medium has been injected around the spinal cord
nas, naso	nose, nasal	**nas**al septum \nā-z*e*l\ bone that separates the right and left nasal cavities
necr	death, those who are dead, corpse	**necr**osis \n*e*-krō-s*es*\ death of living tissue
neur	nerve	**neur**al \nür-*e*l\ pertaining to or affecting a nerve
ocul	eye	**ocu**lar \äk-y*e*-l*e*r\ relating to the eye
odont	tooth	**odont**otomy \ō-dän-tō-mē\ the operation of cutting into a tooth
oophor	ovary	**ooph**oritis \ō-*e*-fe-r_t-es\ inflammation of one or both ovaries
opt	vision	**opt**ic \äp-tīk\ relating to vision

Word Root	Refers to or Means	Example with Pronunciation and Definition
orth, ortho	straight, upright	**orth**opnea \ōr-thăp-nē-*e*\ inability to breathe except in an upright position
oste	bone	**oste**omyelitis \äs-tē-ō-mī-*e*-līt-es\ inflammation of the bone and bone marrow secondary to infection
oto	ear	**oto**plasty \ōt-*e*-plăs-tē\ plastic surgery to the external ear
pancreat	pancreas	**pancreat**ic \pǎn-krē-at-ik\ relating to or produced in the pancreas
ped	foot, feet	**ped**icure \ped-ī-kyūr\ care for the feet
ped	child, children	**ped**iatrician \pēd-ē-*e*-trĭsh-*e*n\ a specialist dealing with the care, development, and disease of children
pharmac	medicine, drug	**pharmac**opsychosis \fär-m*e*-kō-sī-kō-s*e*s\ addiction to a drug
phleb	vein	**phleb**otomist \flĭ-bät-*e*-m*e*st\ one who draws blood from a vein
phobia	abnormal fear	acro**phobia** \ăk-r*e*-fō-bē-*e*\ fear of height
phon	sound, voice, speech	**phon**etic \f*e*-net-ĭk\ relating to spoken language or speech sounds
pneumo	lung	**pneumo**lithiasis \nü-mō-lĭth-ī-*e*-s*e*s\ the formation of calculi in the lungs
polio	relating to the gray matter of the brain	**polio**encephalitis \pō-lē-ō-ĭn-s*e*f-*e*-lī-t*e*s\ inflammation of the gray matter of the brain
poly	many, several, much	**poly**cystic \pǎl-ē-sĭs-tĭk\ having or involving more than one cyst
proct	rectum	**proct**itis \präk-tīt-*e*s\ inflammation of the anus and rectum
pseudo	false, spurious	**pseudo**cyesis \süd-ō-sī-ē-s*e*s\ false pregnancy
psych	mind, mental processes and activities	**psych**opathy \sī-käp-*e*-thē\ mental disorder
pulmon	lung	**pulmon**ary edema \pǔl-m*e*-ner-ē ĭ-dē-m*e*\ abnormal accumulation of fluid in the lungs
pyel	renal pelvis	**pyel**itis \pī-*e*-līt-*e*s\ inflammation of the renal pelvis of the kidney

Word Root	Refers to or Means	Example with Pronunciation and Definition
radi	radiant energy, radiation, radioactive	**radi**ologist \rād-ē-äl-*e*-jest\ a physician specializing in the use of radiant energy for diagnostic and therapeutic purposes
ren	kidney, renal	**ren**al calculus \rēn-l\ kidney stone
rhin	nose, nasal	**rhin**otomy \rī-nät-*e*-mē\ surgical incision of the nose
sacr	sacrum	**sacr**al vertebrae \sāk-r*e*l v*e*rt-*e*-brā\ any of the five fused vertebrae that make up the sacrum
salping	fallopian tube	**salping**ophorectomy \săl-pĭn-gō-f*e*-rek-t*e*-mē\ surgical removal of fallopian tubes and ovaries
scapul	scapula	**scapul**a \skăp-y*e*-l*e*\ shoulder blade
son	sound	**son**ic \sän-ĭk\ utilizing, produced by or relating to sound waves
spiro	respiration	**spiro**metry \spī-räm-*e*-trē\ measurement of the air entering and leaving the lungs
splen	spleen	**splen**omelagy \spl*e*n-ō-m*e*g-*e*-lē\ abnormal enlargement of the spleen
stern	breastbone, sternum	**stern**al \st*e*rn-l\ relating to the sternum
stomat	mouth	**stomat**oscope \st*e*-măt-*e*-skōp\ an instrument used for examination of the mouth
therm	heat	**therm**otherapy \th*e*r-m*e*-th*e*r-*e*-pē\ treatment of disease by heat
thorac	chest, thorax	**thorac**ic \th*e*-răs-ĭk\ pertaining to the rib cage
thromb	blood clot, clotting of blood	**thromb**ophlebitis \thräm-bō-fli-bīt-es\ inflammation of a vein with formation of a thrombus
toxic	poison	**toxi**phobia \täk-s*e*-fō-bē-*e*\ abnormal fear of poisons
trache	trachea	**trache**otomy \trā-kē-ät-*e*-mē\ surgical cutting in the trachea
ureter	ureter	**ureter**ocele \yū-rēt-*e*-re-sēl\ cystic dilation of the lower part of a ureter into the bladder
vascul	vessel, blood vessel	**vascul**ar \vas-kū-l*e*r\ relating to a tube or a system of tubes for carrying blood
ven	vein	**ven**ogram \vē-n*e*-gram\ an x-ray after the injection of an opaque substance into a vein

SUFFIXES

Suffixes, when used, are always attached to the end of the medical term. Suffixes are components that can modify a word root, such as giving clues to the condition, disease, disorder, or procedure affecting the word root. Suffixes are usually attached to a word with a combining vowel. The most commonly used combining vowel is _o_. For example, in the word _hematology_, _hemat_ is the word root, _o_ is the combining vowel, and _logy_ is the suffix.

Suffix	Refers to or Means	Example with Pronunciation and Definition
-al	pertaining to	na**sal** \ nā-z_e_l \ pertaining to the nose
-algia	pain	neur**algia** \nū-ral-jē-_e_\ nerve pain
-blast	immature cells	normo**blast** \nōr-m_e_-blast\ immature red blood cell
-cele	tumor, hernia	cysto**cele** \sĭs-t_e_-sēl\ hernia of the bladder
-centesis	puncture	thora**centesis** \thō-r_e_-s_e_n-tē-s_e_s\ aspiration of fluid from the chest
-cide	kill	germi**cide** \jer-m_e_-sīd\ an agent that destroys germs
-cise	cut	ex**cise** \ĕk-sīz\ remove by cutting
-ectomy	surgical removal	patell**ectomy** \păt-_e_-lek-t_e_-mē\ surgical removal of the patella
-emesis	vomiting	hemat**emesis** \hē-m_e_-te-mē-s_e_s\ vomiting of blood
-emia	condition of having, condition of having blood	an**emia** _e_-nē-mē-_e_\ a low red blood cell count
-gram	record	myelo**gram** \mī-_e_-le-gram\ record of the spinal cord
-graph	instrument for recording	electrocardio**graph** \ĭ-lek-trō-kärd-ē-ō-graf\ an instrument for recording the changes of the electrical potential occurring during the heartbeat
-graphy	process of recording	electrocardio**graphy** \ĭ-lek-trō-kärd-ē-äg-re-fē\ the process of recording the changes of the electrical potential occurring during the heartbeat
-ic	pertaining to	opt**ic** \äp-tĭk\ pertaining to the eye
-itis	inflammation of	appendic**itis** _e_-pen-de-sīt-_e_s\ inflammation of the appendix
-lepsy	seizure	epi**lepsy** \ep-_e_-lep-sē\ a group of nervous system disorders
-lysis	disintegration, reduction	hemo**lysis** \hē-mäl-_e_-s_e_s\ breakdown of red blood cells

Suffix	Refers to or Means	Example with Pronunciation and Definition
-malacia	softening	chondro**malacia** \kän-drō-m*e*-lā-shē-*e*\ softening of cartilage
-megaly	enlargement	spleno**megaly** \splēn-ō-m*eg*-*e*-lē\ enlargement of spleen
-meter	measure	thermo**meter** \th*e*-mäm-*et*-*er*\ an instrument for measuring temperature
-logy	study of	hemato**logy** \hē-m*e*-täl-*e*-jē\ study of blood
-oma	tumor	carcin**oma** \kär-c**ǐ**n-ō-m*e*\ a cancerous tumor
-pexy	fixation, usually surgical	myo**pexy** \mī-ō-p*ex*-ē\ fixation of the muscle
-phobia	irrational fear	hydro**phobia** \hī-dr*e*-fō-bē-*e*\ fear of water
-plasty	surgical repair	arthro**plasty** \är-thr*e*-plas-tē\ repair of a joint
-pnea	breath, breathing	a**pnea** \ăp-nē-*e*\ without a breath
-rrhagia, -rrhea	abnormal or excessive discharge or flow	dia**rrhea** \dī-*e*-rē-*e*\ excessive liquid-type stool
-rrhaphy	suture	cardio**rrhaphy** \kärd-ē-ōr-*e*-fē\ suture of the heart muscle
-rrhexis	rupture, splitting	hystero**rhexis** \hǐs-t*e*-ōr-r*e*ks-ǐs\ rupture of the uterus
-sclerosis	hardening	athero**sclerosis** \ă-th-*er*-ō-skle-rō-s*es*\ hardening of joints
-scopy	visual examination of	procto**scopy** \präk-täs-k*e*-pē\ visual examination of the rectum
-sis	action, process, or condition	diagno**sis** \dī-ig-`nō-ses\ the act of identifying a disease from signs and symptoms
-stomy	artifical or surgical opening	tracheo**stomy** \trāk-ē-äst-*e*-mē\ an artificial opening into the trachea
-tomy	incision, to cut	cranio**tomy** \krā-nē-ät-*e*-mē\ a cut into the skull
-penia	abnormally low number, deficiency	leuko**penia** \lü-kō-pē-nē-*e*\ deficiency of white blood cells
-thermy	heat	dia**thermy** \dī-a-ther-mē\ the generation of heat in tissues caused by electrical currents
-trophy	development	a**trophy** \a-tr*e*-fē\ no development
-uria	presence of, in urine	hema**turia** \hē-m*e*-tü-rē-*e*\ blood in the urine

SUMMARY

The ability to form medical terms is vital for a health unit coordinator. The rules for spelling and pronouncing medical terms are the same as those used in English, but the prefixes, suffixes, and word roots have specialized meanings. Knowledge of what the various word parts mean will give the health unit coordinator confidence. Accuracy in health care is vital. Whenever the health unit coordinator is in doubt as to how to spell or pronounce a medical term he or she should refer to a medical dictionary.

REVIEW QUESTIONS

Fill in the blanks.

1. A word root refers to the _____ of the word.

2. A prefix is a word part that is attached to the _____ of a word to produce a new word with a new meaning.

3. A suffix is a word part that is attached at the _____ of a base word to form a new word with a _____ _____.

4. A combining vowel is used to join a _____ _____ to a _____ and to join two word roots together.

Match the prefixes in the left column to the meanings in the right column.

5. ab   a. under, less than normal

6. ante   b. upon, attached to

7. auto   c. through

8. brady   d. between

9. dys   e. around

10. epi   f. under, below

11. hyper   g. from, away

12. hypo   h. excessive

13. inter   i. in front of

14. intra   j. many

15. neo   k. within

16. peri   l. difficult

17. poly   m. self

18. sub   n. new

19. trans   o. slow

Match the word roots in the left column to the meanings in the right column.

20. angi   a. bladder

21. anter   b. cold

22. arthr   c. heart

23. cardi   d. bone

24. cry   e. marrow or spinal cord

25. cyst   f. blood

26. cyt   g. joint

27. erythr   h. muscle

28. hepat   i. part of the pelvis

29. ileum   j. liver

30. illium   k. stomach

31. my   l. red

32. myel   m. cell

33. oste   n. part of small intestine

34. gastr   o. front

Match the suffixes in the left column to the meanings in the right column.

35. al   a. pain

36. algia   b. tumor

37. cele   c. surgical removal

38. ectomy   d. pertaining to

39. oma   e. enlargement

40. plasty   f. pertaining to

41. pnea   g. softening

42. sclerosis   h. inflammation of

43. scopy   i. tumor

44. stomy   j. surgical repair

45. ic   k. breath

46. itis   l. incision or to cut

47. malacia   m. visual examination

48. megaly   n. hardening

49. tomy   o. artifical or surgical opening

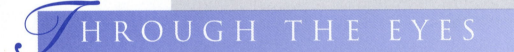

NAHUC CERTIFICATION EXAM

CONTENT AREAS

I. A. 2   Interpret medical symbols, abbreviations, and terminology

THROUGH THE EYES

OF A HEALTH CARE PROFESSIONAL

As a night shift health unit coordinator, I don't use medical terminology very much. However, knowledge of medical terminology helps me to better understand tests that need to be scheduled. It helps me to differentiate between invasive and non-invasive tests. Medical terminology helps when completing procedure consent forms and checklists.

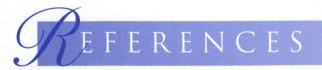

REFERENCES

Chabner, D. E. (2001). *The language of medicine* (6th ed.). Philadelphia: Saunders.

Medical desk dictionary (rev. ed.). (2002). Springfield, MA: Merriam-Webster.

Senisi-Scott, A., & Fong, E. (1998). *Body structures and functions* (9th ed.). Clifton Park, NY: Thomson Delmar Learning.

Simmers, L. (2004). *Diversified health occupations essentials* (6th ed.). Clifton Park, NY: Thomson Delmar Learning.

CHAPTER 21

Body Structure

Learning Objectives

Upon completion of this chapter and review questions, the learner should be able to:

1. List the 10 major systems of the human body.

2. Describe five main functions of the skeletal system.

3. Define three functions of the muscle system.

4. Name two main divisions of the nervous system.

5. Name the two main functions of the cardiovascular system.

6. Describe the two main functions of the lymphatic system.

7. List the 10 major glands of the endocrine system.

8. List five components of the cardiovascular system.

9. Describe the main function of the respiratory system.

10. List the major components of the digestive system.

11. Describe the purpose of the digestive system.

12. State another name for the urinary system.

13. Give another name for the reproductive system.

Key Terms

aldolase   An enzyme that helps muscle turn sugar into energy.

cartilage   A translucent elastic tissue that composes most of the skeleton of embryonic and very young vertebrates and becomes for the most part converted into bone in adult vertebrates.

endoscopic retrograde cholangiopancreatography   Using an endoscope through the mouth and stomach to the duodenum, which is the first part of the small intestine. It examines the bile ducts, pancreas, and gallbladder.

gastroscopy   To look into the inside of the stomach by means of a special instrument.

hematopoiesis   The production of blood cells; mostly takes place in the red marrow of the bones.

ligament   A band of fibrous tissue connecting bones or supporting organs.

lymph   Fluid formed in body tissues and circulated in the lymphatic vessels.

lymphangiogram   An x-ray with the injection of a contrast medium that views lymphatic circulation and the lymph nodes.

Papanicolaou test   Test in which cells are scraped from the cervix and tested for cancer.

tendon   A cord of connective tissue that attaches a muscle to a bone or other structure.

Abbreviations

ABG   Arterial Blood Gases

ACTH   Adrenocorticotropin hormone

AER   Auditory Evoked Response

BAER   Brainstem Auditory Evoked Response

CNS   Central Nervous System

ECG or **EKG**   Electrocardiogram

EEG   Electroencephalogram

EGD   Esophagogastroduodenoscopy

EMG   Electromyography

ERCP   Endoscopic Retrograde Cholangiopancreatography

PAP Papanicolaou Test

PFT Pulmonary Function Test

TSH Thyroid-Stimulating Hormone

U/A Urinalysis

VER Visual Evoked Response

INTRODUCTION TO BODY SYSTEMS

This chapter is an introduction to the body systems. Only basic knowledge of the various systems is included. This chapter should be used as a pictorial view of the human body system. For further information regarding the body systems, body structure, and physiology, a formal medical terminology class is recommended. In transcribing physicians' orders it is important to accurately list the body part and spell it correctly. This chapter will help you understand the different body parts that may be included in the physicians' orders.

There are 10 major systems that make up the human body. They are the skeletal system, muscular system, nervous system, endocrine system, cardiovascular system, lymphatic system, respiratory system, digestive system, urinary system, and reproductive system.

SKELETAL SYSTEM

The human skeletal system consists of 206 individual bones in the adult body and **cartilage**, **ligaments**, and **tendons**. Cartilage provides a strong yet flexible support for the skeleton. A ligament is a band of fibrous tissue connecting bones or supporting organs. A tendon consists of cords of connective tissue that attach a muscle to a bone or other structure. There are five main functions of the skeletal system:

◆ The bones support the body and provide shape to the body.

◆ The bones protect internal organs.

◆ The bones and muscles work together to produce body movement.

◆ Bones contain calcium. When the blood calcium level decreases, the calcium from the bone is released. **Hematopoiesis**, the production of blood cells, mostly takes place in the red marrow of the bones.

Physicians often order imaging views of the various body systems. Table 21-1 lists some common physician orders regarding the skeletal system.

For a better understanding of the body location of those orders see Figures 21-1 and 21-2.

TABLE 21-1   Common Physicians' Orders for Imaging Views

Abbreviated Order	Meaning
PA & LAT CXR	Posterior/back to anterior/front and lateral/side view chest x-ray
CT of C1 to L5	Computerized tomography scan from the first cervical vertebra to the last lumbar vertebra
MRI of R femur	Magnetic resonance imaging scan of right femur

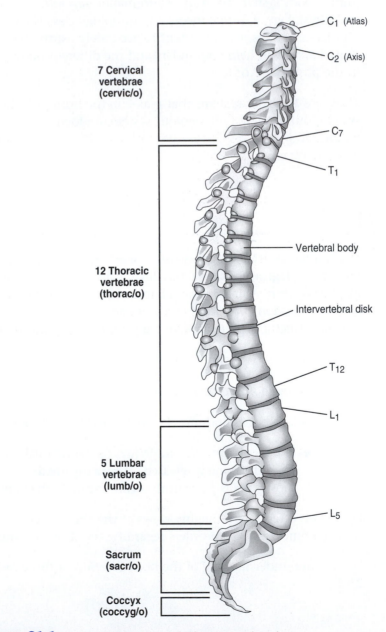

7 Cervical vertebrae (cervic/o)

C_1 (Atlas)
C_2 (Axis)
C_7
T_1

12 Thoracic vertebrae (thorac/o)

Vertebral body

Intervertebral disk

T_{12}
L_1

5 Lumbar vertebrae (lumb/o)

L_5

Sacrum (sacr/o)

Coccyx (coccyg/o)

Figure 21-1 • *Lateral view of the spinal column*

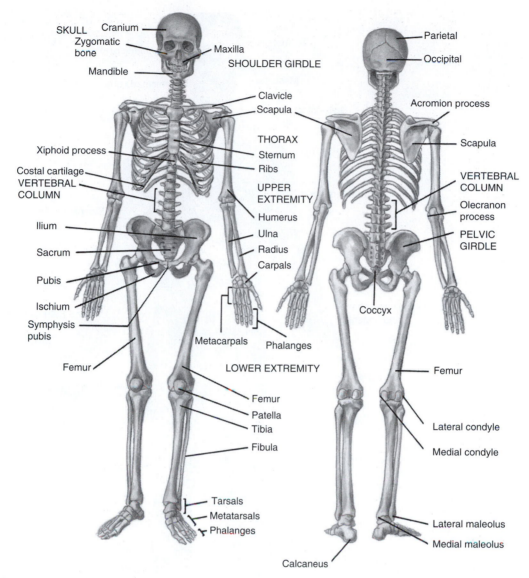

Figure 21-2 • *Bones of the skeleton*

MUSCULAR SYSTEM

There are over 650 muscles in the human body. Muscles are used for all body movement, and they give the body form and shape. There are three main functions of the muscle system:

◆ The muscle system is responsible for all body movement. This body movement is recognized as voluntary because a person has control over the movement.

◆ The muscle system is responsible for body form and shape, and these are also considered voluntary.

◆ The muscle system is responsible for body heat. This function is involuntary, or without conscious thought.

See Figures 21-3 and 21-4 for a view of the major muscles.

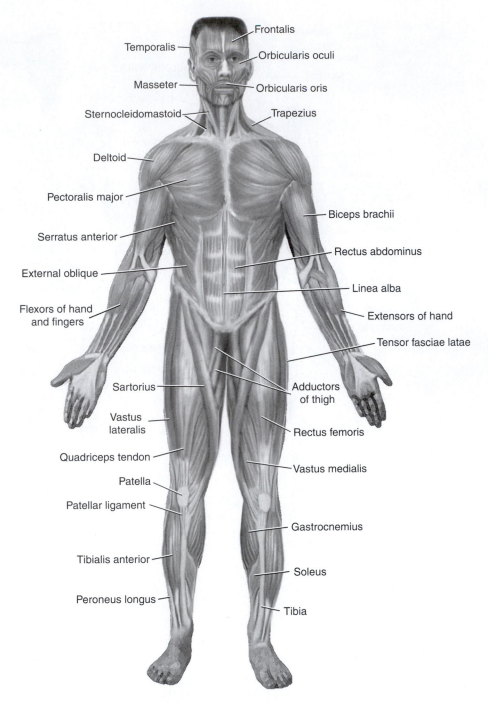

Figure 21-3 • *Principal skeletal muscles of the body, anterior view*

Aldolase is an enzyme that helps muscle turn sugar into energy. An aldolase test may be done to diagnose and monitor skeletal muscle diseases. Electromyography (EMG) is the electrical recording of muscle activity that aids in the diagnosis of neuromuscular disease.

NERVOUS SYSTEM

The nervous system is a complex, organized system of nerve cells that starts, oversees, and controls all the functions of the body. It is the command center for all mental

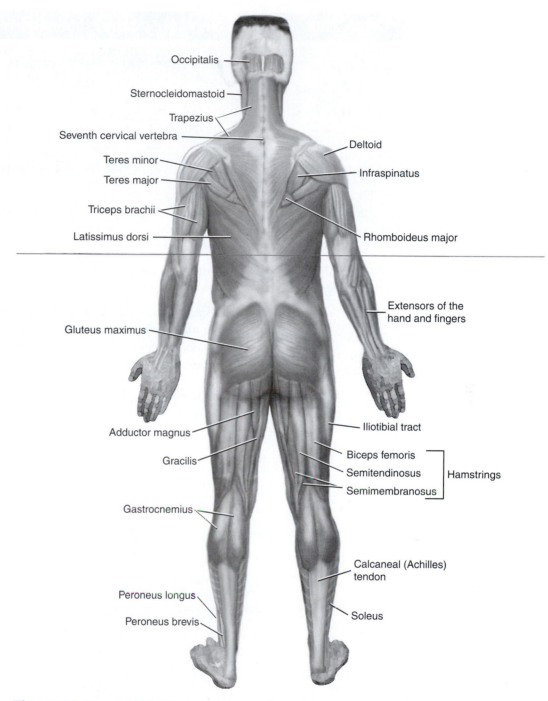

Occipitalis

Sternocleidomastoid

Trapezius

Seventh cervical vertebra

Teres minor

Teres major

Triceps brachii

Latissimus dorsi

Deltoid

Infraspinatus

Rhomboideus major

Extensors of the
hand and fingers

Gluteus maximus

Adductor magnus

Gracilis

Iliotibial tract

Biceps femoris

Semitendinosus

Semimembranosus

Hamstrings

Gastrocnemius

Peroneus longus

Peroneus brevis

Calcaneal (Achilles)
tendon

Soleus

Figure 21-4 · *Principal skeletal muscles of the body, posterior view*

activity, including thought, learning, and memory. It is divided into the central nervous system (CNS), which consists of the brain and spinal cord, and the peripheral nervous system, consisting of cranial nerves and spinal nerves. These nerves combine and communicate with all organs and tissues of the body. Some of the cranial nerves are for special senses such as taste, smell, sight, and hearing.

The spinal nerves carry messages to and from the spinal cord and are mixed nerves of sensory and motor types. Examinations that a health unit coordinator will need to request and schedule are listed in Table 21-2.

Note Figures 21-5 through 21-7 for a view of the nervous system.

TABLE 21-2 Common Nervous System Examinations

Lumbar puncture	Needle puncture into the spinal canal to remove blood or fluid.
VER (visual evoked response) AER (auditory evoked response) BAER (brainstem auditory evoked response)	Evoked potential studies are a group of tests of the nervous system that measure electrical signals along the nerve pathways. Three major types of evoked potential studies are used regularly: ◆ Visual evoked potentials are used to diagnose visual losses due to optic nerve damage, especially from multiple sclerosis. ◆ Auditory evoked potentials are used to diagnose hearing losses. ◆ Brainstem auditory evoked responses can distinguish damage to the acoustic nerve, which carries signals from the ear to the brainstem, from damage to the auditory pathways within the brainstem.
EEG	Electoencephalography is a neurological test that measures the electrical signals the brain sends to the body.

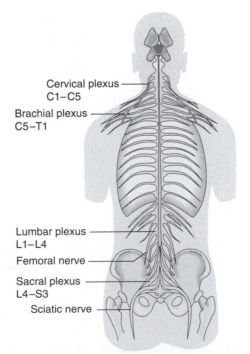

Figure 21-5 • *The spinal cord and nerves*

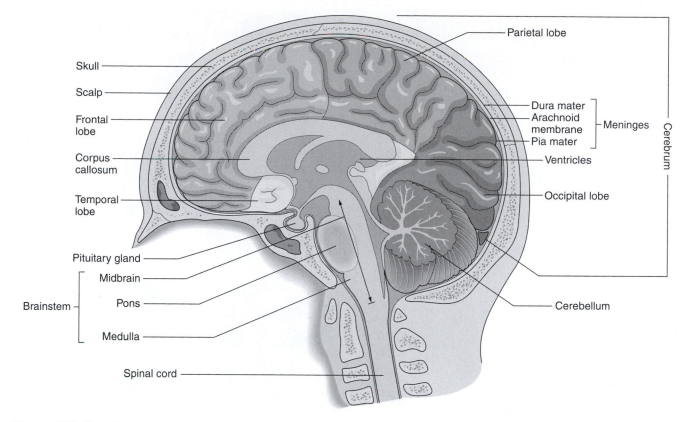

Figure 21-6 • *Cross section of the brain*

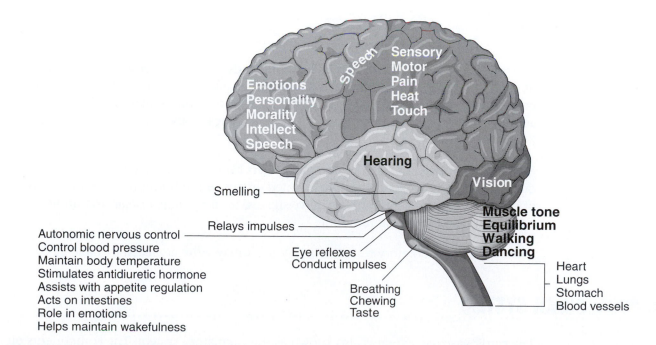

Figure 21-7 • *Cerebral functions*

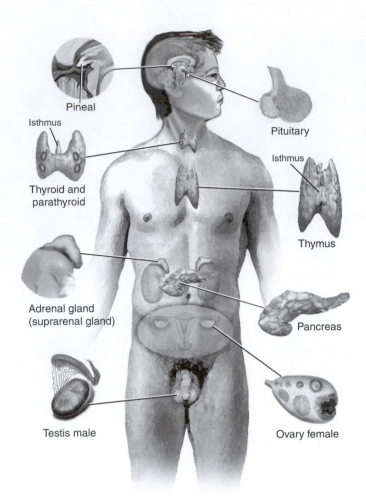

Pineal

Isthmus

Pituitary

Isthmus

Thyroid and
parathyroid

Thymus

Adrenal gland
(suprarenal gland)

Pancreas

Testis male

Ovary female

Figure 21-8 • *Locations of endocrine glands*

ENDOCRINE SYSTEM

The endocrine system consists of a group of glands that secrete or give off substances directly into the bloodstream. The substances are called hormones. The major glands of the endocrine system are the pituitary gland, thyroid gland, parathyroid glands, adrenal glands, pancreas, ovaries, testes, thymus, pineal body, and placenta. See Figures 21-8 and 21-9.

Hormones are often called chemical messengers because they are transported throughout the body by the bloodstream to targeted organs. Some hormones regulate release of other hormones, in response to nerve signals, from the target organ that indicate a need for the stimulating hormone.

Some common laboratory tests that a physician may write are listed in Table 21-3.

CARDIOVASCULAR SYSTEM

The cardiovascular system is also known as the circulatory system. The components of the cardiovascular system are the heart, arteries, veins, and capillaries as well as blood and the lymphatic system. The cardiovascular system is the longest system of the body. It

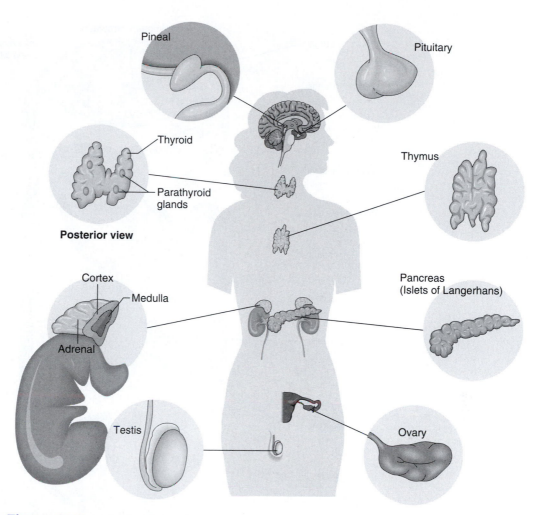

Pineal

Pituitary

Thyroid

Thymus

Parathyroid glands

Posterior view

Cortex

Medulla

Adrenal

Pancreas
(Islets of Langerhans)

Testis

Ovary

Figure 21-9 • *Endocrine glands*

TABLE 21-3	Common Endocrine System Laboratory Tests
ACTH	Adrenocorticotropin hormone to check for adrenal insufficiency
TSH	Thyroid-stimulating hormone to check for hyper- or hypothyroidism
Urine estrogen	Used in evaluating menstrual and fertility problems

goes throughout the body. The cardiovascular system passes blood, oxygen, and nutrients *to* body cells as well as passing carbon dioxide *away* from body cells. Figure 21-10 is an illustration of the pattern of circulation in the cardiovascular system. Figure 21-11 shows how blood is carried *into the heart by veins* and *away from the heart by arteries*. Figure 21-12 shows a more detailed view of the arteries and Figure 21-13 shows the veins. Capillaries are the smallest of the blood vessels. They allow for the exchange of nutrients and gases between the blood and the body cells. Table 21-4 shows common heart circulation studies.

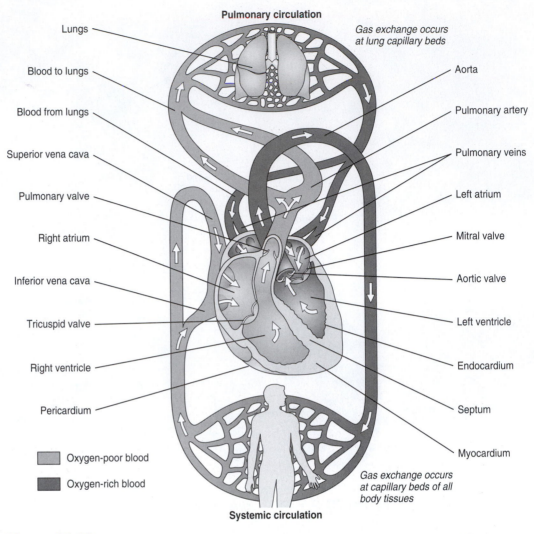

Figure 21-10 labels:

Pulmonary circulation

Lungs

Blood to lungs

Blood from lungs

Superior vena cava

Pulmonary valve

Right atrium

Inferior vena cava

Tricuspid valve

Right ventricle

Pericardium

Gas exchange occurs at lung capillary beds

Aorta

Pulmonary artery

Pulmonary veins

Left atrium

Mitral valve

Aortic valve

Left ventricle

Endocardium

Septum

Myocardium

Oxygen-poor blood

Oxygen-rich blood

Gas exchange occurs at capillary beds of all body tissues

Systemic circulation

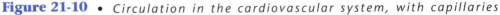

Figure 21-10 • *Circulation in the cardiovascular system, with capillaries*

LYMPHATIC SYSTEM

The lymphatic system consists of lymph fluid, lymph vessels, lymph nodes, and the spleen and thymus gland. The lymphatic system is mentioned as part of the cardiovascular system because it works in conjunction with the circulatory system since it has no pump of its own. Its main function is to remove waste and excess fluids from the tissues. **Lymph** is a watery fluid formed in body tissues and circulated in the lymphatic vessels. Figure 21-14 (page 364) shows the main components of the lymphatic system. See Table 21-5 (page 364) for tests related to the lymphatic system.

RESPIRATORY SYSTEM

The main functions of the respiratory system are to provide for the exchange of oxygen and carbon dioxide in the body and to produce sound from the larynx. The respiratory system consists of the nose, pharynx, larynx, trachea, bronchi, alveoli, and the lungs.

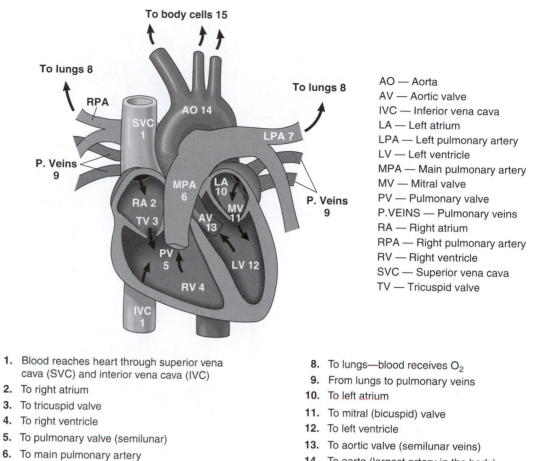

To body cells 15

To lungs 8

RPA

SVC 1

AO 14

To lungs 8

LPA 7

P. Veins 9

MPA 6

LA 10

RA 2

TV 3

MV 11

AV 13

P. Veins 9

PV 5

LV 12

RV 4

IVC 1

AO — Aorta
AV — Aortic valve
IVC — Inferior vena cava
LA — Left atrium
LPA — Left pulmonary artery
LV — Left ventricle
MPA — Main pulmonary artery
MV — Mitral valve
PV — Pulmonary valve
P.VEINS — Pulmonary veins
RA — Right atrium
RPA — Right pulmonary artery
RV — Right ventricle
SVC — Superior vena cava
TV — Tricuspid valve

1. Blood reaches heart through superior vena cava (SVC) and interior vena cava (IVC)
2. To right atrium
3. To tricuspid valve
4. To right ventricle
5. To pulmonary valve (semilunar)
6. To main pulmonary artery
7. To left pulmonary artery and right pulmonary artery

8. To lungs—blood receives O_2
9. From lungs to pulmonary veins
10. To left atrium
11. To mitral (bicuspid) valve
12. To left ventricle
13. To aortic valve (semilunar veins)
14. To aorta (largest artery in the body)
15. Blood with oxygen then goes to all cells of the body

Figure 21-11 • *Normal heart function*

TABLE 21-4	Heart Circulation Studies
ECG/EKG	Electrocardiogram, a test to detect abnormal electric activity of the heart
Echo	Echocardiogram, an examination to study the structure and motion of the heart
Holter monitor	Method of 24-hour continuous electrocardiogram to diagnose suspected rhythm disturbances

See Figure 21-15 (page 365) for a view of the respiratory system. The health unit coordinator may need to order the following tests regarding the respiratory system:

ABG: Arterial blood gases, to test oxygen intake and distribution

PFTs: Pulmonary function tests, a series of tests studying the ability of the lungs to exchange oxygen and carbon dioxide

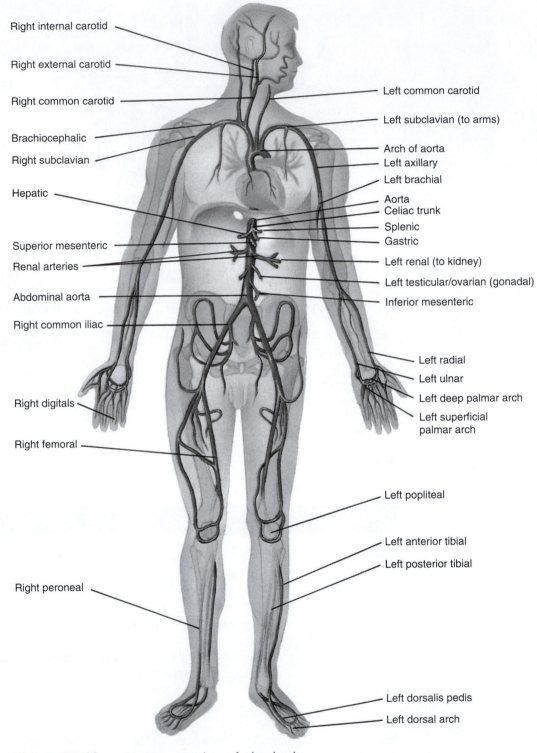

Right internal carotid

Right external carotid

Right common carotid

Brachiocephalic

Right subclavian

Hepatic

Superior mesenteric

Renal arteries

Abdominal aorta

Right common iliac

Right digitals

Right femoral

Right peroneal

Left common carotid

Left subclavian (to arms)

Arch of aorta

Left axillary

Left brachial

Aorta

Celiac trunk

Splenic

Gastric

Left renal (to kidney)

Left testicular/ovarian (gonadal)

Inferior mesenteric

Left radial

Left ulnar

Left deep palmar arch

Left superficial palmar arch

Left popliteal

Left anterior tibial

Left posterior tibial

Left dorsalis pedis

Left dorsal arch

Figure 21-12 • *Major arteries of the body*

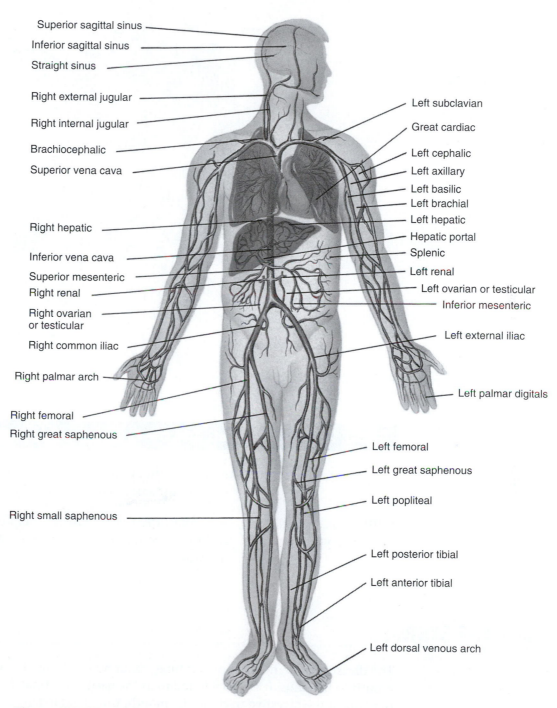

Superior sagittal sinus

Inferior sagittal sinus

Straight sinus

Right external jugular

Right internal jugular

Brachiocephalic

Superior vena cava

Right hepatic

Inferior vena cava

Superior mesenteric

Right renal

Right ovarian
or testicular

Right common iliac

Right palmar arch

Right femoral

Right great saphenous

Right small saphenous

Left subclavian

Great cardiac

Left cephalic

Left axillary

Left basilic

Left brachial

Left hepatic

Hepatic portal

Splenic

Left renal

Left ovarian or testicular

Inferior mesenteric

Left external iliac

Left palmar digitals

Left femoral

Left great saphenous

Left popliteal

Left posterior tibial

Left anterior tibial

Left dorsal venous arch

Figure 21-13 • *Major veins of the body*

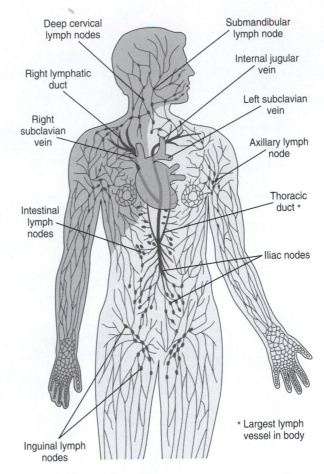

Deep cervical lymph nodes

Submandibular lymph node

Internal jugular vein

Right lymphatic duct

Left subclavian vein

Right subclavian vein

Axillary lymph node

Intestinal lymph nodes

Thoracic duct *

Iliac nodes

* Largest lymph vessel in body

Inguinal lymph nodes

Figure 21-14 • *Lymphatic system*

TABLE 21-5	Tests Related to the Lymphatic System
Lymphangiogram	An x-ray with an injection of a contrast medium that views lymphatic circulation and the lymph nodes
T(thymus derived) lymphocyte count	A count of the T cells, which is helpful in the diagnosis and treatment of immunodeficiency and lymphocytic diseases

DIGESTIVE SYSTEM

The digestive system is a muscular tube, about 30 feet long, that extends from the mouth to the anus. It is also referred to as the gastrointestinal system. The major components of the digestive tract are the mouth, throat, stomach, small intestine, and large intestine. The main purpose of the digestive system is to break down food both physically and chemically. Figure 21-16 shows the structure of the digestive system. Since health unit coordinators on a medical and surgical unit order many tests regarding the digestive system, Table 21-6 lists a few diagnostic examinations regarding the digestive system.

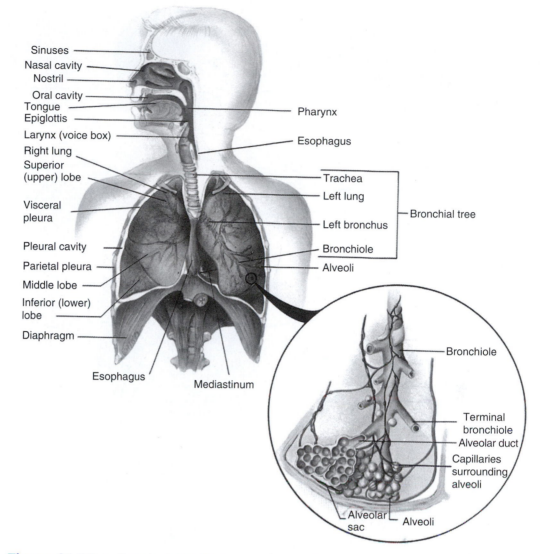

Sinuses
Nasal cavity
Nostril
Oral cavity
Tongue
Epiglottis
Larynx (voice box)
Right lung
Superior (upper) lobe
Visceral pleura
Pleural cavity
Parietal pleura
Middle lobe
Inferior (lower) lobe
Diaphragm
Esophagus
Mediastinum

Pharynx
Esophagus
Trachea
Left lung
Left bronchus
Bronchiole
Alveoli
Bronchial tree

Bronchiole
Terminal bronchiole
Alveolar duct
Capillaries surrounding alveoli
Alveolar sac
Alveoli

Figure 21-15 • *Respiratory organs and structure*

URINARY SYSTEM

The urinary system is also known as the excretory system, or the system that eliminates waste from the body. Figure 21-17 illustrates the many components of the urinary system. The most common test of the urinary system is a urinalysis (U/A); other tests are listed in Table 21-7.

Urinalyses reveal many diseases and chemical imbalances. At times, the physician will be very specific with the test that should be performed, such as urine for protein or urine drug screen. Examples of problems detected by urine system tests include diabetes mellitus and chronic urinary tract infections. Other types of urine studies include 24-hour urine collection.

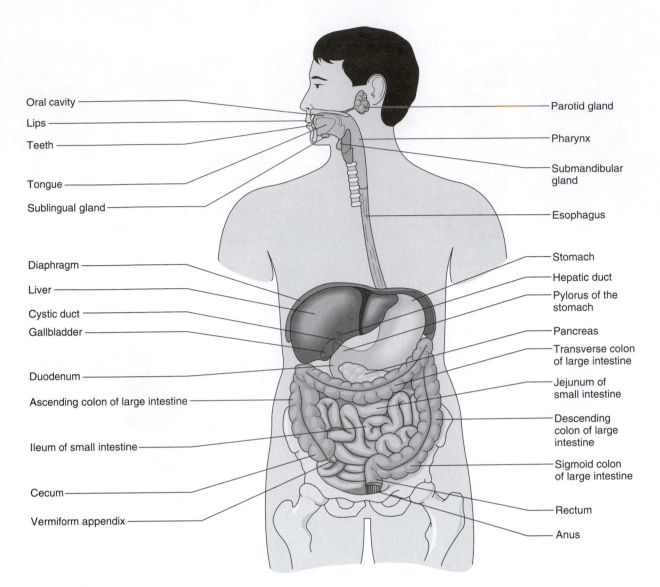

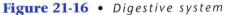

Figure 21-16 • *Digestive system*

TABLE 21-6	Digestive System Diagnostic Examinations
EGD	Esophagogastroduodenoscopy, allows visualization of the interior of the upper gastrointestinal tract to diagnose many irregularities of the digestive system.
ERCP	**Endoscopic retrograde cholangiopancreatography**, using an endoscope through the mouth and stomach to the duodenum, which is the first part of the small intestine, to examine the bile ducts, pancreas, and gallbladder
Gastroscopy	An inspection of the inside of the stomach by means of a special instrument.

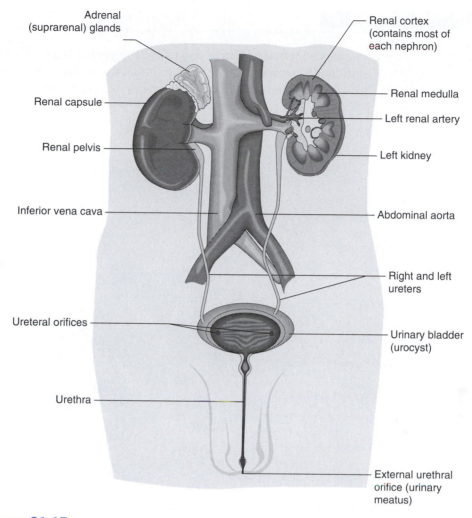

Adrenal
(suprarenal) glands

Renal cortex
(contains most of
each nephron)

Renal capsule

Renal medulla

Left renal artery

Renal pelvis

Left kidney

Inferior vena cava

Abdominal aorta

Right and left
ureters

Ureteral orifices

Urinary bladder
(urocyst)

Urethra

External urethral
orifice (urinary
meatus)

Figure 21-17 • *Urinary system*

TABLE 21-7 Urinary System Laboratory Tests

U/A	A chemical analysis to identify and quantify any large number of substances, most often ketones, sugar, proteins, and blood. Macroscopic urinalysis is the direct visual observation of the urine, noting its quantity, color, clarity or cloudiness, and much more. The microscopic urinalysis is the study of the urine under the microscope.
Urine for O B	Urine for occult blood, such a small amount that it is undetectable by just the clinical method.
Urine for C & S	Urine culture and sensitivity; a urine culture is a method to grow and identify bacteria that may be in the urine. Bacteria are germs that cause infections. The sensitivity test helps caregivers pick the best medicine to treat the infection.

REPRODUCTIVE SYSTEM

The reproductive system is also called the genital tract. The purpose of the reproductive system is to reproduce. The male reproductive system consists of the testicles, epididymis, vas deferens, seminal vesicles, ejaculatory ducts, urethra, prostate gland, and penis.

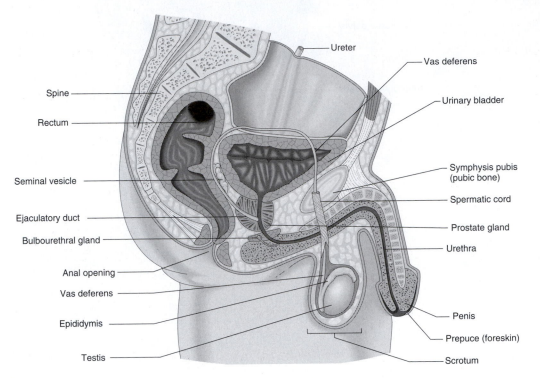

Spine
Rectum
Seminal vesicle
Ejaculatory duct
Bulbourethral gland
Anal opening
Vas deferens
Epididymis
Testis

Ureter
Vas deferens
Urinary bladder
Symphysis pubis (pubic bone)
Spermatic cord
Prostate gland
Urethra
Penis
Prepuce (foreskin)
Scrotum

Figure 21-18 • *Structures of the male reproductive system*

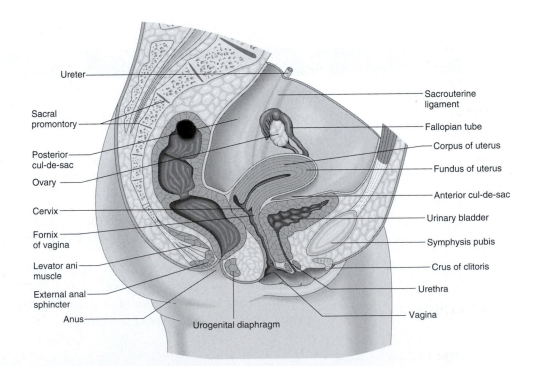

Ureter
Sacral promontory
Posterior cul-de-sac
Ovary
Cervix
Fornix of vagina
Levator ani muscle
External anal sphincter
Anus
Urogenital diaphragm

Sacrouterine ligament
Fallopian tube
Corpus of uterus
Fundus of uterus
Anterior cul-de-sac
Urinary bladder
Symphysis pubis
Crus of clitoris
Urethra
Vagina

Figure 21-19 • *Structures of the female reproductive system*

The female reproductive system consists of the ovaries, fallopian tubes, uterus, vagina, clitoris, vulva, and breasts. See Figure 21-18 for the structures of the male reproductive system, and Figures 21-19 through 21-21 for the female reproductive structures. Some exams ordered for the reproductive system are listed in Table 21-8.

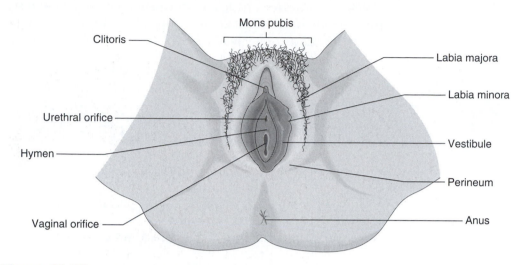

Figure 21-20 • *External female genitalia*

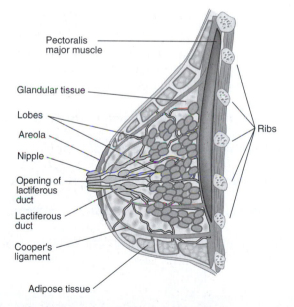

Figure 21-21 • *Sagittal section of the female breast*

TABLE 21-8 Reproductive System Laboratory Tests	
U/A for pregnancy	Urinalysis test to determine if the female is pregnant
PAP, or Pap smear	Papanicolaou test, in which cells are scraped from the cervix and tested for cancer
US for gestation	Ultrasound to show a picture of an unborn baby; also shows images of the uterus, amniotic sac, placenta, and ovaries

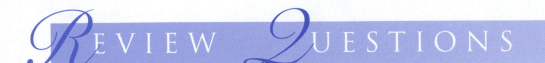

SUMMARY

This brief overview of the body system has illustrated the major parts of the body systems. It provides a basic idea of where many organs and systems are located and the function of each system. It is hoped that this has generated enough interest for you to pursue a complete separate course on medical terminology.

REVIEW QUESTIONS

1. List the 10 major systems of the human body.

2. Describe five main functions of the skeletal system.

3. Define three functions of the muscle system.

4. Name two main divisions of the nervous system.

5. Name the two main functions of the cardiovascular system.

6. Describe the two main functions of the lymphatic system.

7. List the 10 major glands of the endocrine system.

8. List five components of the cardiovascular system.

9. Describe the main function of the respiratory system.

10. List the major components of the digestive system.

11. Describe the purpose of the digestive system.

12. State another name for the urinary system.

13. Give another name for the reproductive system.

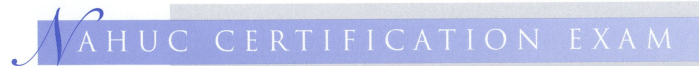

NAHUC CERTIFICATION EXAM

CONTENT AREAS

I. A. 2   Interpret medical symbols, abbreviations, and terminology

THROUGH THE EYES

OF A HEALTH CARE PROFESSIONAL

A unit coordinator shares his thoughts.

Medical terminology is the foundation to transcribing orders. Medical terminology gives insight when coordinating tests so all the tests are completed in a timely manner. Knowing medical terminology gives a coordinator a basic knowledge of tests and some logic as to why they are ordered.

REFERENCES

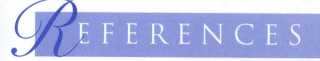

http://www.healthatoz/atoz Accessed October 2003.

http://www.web.md Accessed October 2003.

Senisi Scott, A., & Fong, E. (1998). *Body structure and functions* (9th ed.) Clifton Park, NY: Thomson Delmar Learning.

Simmers, L. (2004). *Diversified health occupations essentials* (6th ed.). Clifton Park, NY: Thomson Delmar Learning.

Mosby Medical Encyclopedia. (1992). New York: Plume Publishing.

Abbreviations and Symbols

Learning Objectives

Upon completion of this chapter and review questions, the learner should be able to:

1. Explain why abbreviations are used in health care.

2. Describe three ways abbreviations evolve from the medical term.

3. Memorize the abbreviations and symbols listed.

Key Terms

abbreviation   a shortening of a word.

symbol   a written sign or character that is used to represent a word.

ABBREVIATIONS

Time-saving measures are usually of interest to busy people. People may look for ways to prepare meals more quickly, to drive to school on a shorter route, or to implement shortcuts in their daily routines. People also look for ways to communicate more quickly. In writing, **abbreviations** are used to speed the process of completing a message. An abbreviation is a shortening of a word. The abbreviations can be a letter or group of letters that are used to represent the whole word. If one has sent a text message, one has probably used an abbreviation. For example, one might write "c u later" to abbreviate the words "see you later." Abbreviations save time.

ABBREVIATIONS IN HEALTH CARE

Many medical terms are long and difficult to spell and pronounce. Because abbreviations save time, they are commonly used in health care. Even though abbreviations are widely used in health care, there are risks involved. The danger in using abbreviations is in the interpretation. One person may write the abbreviation to represent one word, and another person may read the abbreviation to represent another word. To eliminate misinterpretation of abbreviations, health care facilities have a list of approved abbreviations. The health care facility may use an approved abbreviation list from another source, such as the American Association for Medical Transcriptionists or the Institute for Safe Medical Practices, or they may create their own list. The list of approved abbreviations should be available and understood by all who write and read abbreviations.

JCAHO NATIONAL PATIENT SAFETY GOALS

Regulatory agencies such as the Joint Commission on Accreditation of Healthcare Organizations (JCAHO) are concerned with safety issues regarding abbreviations. According to the JCAHO Web site, the Joint Commission's Board of Commissioners approved the 2004 National Patient Safety Goals. One of the safety goals is to improve the effectiveness of communication among caregivers. Part of the JCAHO patient safety goals reads, "Standardize the abbreviations, acronyms and symbols used throughout the organization, including a list of abbreviations, acronyms and symbols *not* to use." A minimum list of dangerous abbreviations, acronyms, and symbols has been approved by JCAHO. Beginning January 1, 2004, the following items must be included on each accredited organization's "Do not use" list:

- u for unit
- iu for international unit
- qd for every day
- qod for every other day
- M.S., MS04, MgS04 for magnesium sulfate or morphine sulfate
- Trailing zeros or lack of leading zero when writing decimals

It is expected that the Do-not-use abbreviation list will be lengthened. Check with your facility and the JCAHO Web site for the most current list of approved abbreviations and prohibited abbreviations.

PREVENTING ERRORS

A general rule for preventing errors due to abbreviations is, "When in doubt, write it out." If you are unsure of how an abbreviation is written or think the written abbreviation could be read as another abbreviation, you should write out the entire term. If you are reading an abbreviation and are unsure of what it means, you should clarify the abbreviation with the person who wrote it. In the case of clarifying abbreviations in physicians' orders, the health care facility policy should be followed. In many health care facilities, order clarification must be sought by a licensed health care worker only. In such a case, the health unit coordinator would bring the abbreviation in question in the physician's order to the attention of a licensed health care worker such as a registered nurse and ask that person to seek clarification.

INCONSISTENCIES IN ABBREVIATIONS

To complicate matters for those new to medical terminology, some abbreviations are written only in lower case letters, and some abbreviations only in upper case letters, and, for some abbreviations, either lower or upper case letters are acceptable. Some abbreviations may have more than one meaning depending on the context in which they are used. And some words may have more than one acceptable abbreviation. Experience with reading physicians' orders and other health care documents will help one become more familiar with the proper way to write abbreviations. Memorization of abbreviation lists is also helpful.

TYPES OF ABBREVIATIONS

Medical abbreviations evolve in a number of ways. An abbreviation could be a shortened version of the word, it could be a selection of letters that form the term, or it could be based on the original Latin or Greek terminology.

SHORTENED WORDS

Sometimes a word is abbreviated simply by shortening the word. For example *temperature* may be abbreviated by shortening to "temp." *Continuous* may be shortened to "cont." Table 22-1 lists some abbreviations that are formed by shortening the word.

INITIAL LETTERS

Some abbreviations are formed by the initial letters in the expression or name. For example, one may write FAQ to represent *frequently asked questions* or PC to abbreviate *personal computer*. Job titles in health care are often abbreviated by using the initial letters of the title. For example, registered nurse is abbreviated RN; medical doctor is

TABLE 22-1   Shortened Words

Medical Term	Shortened Word
Technician	tech
Catheter	cath
Calorie	cal
General	gen

TABLE 22-2 Abbreviations Formed by Initial Letters

Medical Term	Abbreviation
BRP	Bathroom privileges
IV	Intravenous
US	Ultrasound
MRI	Magnetic resonance imaging

abbreviated MD; and health unit coordinator may be abbreviated HUC. In health care, when words are abbreviated by the initial letters, the abbreviation is usually pronounced by stating the letters rather than blending them into a new word of their own. For example, the pronunciation of RN is "Ahr-en" as two separate letters, not "arn," a blending of the letters. MD is pronounced "em-dee," not "emd"; and HUC is pronounced "aich-you-see." not "huck."

As stated earlier, there are inconsistencies in the rules of writing and pronouncing abbreviations. Some are pronounced as if the letters form a word. For example, the abbreviation for the procedure *coronary artery bypass graft* may be abbreviated on a surgery schedule as CABG. CABG is usually pronounced "cabbage," as if it were a new blended word. Many abbreviations for medical terms are abbreviated by using initial letters, as shown in Table 22-2.

ABBREVIATIONS WITH LATIN ROOTS

Words that are abbreviated by initial letters and by shortening the word may be the easiest to remember because the abbreviation bears some resemblance to the meaning of the word. For example, when trying to figure out the meaning of the abbreviation LPN, one can remember that this abbreviation is for three words beginning with an *l*, a *p*, and an *n*. When trying to remember the abbreviation nec, one can think of familiar words that can be shortened by nec, such as necessary. However, many abbreviations used in health care come from Latin words.

Much of medical terminology has it roots in Latin. Therefore, many abbreviations also have Latin roots. The word *abbreviation* itself is based on the Latin root *brevis*, which means "short."

A medical abbreviation commonly heard in popular culture, as well as in health care, is "stat." *Stat* means "immediately." *Stat* is not formed by initial letters, nor is it a shortened version of a word meaning immediately. *Stat* is an abbreviation that has its roots in the Latin language. The Latin word *statim* means "immediately" or "without delay." Health care recognizes the abbreviation stat to mean immediate. Another common abbreviation is prn. In health care, prn means "as necessary." It comes from the Latin term *pro re nata* meaning "as the occasion arises." There are many examples of medical abbreviations with Latin roots. Some are given in Table 22-3.

TABLE 22-3 Abbreviations with Latin Roots		
Abbreviation	**Latin Root**	**Meaning**
ad lib	ad libitum	freely, as desired
bid	bis in die	two times a day
NPO	non per os	nothing by mouth
qd	quaque die	once a day
qid	quarter in die	four times a day
tid	ter in die	three times a day

ABBREVIATION LIST

There are hundreds of medical abbreviations. This chapter is an introduction to a few of the most common ones. Additional abbreviations will be introduced in future transcription chapters.

ABBREVIATIONS ASSOCIATED WITH JOB TITLES

CNA, certified nursing assistant

DO, doctor of osteopathy

HUC, health unit coordinator

LPN, licensed practical nurse

LVN, licensed vocational nurse

MD, medical doctor

PCT, patient care technician

RN, registered nurse

Tech, technician

ABBREVIATIONS ASSOCIATED WITH TIME AND FREQUENCY

These abbreviations may be used to indicate when or how often a treatment, observation, or therapy is to be performed or when a medication is to be administered.

ac, before meals

ad lib, as desired

asap, as soon as possible

as tol, as tolerated

bid, 2 times a day

cont, continuous

dc, discontinue

h, **hr**, **hrs**; hour(s)

hs, bedtime

midnoc, midnight

min, minute

MN, midnight

MR, may repeat

nec, necessary

pc, after meals

prn, as necessary

q, every

q day, everyday

qh, every hour

qid, 4 times a day

qod, every other day

rt, routine

stat, immediately

tid, 3 times a day

ABBREVIATIONS ASSOCIATED WITH ACTIVITY

These abbreviations may be used to indicate what level of activity the patient may have.

amb, ambulatory

BR, bedrest

BRP, bathroom privileges

BSC, bedside commode

CBR, complete bedrest

OOB, out of bed

ABBREVIATIONS ASSOCIATED WITH OBSERVATION AND MONITORING

These abbreviations may be used for various types of nursing observation tasks.

ax, axillary

BP, blood pressure

CMS, circulation, motion sensation

I/O, intake/output

NVS, neurological vital signs

P, pulse

R, respiration

T, Temp; temperature

VS, vital signs

wt, weight

ABBREVIATIONS ASSOCIATED WITH POSITIONS

These abbreviations may be used to indicate positions or locations.

HOB, head of bed

lt, L; left

rt, R; right

ABBREVIATIONS ASSOCIATED WITH TREATMENTS

These abbreviations may be used for the various treatments a patient may receive.

AE, antiembolism

cath, catheter

CBI, contiunous bladder irrigation

drsg, dressing

irrig, irrigation

NG, nasogastric

SSE, soap suds enema

st, straight

TCDB, turn, cough, deep breathe

TEDs, AE hose

TWE, tapwater enema

WMC, warm moist compress

ABBREVIATIONS ASSOCIATED WITH MEASUREMENTS

These abbreviations may be used to indicate medication measurements.

cc, cubic centimeter

cm, centimeter

gtts, drops

g, gram

gr, grain

mEq, milliequivalent

mg, milligram

ml, **mL**; milliliter

ABBREVIATIONS ASSOCIATED WITH DIETS

These abbreviations may be used in diet orders.

cal, calorie

cl, clear

DAT, diet as tolerated

FF, force fluids

gen, general

liq, liquid

MN, midnight

NAS, no added salt

NPO, nothing by mouth

reg, regular

ABBREVIATIONS ASSOCIATED WITH MEDICATIONS

These abbreviations may be used to indicate how the patient will be receiving medication.

IM, intramuscular

INT, intermittent

IVPB, intravenous piggyback

po, by mouth

subl, sublingual

subq, subcutaneous

ABBREVIATIONS ASSOCIATED WITH IVs AND SOLUTIONS

These abbreviations may be used to indicate the type of intravenous fluid or the rate of an intravenous infusion.

D/RL, dextrose lactated Ringers

D5W, dextrose 5% water

DW, dextrose/water

H₂O₂, hydrogen peroxide

IV, intravenous

LR, **RL**; lactated Ringers

NS, normal saline

soln, solution

TKO, to keep open

SYMBOLS

In addition to shortened words, initial letters, and Latin terms, **symbols** are also used in health care. A symbol is a written sign or character that is used to represent a word. For example, the symbol for dollar is $. In daily life, symbols are can be seen on traffic signs, keyboards, menus, and billboards. There are a variety of symbols used in health care, as shown in Table 22-4.

TABLE 22-4   Symbols

Symbol	Word Represented
p̄	after
c̄	with
/	per
✓	check
↑	up
↓	down
△	change
@	at

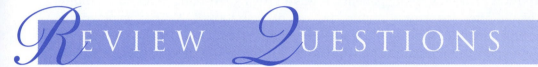

SUMMARY

Abbreviations are shortened words. Abbreviations are popular in health care because they save time. Memorize as many abbreviations as possible before transcribing orders. Be sure to have access to the facility's approved list of abbreviations to assist in interpretation. When in doubt, write it out.

REVIEW QUESTIONS

1. List three different ways abbreviations are formed.

2. Write the abbreviation for the following times and frequencies:
   a. Every day
   b. Two times a day
   c. Three times a day
   d. Four times a day
   e. Before meals
   f. After meals
   g. Bedtime

3. Write the full terms for the following abbreviations:
   a. BRP
   b. BP
   c. I/O
   d. HUC
   e. RN
   f. LPN
   g. PCT

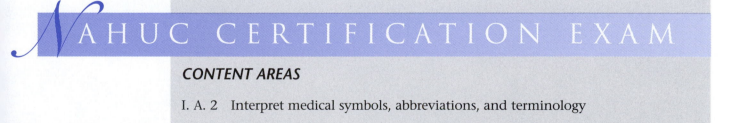

NAHUC CERTIFICATION EXAM

CONTENT AREAS

I. A. 2   Interpret medical symbols, abbreviations, and terminology

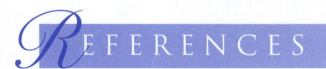

OF A HEALTH CARE PROFESSIONAL

A hospital chaplain shares her thoughts.

Before working in the pediatric unit in a health care facility, I had years of experience ministering to children and their families. Although I was very confident in the service I was providing to the patients, it was a little like working in a foreign country. I would often see signs posted by the patients that looked like they were written in another language. Signs would read NPO or I/O. When I asked for the location of a patient and was told that the patient was in OT doing ADL, it sounded like an unfamiliar language. Even though I did not need to know details about the patient's plan of care, it was helpful to learn what these abbreviations and terms meant. Just as if I was working in another country, I strived to learn more about the written and spoken language of the residents. That is why it was important to me to become familiar with medical abbreviations and terminology.

REFERENCES

jcaho.org/accredited+organizations/patient+safety/04+npsg/facts+about+the+04+npsg.htm Accessed April 2004.

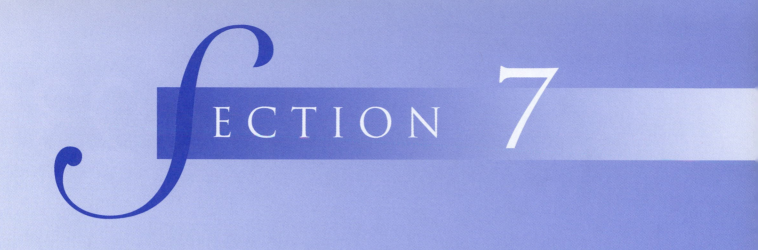

SECTION 7

Order Transcription

CHAPTER 23

Transcription: The Process

Learning Objectives

Upon completion of this chapter and review questions, the learner should be able to:

1. Define transcription of physicians' orders.

2. Compare the term *transcription* as it applies to health unit coordinating with the health unit coordinator and with the medical transcriptionist.

3. Name the components of the physician's order.

4. Describe how to recognize an order that needs to be transcribed.

5. List and describe the four order categories.

6. List the tools used in transcription of physicians' orders.

7. List the steps of the transcription process.

8. List methods to avoid errors.

Key Terms

Kardex A profile of all current physicians' orders for a patient.

medical staff The licensed physicians who have privileges to admit and attend to patients in the health care facility.

medical transcription Translating from oral to written (on paper or electronically) the record of a person's medical history, diagnosis, prognosis, and outcome.

physician's order sheet A specific chart form used by the physician to record orders for the patient.

transcription The procedure involving activating or communicating the plan of care that the physician determines for the patient.

Abbreviations

ASAP As Soon As Possible

HIM Health Information Management

MAR Medication Administration Record

PRN As Necessary

Stat Immediately

T.O. Telephone Order

V.O. Verbal Order

WHAT IS TRANSCRIPTION?

Transcription is the procedure involving activating or communicating the plan of care that the physician determines for the patient. It is the key responsibility of the health unit coordinator. When transcribing physicians' orders, the health unit coordinator acknowledges or recognizes, processes, and communicates the diagnostic and therapeutic orders of the **medical staff**.

TRANSCRIPTION IN HEALTH UNIT COORDINATING AND MEDICAL TRANSCRIBING

The term *transcription* has two meanings within the health care setting. It applies to both the health unit coordinating and the medical transcribing professions. Transcription has separate meanings for the separate professions. If just beginning training in health unit coordinating, one may encounter this situation of dual definitions when telling people about going to school to learn how to transcribe physicians' orders. Transcription, as it applies to health unit coordinating, is the procedure of acknowledging, processing, and communicating the orders of the medical staff. **Medical transcription**, as defined by the American Association for Medical Transcription, "is translating from oral to written (on paper or electronically) the record of a person's medical history, diagnosis, prognosis, and outcome."

The Differences

There are both differences and similarities between health unit coordinator transcription and medical transcription. The medical transcriptionist in the health care setting works for the health information management (HIM) department, also known as the clinical information department (Figure 23-1). The physician dictates the reports. The dictated information is saved for the medical transcriptionist. The medical transcriptionist, at a later time, listens to physician's dictated reports and, using a keyboard, transcribes the information onto a paper or electronic file. The medical transcriptionist typically works in a home setting, business, or in the HIM department and has limited contact with patients and other health care workers.

The health unit coordinator in the health care setting works in the nursing or unit service department (Figure 23-2). The health unit coordinator reads the diagnostic and therapeutic orders in the patient's current medical record and utilizes a variety of tools to process and communicate the orders to ensure that the patient receives the plan of care ordered by the physician. The physician may give the order in oral, written, or

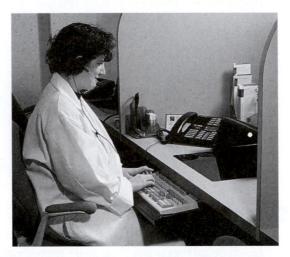

Figure 23-1 • *A medical transcriptionist in the work environment*

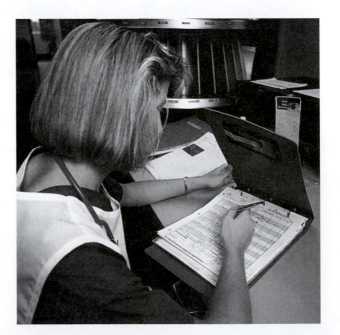

Figure 23-2 • *A health unit coordinator in the work environment*

TABLE 23-1	Health Unit Coordinating Transcription and Medical Transcription	
	Health Unit Coordinating	**Medical Transcribing**
Transcription definitions	The procedure of acknowledging, processing, and communicating the orders of the medical staff	Translating from oral to written (on paper or electronically) the record of a person's medical history, diagnosis, prognosis, and outcome
Work area	Nursing or unit service department	Health information management department or clinical information department
Basic knowledge	Anatomy, physiology, disease processes, medical terminology, and abbreviations	Same
Knowledge application	To accurately process physicians' orders for the treatment and care of the patient	To accurately transfer the physician's oral dictation to a written report
Interacts with	Nurses, physicians, patients, visitors, ancillary staff	Physicians

electronic form. The order is then processed as soon as possible. Transcription is the transferring of data from one form to another. Health unit coordinators transfer the data from the physician order sheet to a number of different areas via written forms, phone calls, and computer entries. The health unit coordinator, who works in the center of the patient care delivery area, interacts with patients, visitors, nurses, physicians, and ancillary staff.

The Similarities

Both the medical transcriptionist and the health unit coordinator use the basic knowledge of anatomy, physiology, disease processes, medical terminology, and abbreviations. The medical transcriptionist applies that knowledge to accurately transfer the physician's oral dictation to a written report. The health unit coordinator applies that same knowledge to accurately process physician's orders for the treatment and care of the patient. The roles are compared in Table 23-1.

THE PHYSICIAN'S ORDER

The physician's order is the physician's instructions for the patient's health care. In simple terms, a physician's order is something that the physician wants the patient to have or undergo. Before anything can be done for a patient, the physician must order it. The patient may not eat, drink, or move or be given a medication, treatment, therapy, or diagnostic test until the physician puts it in the form of an order. The physician may give the order in a written, verbal, or electronic form. As health care facilities move toward a paperless, or electronic, chart, the practice of the physician's submitting the order electronically will become widely used.

The majority of physician orders are written. The physician assesses the patient and determines what needs to be done and writes the orders in the patient's chart. The order is written on a specific chart form called the **physician's order sheet**. The physician's order sheet may be on carbon or NCR© (No Carbon Required) paper to provide duplicate copies of the order. Health unit coordinators transcribe only orders that are on the physician's order sheet.

The physician may also give a verbal order, or V.O. The verbal order may be given in person or over the telephone. When given over a telephone, the order is termed a T.O. As stated earlier, health unit coordinators transcribe only those orders that are written on the physician's order sheet. Therefore, the verbal order must still be written on the physician's order sheet. State legislation and employer policy dictate which health care professionals may accept verbal orders from physicians. In some facilities, orders must be given from a licensed professional to a licensed professional; in other words from a physician to a registered nurse. In other facilities, health unit coordinators may accept all verbal physician orders with the exception of medication orders. It is important for the health unit coordinator to know and understand the employer's policy regarding verbal physician orders.

JCAHO READ-BACK REQUIREMENTS

There is always room for error when one person gives another person verbal instructions. Most health care facilities have procedures in place to ensure that verbal instructions are given and received properly. The Joint Commission on Accreditation of Healthcare Organizations (JCAHO) has developed a national patient safety goal regarding the verbal exchange of critical information. According to the JCAHO Web site, one of the goals is to "implement a process for taking verbal or telephone orders or critical test results that require a verification read-back of the complete order or test result by the person receiving the order or test result." JCAHO recommends "whenever possible, the receiver of the order should write down the complete order or enter it into a computer, then read it back, and receive confirmation from the individual who gave the order." As stated in Chapter 15, the receiver must receive the message sent by the sender in order for communication to happen. When the receiver repeats the information back to the sender, the sender hears what message the receiver heard. This type of feedback or response allows both parties, the receiver and the sender, to clarify the message.

Within the heath care setting, it is not unusual to have an emergency situation. In an emergency situation, such as cardiac arrest, a physician may call out a medication order, the nurse may repeat it back before administering the drug, and another health care professional may document the order and its administration. JCAHO says, "In certain situations such as a code, it may not be feasible to do a formal read-back. In such cases, repeat-back is acceptable."

COMPONENTS

Physician orders have general components that are a part of any order. Physician orders must include the following components:

◆ *Date.* The date the order was written, and the time may also be included.

◆ *Content of order.* What the physician determines the patient needs.

◆ *Physician's signature.* The physician who writes the order signs the order. In the event of a verbal or telephone order, the individual taking the order will write the ordering physician's name and his or her own name and title. The physician must co-sign in person within 72 hours of when the verbal order was written.

◆ *Patient identification.* The proper patient identification, consisting of the patient's name, patient or medical record number, patient's birth date, and admitting physician.

◆ *Transcriptionist's signature.* Signature and title of the person transcribing the order and date and time.

Usually, physician orders consist of multiple ideas or instructions for different treatment or patient care. A group of orders written for the patient at one time is referred to as a set of orders (Figure 23-3).

PHYSICIAN'S ORDERS		Patient Number Medical Records Number Patient Name
(START WRITING AT TOP OF FIRST BLANK SECTION) USE BALL POINT ONLY		DOB Sex Age Physician

DATE 11/20/XX	TIME 1145	☐ A.M. ☐ P.M.
ALLERGIES		
BRP		
1800 cal ADA diet		
VS q 4°		
CXR		
CBC, lytes		
Dr. Pepper		
DATE	TIME	☐ A.M. ☐ P.M.

Figure 23-3 • *The physician's order form must include the date, the order content, and the physician's signature. The form must also be labeled with proper patient identification.*

RECOGNIZING ORDERS THAT NEED TO BE TRANSCRIBED

After the order has been written on the physician's order sheet, the health unit coordinator must transcribe it. Ideally, the person writing the order will bring the order to the attention of the health unit coordinator. Facilities may use several methods to indicate an order has been written. The most common method is called flagging. Flagging is the process of drawing attention to new orders in the chart by inserting a brightly colored marker or card into the patient's medical record (Figure 23-4). Some medical record binders have built-in flags. Some health care facilities have a light system just outside the patient's room that may be activated to alert the staff there are orders to be transcribed. Some of these light systems even indicate the category of the order, such as stat (immediate).

It is important for the health unit coordinator to recognize orders that need to be transcribed even when they are not flagged. The physician may write but not flag the order. Because the transcription of the physician's orders must be completed in a timely fashion, the health unit coordinator must have a process to ensure that unflagged orders are not missed. A missed or nontranscribed physician's order may result in anything from a small inconvenience to a life-threatening consequence. Therefore, the health

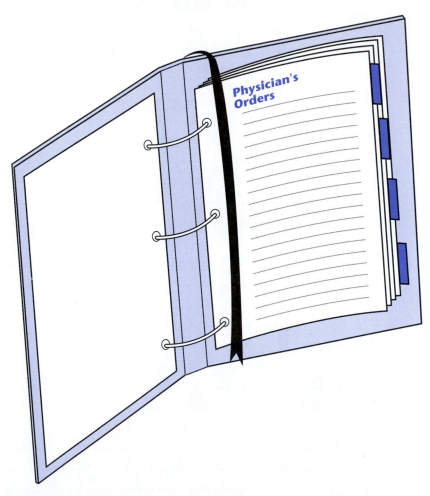

Figure 23-4 • *Flagging is the process of drawing attention to new orders.*

unit coordinator must frequently check all patient medical records in the patient care areas for orders that need to be transcribed.

To determine if an order needs transcribing, the health unit coordinator looks for physician orders that are lacking a sign-off signature. After the orders have been transcribed, the health unit coordinator signs off on the order with his or her name, title, date, and time (Figure 23-5). Some facilities also require the signature of a nurse to indicate that a registered nurse has also read the physician's order (Figure 23-6). In these facilities, a health unit coordinator who discovers a physician's order without a sign-off signature should immediately check with the nurse caring for that patient to determine if the order was missed or if someone neglected to sign off. Depending on the severity of the missed order, the order may be processed as written, or the physician may be notified. In most cases, an incident report will also be completed. In the incident report, the nurse or health unit coordinator will describe the discovery of the missed order and the actions taken.

PHYSICIAN'S ORDERS

| Patient Number |
| Medical Records Number |
| Patient Name |
| DOB   Sex   Age |
| Physician |

(START WRITING AT TOP OF FIRST BLANK SECTION)
USE BALL POINT ONLY

DATE 11/20/XX	TIME 1145	☐ A.M. ☐ P.M.

ALLERGIES

✓ BRP

✓ 1800 cal ADA diet

✓ VS q 4°

✓ CXR

✓ CBC, lytes

✓ Dr. Pepper

11/20/xx   12:20   Jane Doe, CHUC

DATE	TIME	☐ A.M. ☐ P.M.

Figure 23-5 • *After the orders have been transcribed, the health unit coordinator signs off on the order with the name, title, date, and time.*

PHYSICIAN'S ORDERS

(START WRITING AT TOP OF FIRST BLANK SECTION)
USE BALL POINT ONLY

| Patient Number |
| Medical Records Number |
| Patient Name |
| DOB   Sex   Age |
| Physician |

DATE 11/20/XX	TIME 1145	☐ A.M. ☐ P.M.
ALLERGIES		

✓ BRP

✓ 1800 cal ADA diet

✓ VS q 4°

✓ CXR

✓ CBC, lytes

✓ Dr. Pepper

     11/20/xx   12:20   Jane Doe, CHUC

     11/20/XX   1300   Bob Johnson, RN

DATE	TIME	☐ A.M. ☐ P.M.

Figure 23-6 • *Some health care facilities may also require the co-signature of a registered nurse.*

RECOGNIZING ORDERS THAT NEED TO BE CLARIFIED

Some physicians' orders need to be clarified before they can be transcribed. Examples of orders that need to be clarified include orders that are missing any of the required components, orders that are unclear or difficult to read, and orders that may contain errors. The health unit coordinator is the front-line defense against orders that require clarification. Even the novice health unit coordinator should recognize orders that are missing components or that are difficult to read. It will require training and experience for the health unit coordinator to recognize orders that have other errors such as dosage errors or conflicting treatments and therapies.

A health unit coordinator who recognizes that an order needs clarification must follow the facility's protocol for order clarification. Order clarification always requires communication with the physician. In most facilities, the health unit coordinator must place a call to the physician. In a few facilities, a nurse must make the call. Whether the nurse or health unit coordinator obtains the clarification instructions depends on the facility's policy for taking physicians' verbal orders.

ORDER PRIORITY

In addition to transcribing accurately, the health unit coordinator must transcribe efficiently. The health unit coordinator does not necessarily transcribe the orders in the sequence in which they were received. Often, there will be several physician's order sheets (or charts) requiring transcription of orders at the same time. The health unit coordinator needs to know how to prioritize orders.

Sometimes the physician will write the priority as part of the order. For example, the physician may indicate that an order is stat or asap. A stat order is one that has to be done immediately. Asap is the abbreviation for *as soon as possible*, meaning the order has a high priority but does not have to be done immediately. The physician may indicate if the order is to be done today or the next morning. If the physician writes "in am," it usually means the next morning as opposed to "this am" which means today.

Orders that are not stat or asap may be prioritized as routine. There will be times when the health unit coordinator determines the priority of the routine orders on the basis of facility protocol. For example, the physician may order a series of tests and not indicate a time for any of the orders. The health unit coordinator will use knowledge of facility protocol to order the tests as efficiently as possible. For example, the health unit coordinator will utilize his or her knowledge of diagnostic tests to determine what tests can be performed on the same day and what tests have to be performed at a later date because of preparation or scheduling protocol.

ORDER CATEGORY

Physician orders can be categorized by the time frame, or duration, of the order (Table 23-2). Order categories include:

◆ *Stat.* Orders that are activated immediately. The orders are done one time, then discontinued. For example, "Heparin 5000 units subq stat."

TABLE 23-2 Order Category

Order Category	Activation and Duration	Example
Stat	Orders are activated immediately.	Chest x-ray stat.
Standing	Orders remain active or in place until orders are written to change or discontinue.	Bathroom privileges.
Standing PRN	Orders remain active or in place until orders are written to change or discontinue, but are only administered as necessary.	Heating pad to lower back prn.
One time or short-order series	Orders are active or in place only once or for just a specified short amount of time.	Nothing by mouth until gag reflex returns.

◆ *Standing.* Orders that remain active or in place until further orders are written to discontinue or change. For example, "Clear liquid diet."

◆ *Standing prn.* Orders that remain active or in place until further orders are written to discontinue or change but are only as necessary. For example, "Up as tolerated with help prn."

◆ *One-time or short-order series.* Orders that are active or in place only once or just for the specified amount of time. For example, "Tapwater enema in am," or "Vitals signs every hour times four."

ORDER CLASSIFICATION

Orders can be classified by the department that will be involved with the execution of the orders.

◆ Nursing Care:

　　Activity

　　Observation

　　Treatment

◆ Food and nutrition services

◆ Diagnostic procedure

　　Laboratory

　　Diagnostic imaging

　　Cardiology

　　Neurophysiology

◆ Therapy

　　Respiratory care

　　Physical medicine and rehabilitation

◆ Intravenous therapy

◆ Medication

◆ Miscellaneous

Transcribing the different classifications of orders will be discussed in greater detail in future chapters.

TRANSCRIPTION TOOLS AND STEPS

Transcribing physicians' orders is a process of acknowledging and communicating. The health unit coordinator may use a variety of tools and follows a standard procedure to communicate the orders to the appropriate parties to ensure that the physician's plan of care is implemented for the patient.

TRANSCRIPTION TOOLS

The health unit coordinator may use any or all of the following tools:

- Physician's order sheet
- Patient medical record
- Medication administration record (MAR)
- Kardex
- Note cards
- Specimen cards
- Prep cards
- Telephone
- Computer
- Facsimile machine
- Pneumatic tube

The **Kardex** is a profile of all current physicians' orders for a patient. It serves as one document where all of the current orders are consolidated. The Kardex identifies all activities and treatments for a patient, including all active ancillary and diagnostic testing orders. The Kardex eliminates the need to frequently read through the patient's entire chart to learn of the current orders. It is used by the staff caring for the patient.

Kardexes come in a variety of sizes and styles. Kardexes may even vary from department to department depending on the needs. Kardexes are usually divided into sections with headings to describe the various components. Kardex sections may include:

- Patient data (name, age, physician, religion, room number, admission date, code or resuscitation status, allergies, contact persons)
- Medical diagnosis
- Nursing diagnosis or patient acuity assessment
- Diet
- Activity
- Nursing treatment and observation
- Medications
- Laboratory
- Diagnostic tests and procedures
- Therapies and treatments

The Kardex may be on a hard-copy form on which documentation is written by hand (Figure 23-7), or it may be an electronic form on which documentation is made via

MARQUETTE GENERAL HOSPITAL—Patient Information Kardex

Diagnosis				Patient Label			Room #
Code Status:				OR/Procedure Date:			
Daily Weights							
Activity:				Isolation:			
				Other:			
Fluid Restriction: Diet:							
Contrast Allergy: ☐ YES ☐ NO				Social Security #:			

Date	To Be Done	Test/Labs	Date	To Be Done	Test/Labs

Daily Labs:

Contact Person:

Place Staying:

Phone #:

Figure 23-7 · *Sample Kardex form (Courtesy of Marquette General Health System, Marquette, MI)*

MARQUETTE GENERAL HOSPITAL—Patient Information Kardex

Name: _____ Room: _____ Age: _____

Date Admitted: _____ | **Code Status:** _____

Diet: _____ | *Tele:* _____ | *Allergies:* _____

Fluid Restriction: _____ *cc/day* | | *Isolation:* _____
D   E   N | | *RT:* _____

I&O | |
Foley: ____ *IV:* ____ | |
VS: _____ | |

Neuro: _____ | |
Chem: _____ | |
Weights: _____ | |
Activity: _____ | | *SS Consult:* _____

| | *Sp Equip:* _____
| | *Med. Update:* _____
| | *Daily Chgs:* _____

| | *Consult:* _____
| | *Dr.:* _____
| | *Diag:* _____

- -

SS# _____

Date Ordered	Date To Be Done	Tests To Be Done	Date Ordered	Date To Be Done	Tests To Be Done

Daily Labs: _____

Person(s) to Contact: _____

Figure 23-7 • *Sample Kardex form (Courtesy of Marquette General Health System, Marquette, MI)*

computer entry. If the Kardex is a hard copy form, it may be filed at a central location at the workstation. The Kardexes may be filed in room order in a metal or plastic Kardex holder. Electronic Kardexes are accessed via the information system. In some facilities, the staff caring for the patient can review and document on the Kardex on a portable device at the patient's bedside or at other remote terminals. Even though electronic Kardexes can be viewed on a computer screen, a hard copy may be printed at the beginning of each shift.

Because it represents only current orders, the Kardex is dynamic, or always changing. For example, if a patient was on strict bed rest when he was admitted but has since progressed to being ambulatory, the activity section of the Kardex will reflect the current ambulatory status, not the strict bed rest. Information or orders that may change may be documented in pencil on the handwritten Kardex. Information not subject to change, such as the patient's name, age, and diagnosis may be written in ink. Information that requires special attention, such as allergies, may be written in red. Because the Kardex is not traditionally part of the patient's medical record, writing in pencil and erasures are allowed. The Kardex is normally discarded after the patient is discharged.

TRANSCRIPTION STEPS

1. Read the entire order set thoroughly.

2. Prioritize orders.

3. If medications are included in order set, send order carbon or copy to Pharmacy.

4. Communicate order to individual or department that will be performing order—communication may be via any of the tools listed in the section titled Transcription Tools.

5. Record orders on patient Kardex.

6. Record medication orders on medication administration record.

7. Check off each order in the set as completed.

8. Re-read and check all work for accuracy.

9. Sign off order with name, title, date, and time (Table 23-3).

ERROR PREVENTION

Accuracy in transcribing physicians' orders is imperative. The consequences of incorrectly transcribing physicians' orders can range from a minor inconvenience to life threatening. Two common types of error are patient identification errors and order misinterpretation. Both types of error can be avoided by being cautious.

TABLE 23-3 Transcription Steps

Transcription Step	Key Points
1. Read the entire order set thoroughly.	Careful reading of the orders allows the health unit coordinator to review, prioritize, and check for incomplete or illegible orders.
2. Prioritize orders.	Determine the urgency of the orders in all the charts needing transcription. Decide what orders in the order set need to be transcribed first.
3. If medications are included in the order set, send the order carbon or a copy to the pharmacy.	The pharmacy requires a copy of a signed order.
4. Communicate the order to the individual or department that will be performing the order. Communication may be via any of the tools listed in the section titled Transcription Tools.	The health unit coordinator may schedule tests and appointments, notify ancillary departments of needs, order equipment necessary to perform the order, and contact the nursing personnel responsible for the patient.
5. Record the orders on the patient Kardex or care plan.	Most health care facilities have a form used to keep track of current orders and the plan of care for a patient.
6. Record medication orders on the medication administration record (MAR).	Most health care facilities automatically generate medication administration records every 24 hours based on orders entered into a computer. Orders that are received after the record has been generated may require that the order be added or handwritten on the MAR.
7. Check off each order in the set as completed.	Placing a check mark by each order as it is transcribed can help the health unit coordinator track orders even when interrupted. Some facilities use symbols other than check marks by each order to indicate what has been done in the transcription process. For example, a *K* may be written next to orders that have been transcribed to the Kardex. An *M* may be written next to medication orders that have been forwarded to the pharmacy. *Called* or *P* may be written next to orders for which a phone call has been made.
8. Re-read and check all work for accuracy.	Because of multiple requests received by the health unit coordinator, re-reading and checking work is a necessity.
9. Sign off the order with name, title, date, and time.	The health unit coordinator is accountable for the orders transcribed. Orders should never be checked off or signed off before the transcription process has been completed.

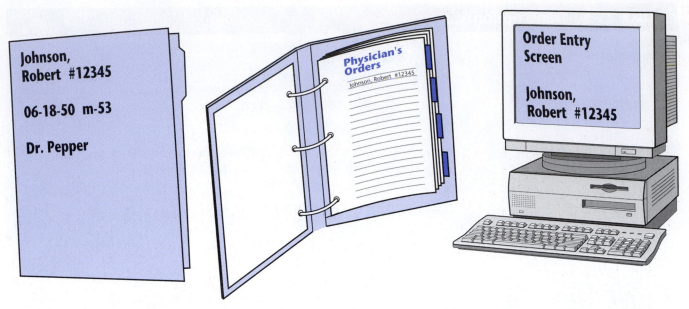

Figure 23-8 • *To prevent errors, carefully check the patient name and identification number on the medical record binder, chart forms, and all computer entries.*

When transcribing orders, carefully check the patient name and identification number on the physician's order sheet and the medical record binder cover. Make sure the patient name and number match exactly on all computer entries, phone calls, and chart forms, including the Kardex, medication administration record, and patient care plan (Figure 23-8).

Many errors can be prevented by avoiding assumptions. Health unit coordinators should not assume that they know what the physician's intent was on an order that does not sound or look right. An order should be transcribed exactly as it appears on the physician's order sheet. If the order is illegible or incomplete or if an error is found, seek clarification, following the facility's order clarification policy.

INDEPENDENT TRANSCRIPTION

Independent transcription refers to the practice of health unit coordinators' taking full accountability for the transcription of physicians' orders. With independent transcription, the health unit coordinator completes and signs off the order without a nurse double-checking the work. In most independent transcription scenarios, the registered nurse still reads the orders but verifies only orders pertaining to medications or transfusions. With independent transcription, the nurse may still sign the order to indicate the orders have been reviewed but does not verify the transcription process.

Some facilities consider that the transcription process begins at the time the physician gives the orders. In such cases, health unit coordinators may take verbal and telephone orders. The exception in most cases is medication orders, which must be checked and co-signed. This is *complete independent transcription*, in which the health unit coordinator is responsible for taking verbal orders as well as being accountable for the transcription process. In *partial independent transcription*, the health unit coordinator does not take verbal orders yet is accountable for the accuracy of the transcription process.

Because many health unit coordinators enter orders into the information system before the nurse has read the order, an informal process of independent transcription is often practiced yet not recognized by facilities. For example, a stat order is written, and the order is transcribed and acted upon hours before the nurse double-checks the order.

Independent transcription is supported by the Standards of Practice set forth by the National Association of Health Unit Coordinators (NAHUC) which include the following, "Health Unit Coordinator personnel shall be prepared through the appropriate education and training programs for their responsibility in the provision of non-direct patient care and non-clinical services." Another NAHUC guideline that supports independent transcription states, "Standards of performance shall define functions, responsibilities, qualifications, and accountability reflecting autonomy of practice." In her article in *Nursing Management*, Nancy C. Komjathy-Salyer summarizes that independent transcription gives recognition and value to unit coordinators who are knowledgeable and capable and that it permits them to do the job for which they are educated and paid.

SUMMARY

Transcription of physicians' orders is a key responsibility of the health unit coordinator. It is important for the health unit coordinator to recognize orders that need to be transcribed or that need to be clarified. The health unit coordinator needs to know how to prioritize orders. The health unit coordinator applies the basic knowledge of anatomy, physiology, disease processes, medical terminology, and abbreviations to the accurate processing and communication of the treatment and care received by the patient.

REVIEW QUESTIONS

1. Define transcription as it pertains to health unit coordinating.

2. If a patient's chart is not flagged, how will the health unit coordinator know if there are orders to be transcribed?

3. List the nine steps of transcription.

4. "The consequences of a missed or nontranscribed physician's order may range from a small inconvenience to a life-threatening situation." Is this statement true or false?

5. "The health unit coordinator is the front-line defense for orders that require clarification." Is this statement true or false?

6. "The health unit coordinator does not need to know how to prioritize orders." Is this statement true or false?

7. "At times, the health unit coordinator will determine the priority of the routine orders on the basis of facility protocol." Is this statement true or false?

8. Indicate the category of the following orders:

   a. Bed rest

   b. Soft diet

   c. Blood cultures now

   d. Chest x-ray today

   e. Use k-pad prn

TRANSCRIPTION PRACTICE

Go to the CD-ROM for transcription exercises that support the content in this chapter.

NAHUC CERTIFICATION EXAM

CONTENT AREAS

I. A. 1	Check charts for orders that need to be transcribed
I. A. 2	Interpret medical symbols, abbreviations, and terminology
I. A. 3	Clarify questionable orders
I. A. 4	Prioritize orders and tasks
I. A. 5	Process orders according to priority
I. A. 6	Enter orders on a Kardex
I. A. 19	Recognize order categories (i.e., standing, one-time, prn, and stat)
I. B. 1	Notify staff of new orders
I. B. 3	Indicate on the order sheet that each order has been processed
I. B. 4	Sign off orders (e.g., signature, title, date, and time)
I. B. 5	Flag charts for co-signature
II. E. 9	Perform quality assurance on charts (i.e. verify that chart forms are filed and labeled correctly, all orders have been transcribed, allergies are noted in appropriate places, prepare incident reports, etc.)
III. B. 4	Enter orders via computers

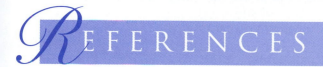

THROUGH THE EYES

OF A HEALTH CARE PROFESSIONAL

A physician shares his thoughts.

When I write orders for my patients, I give their charts to the health unit coordinator. At that point, I assume the orders will be communicated and activated exactly as I intended. When I give the health unit coordinator multiple patient charts with orders, I trust he will read through the orders and prioritize his transcription. I am confident that he will communicate the orders as written and order the supplies and additional forms that are needed to complete the orders. If I order a series of tests, I expect that all of the tests will be scheduled properly and that the results will be filed in the patient's chart. I know if there are questions about the orders, the health unit coordinator will bring them to the attention of the registered nurse. I know the health unit coordinator will know how to contact me if the registered nurse needs to talk to me for clarification. All of us in health care rely on each other to perform our duties to the best of our ability to ensure the patient receives the best care possible.

REFERENCES

American Association for Medical Transcription. *http://www.aamt.org* Accessed January 2004.

Joint Commission on Accreditation of Healthcare Organizations. *http://www.jcaho.org/accredited+organizations/2004 National Patient Safety Goals.htm* Accessed January 2004.

Komjathy-Salyer, N. C. (1992). Why are RNs continuing to cosign for ward clerks? *Nursing Management, 23*(5), 76, 80.

National Association of Health Unit Coordinators (NAHUC). *Standards of Practice.* Accessed August 2004.

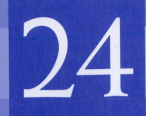
Laboratory Orders

Learning Objectives

Upon completion of this chapter and review questions, the learner should be able to:

1. Discuss the importance of laboratory testing in diagnosing patients.

2. Describe the role of the laboratory departments.

3. Describe ordering priorities and reporting of test results.

4. Name three methods of obtaining random urine specimens.

5. List the tests that are in a coronary risk panel.

6. Name the test that must be performed to order blood for transfusion.

7. Explain the difference between fasting and NPO.

Key Terms

bacteriology   The study of bacteria that cause diseases.

blood bank   A department of the laboratory (transfusion services) that is responsible for testing, preparing, and providing blood and blood products for a patient's need.

chemistry department   Performs tests to determine chemical changes in body fluids.

culture medium   A special substance that the specimen is placed upon or in to allow bacteria to grow and multiply.

culturette   A prepackaged sterile swab and culture medium in a tube.

cytology   The study of cells.

donor services   A department of the laboratory responsible for testing and collecting blood from donors.

hematology   The study of blood cells, coagulation, and bleeding disorders.

laboratory   The department that provides testing to help health care professionals diagnose and evaluate patient health conditions.

microbiology   The study of microscopic organisms.

mycology   The study of fungi that cause diseases.

parasitology   The study of parasites that cause diseases.

pathology   The study of disease.

point-of-care stations   An area set up with basic laboratory testing equipment to provide test results quickly, where the patient is located.

serology department   The department responsible for the testing of specimens that produce a recordable reaction between an antibody and an antigen.

specimen collection department   The department that obtains and processes all the specimens that arrive in the laboratory for testing.

transport medium   A broad term used to describe what the specimen will be placed in to be sent to the laboratory.

urinalysis department   Processes the tests requested on urine specimens.

virology   The study of viruses that cause diseases.

Abbreviations

Acid Phos   Acid Phosphate

ACTH   Adrenocorticotropic Hormone

AFB   Acid-Fast Bacilli

AGAP   Anion Gap

AHEPP   Acute Hepatitis (Hepatitis Profile)

AIDS   Acquired Immunodeficiency Syndrome

Alk Phos   Alkaline Phosphate

ALT   Alanine Aminotransferase

ANA   Antinuclear Antibody

ASO Antistreptolysin O

AST Aspartate Transaminase

Bili Bilirubin

BMP Basic Metabolic Panel

BS Blood Sugar

BUN Blood Urea Nitrogen

Ca Calcium

CBC Complete Blood Count

CC Colony Count

CEA Carcinoembryonic antigen

CSF Cerebrospinal Fluid

Chol Cholesterol

CK Creatine kinase

Cl Chloride

CMP Comprehensive Metabolic Panel

CO$_2$ Carbon Dioxide

COR Coronary Risk

CPK Creatine phosphokinase

Creat Creatine

C & S Culture and Sensitivity

Diff Differential

EDTA Ethylenediaminetetra-acetic acid

FBS Fasting Blood Sugar

Fe Iron

Fib Fibrinogen Level

FSH Follicle-Stimulating Hormone

GTT Glucose Tolerance Test

HbA$_{1C}$, HgbA$_1$C Glycosylated Hemoglobin

HBsAG Hepatitis B Surface Antigen

hCG Human Chorionic Gonadotropin

HCO₃ Bicarbonate

Hct Hematocrit

HDL High-Density Lipoprotein

HEPF Hepatic Function

Hgb Hemoglobin

HIV Human Immunodeficiency Virus

INR International Normalized Ratio

Iso's Isoenzymes

K Potassium

LDH Lactic Dehydrogenase

LDL Low-Density Lipoprotein

LH Luteinizing Hormone

Lytes Electrolytes

Mg Magnesium

Na Sodium

NH₃ Ammonia

NPO Nothing by Mouth

O & P Ova and Parasites

PLT CT Platelet Count

PSA Prostatic Specific Antigen

PT Prothrombin Time

PTT Partial Thromboplastin Time

RA Rheumatoid Arthritis

RBC Red Blood Count

RFP Renal Function Panel

SGOT Serum Glutamic-oxaloacetic

TBG Thyroid Binding Globulin

TCT Thrombin Clotting Time

TIBC Total Iron Binding Capacity

TSH Thyroid-Stimulating Hormone

T3 Triiodothyronine Resin Uptake

T4 Thyroxine

Trig Triglycerides

U/A Urinalysis

VDRL Venereal Disease Research Laboratory

WBC White Blood Count

LABORATORY

A **laboratory** provides testing to help health care professionals diagnose and evaluate patient health conditions. The laboratory is an important department with which the health unit coordinator communicates frequently. The communication includes ordering laboratory tests as requested by the physician, or designee, and receiving the results of those tests. For every laboratory test that is ordered, the health unit coordinator needs to know the type of specimen that is needed, who will collect the specimen, if a consent form is required, and in what type of container the specimen will be transported.

LABORATORY DEPARTMENT

The laboratory may be a department within the health care facility, or it may be a private business that the health care facility contracts with to perform the laboratory tests requested by the physician. The size of the laboratory is dictated by the amount of business that it performs. A health care facility that has fewer than 50 inpatient beds will request fewer specialized laboratory tests than will a health care facility with 1,000 inpatient beds. Most health care facilities do not perform all the laboratory testing requested. They usually send a certain amount of tests out to larger laboratories.

The laboratory is divided into departments that specialize in certain diagnostic tests. It is important for the health unit coordinator to know which tests are performed in the different departments of the laboratory to order and retrieve the results correctly and efficiently. The length of the patient stay could be affected by the laboratory results.

POINT-OF-CARE LABORATORY STATIONS

The health care facility may have laboratory staff members working on the patient care units in small laboratory stations where they can collect the patient specimens and run the tests, providing the test results at the point of care where the patient is located. The **point-of-care stations** are set up with basic laboratory testing equipment to provide test results quickly so that the health care team can use the results to plan the care of the patient. On a patient care unit, if the staff has been trained in collection techniques, the staff may collect the specimen and send it to the laboratory

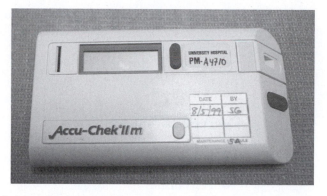

Figure 24-1 • *A blood glucose meter*

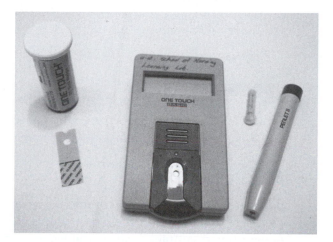

Figure 24-2 • *Blood glucose meter supplies*

for processing. Some tests may be completed on the patient care unit by the nursing staff. For example, a blood glucose fingerstick would be done at a point-of-care station and the blood specimen would be processed using a blood glucose meter (Figures 24-1 and 24-2). Another test done at a point-of-care station is a stool test for occult, or hidden, blood. A member of the patient care staff collects and tests the stool specimen using a hemocult slide test.

SPECIMEN COLLECTION

Testing done in the laboratory department requires that a specimen be collected. The type of specimen required depends on the test requested. Common types of specimens collected include blood, stool, urine, and tissue.

TRANSPORT MEDIUM

Transport medium is a broad term used to describe what the specimen will be placed in to be sent to the laboratory. The transport medium is the container in which the specimen is collected and delivered to the laboratory. Examples of transport media include:

- Culture bottles

- Culturettes

- Dipstick containers

- Jars

- Petri dishes

- Plastic bags

- Plastic cups

- Slides

- Tubes

- Vials

Table 24-1 lists several specimens, who collects them, how the specimen is transported, and if a consent is required.

BLOOD SAMPLES

Blood samples are the most common type of specimens collected. Laboratory staff members usually collect the blood sample. The laboratory staff person who draws the patient blood samples is called a phlebotomist. Blood specimens may be obtained via a venipuncture, capillary puncture, or arterial puncture or through a central venous line. For a venipuncture, blood is drawn from the vein and flows into the attached blood containers. The blood containers are small tubes with colored tops. The colored top defines what is added to the tube. By knowing what is added to the tube, the person drawing the blood sample knows which tube is to be used for the specific tests ordered. The amount of blood drawn is defined by the amount required to perform the testing requested. More than one container can be filled by the initial venipuncture by attaching another container after the first container is filled.

Colored tops include:

- Red top—nothing added to tube

- Red and black top—silicone gel added to tube

- Green top—heparin added to tube

- Lavender top—EDTA added to tube

- Blue top—sodium citrate added to tube

- Gray top—glycolytic inhibitor such as oxalate and fluoride added to tube

For a capillary puncture, the skin is punctured to draw blood. The skin on the heel, toe, or finger may be punctured. A capillary heel puncture is a common way to draw

TABLE 24-1 Specimen Collection

Specimen	Collected By	Transport Media	Consent Required
Blood/serum	Phlebotomist or specially trained staff performs a venipuncture or fingerstick or draws blood from a central line port	Vials, tubes, culture bottles	No
Urine	Patient care staff provides instructions to patient to void or inserts urinary catheter to obtain specimen	Plastic cups, dipstick containers	No
Cerebrospinal fluid (CSF)	Physician performs lumbar puncture, also known as spinal tap	Vials	Yes
Bone marrow	Physician performs bone marrow biopsy or sternal puncture	Vials	Yes
Sputum	Patient care staff or respiratory therapist	Plastic cups	No
Stool	Patient care staff	Plastic cups	No
Cervical smear	Physician performs cervical exam	Slides, Pap smear jars, **culturette** (a prepackaged sterile swab and culture medium in a tube)	No
Throat swab	Patient care staff	Culturette	No
Wound drainage	Patient care staff	Culturette, vials	No
Amniotic fluid	Physician performs amniocentesis	Light-resistant sterile glass container	Yes
Thoracic cavity or pleural fluid	Physician performs thoracentesis	Plastic bags and vials	Yes
Abdominal cavity fluid	Physician performs thoracentesis	Plastic bags and vials	Yes
Biopsy	Physician performs biopsy of a part of the body tissue	Vial, slides	Yes

blood from infants. A capillary finger puncture may be used to draw blood for a glucose level monitor. A sample of arterial blood requires special skills and may be performed by the physician or a respiratory therapist.

Blood may also be drawn from a central venous line. A central venous line is a catheter or tube inserted through the subclavian vein. More information about venous access devices is in Chapter 28.

Timed Blood Specimens

Blood for laboratory tests may be collected randomly or at a specific time. Many laboratory test results can be affected by the patient's food or fluid intake. Two examples are blood glucose and cholesterol tests. To control the test results, a patient may have to fast or have nothing by mouth (NPO) before the test. If the patient is to fast, the patient's breakfast will be held. If the patient is to be NPO, the patient will not be able to drink or eat anything from midnight until the blood is collected. The blood for these tests is usually collected the first thing in the morning. Some tests may be performed specifically to see how the patient's intake is affecting him or her. These tests may be ordered at a specific time. One such test is a 2-hour postprandial blood glucose. *Postprandial* means after meals. Therefore, a 2-hour postprandial blood glucose would be collected 2 hours after the patient finishes a meal.

Peak and Trough Levels

Sometimes, a physician needs to know how a specific medication is being absorbed by the patient. For this type of test, a blood specimen will be collected at specific times before and after a medication is given. The blood collected before the medication is administered is called the trough level, and the blood drawn after the medication is given is called the peak level. Peak and trough levels are commonly drawn when a patient is receiving an antibiotic such as Gentamycin or Tobramycin. Careful coordination with the pharmacy, medication nurse, and laboratory is required for accurate peak and trough levels.

Absorption Tests

Absorption tests are performed to measure how the patient is absorbing specific chemicals or substances. For example, a lactose tolerance test may be ordered to diagnose a carbohydrate malabsorption; a D-Xylose test may be ordered as an indirect measure of intestinal absorption; and a glucose tolerance test may be order to study carbohydrate metabolism. For these tests, a patient may have to ingest a specific chemical or substance and then have a series of timed blood specimens collected. Again, careful coordination is required for these tests.

STOOL SPECIMENS

Stool specimens are usually collected on the patient care units by the nursing staff. The specimen is collected and placed in a sealed container before being sent to the laboratory department for testing. The container is labeled with the information identifying the specimen as required by the laboratory. Depending on the tests ordered, the specimen may need to be brought to the laboratory department within a specific time frame. If this is the case, the health unit coordinator may be asked to transport the stool specimen to the laboratory.

URINE SPECIMENS

The nursing staff or patient care staff usually collects urine specimens. The patient care or nursing staff will provide instruction to the patient on how to collect the urine sample. The patient is asked to urinate into a container. The patient care provider collects the sample from the container and places the sample into the correct container to transport it to the laboratory (Figure 24-3). Some urine samples can be transported to the laboratory via the pneumatic tube system; others need to be delivered to the laboratory within a certain amount of time after being collected. The amount of urine required for the specific test varies, as does the collection container and whether the container contains any additives. The health unit coordinator may be asked to either deliver the urine specimen to the laboratory personally or to send it through the health system delivery system.

Timed Urine Specimens

For the majority of laboratory tests performed on urine, one randomly voided specimen is collected. However, some laboratory urine tests require that a specimen be collected at a certain time or for a certain length of time. Examples of tests that have to be collected at a certain time are a pregnancy test and a 24-hour specimen collection. A urine test for pregnancy, or human chorionic gonadotropin (hcg), usually requires that the urine be collected from the first morning voiding. A creatinine clearance test requires all urine to be collected and saved for a 24-hour period. Additional information about timed urine specimens can be found in the section of this chapter titled Chemistry.

24-Hour Urine Collections

The length of time the urine is collected is determined by the test ordered. Some samples are collected just one time; others are collected for a period of time. A common collection time is 24 hours. This means that all the urine voided in that 24-hour period is collected in a container labeled as such. The nursing staff generally collects urine specimens, and the health unit coordinator requests the test ordered by the physician. The health unit coordinator does not request the test until the collection is completed. Some testing requires that the urine container contain an additive. If this

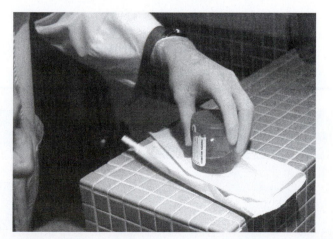

Figure 24-3 • *Urine specimen containers are sent to the laboratory.*

is the case, the health unit coordinator needs to request the container before ordering the test.

TISSUE SPECIMENS

The physician usually collects tissue specimens from patients. Depending on where the collection site is located, the specimen may collected in the patient room or in a specialty area such as the operating room or the endoscopy department. Tissue specimens can be collected during an invasive procedure, or a sample may be collected using a skin scraping in the treatment room. The size of the specimen depends on the area it is being collected from and how big a sample is needed to perform the test requested.

LABORATORY DEPARTMENTS

The laboratory can be divided into many different departments. The departments, in turn, may be divided into divisions. The number and uniqueness of tests processed, as well as the staff members employed in the laboratory, determine the size and function of the departments and divisions (Figure 24-4). Common departments within a laboratory include specimen collection, microbiology, serology, cytology, chemistry, hematology, urinalysis, blood bank, and pathology.

SPECIMEN COLLECTION DEPARTMENT

The laboratory may include a department called **Specimen Collection**. The function of this department is to obtain and process all the specimens that arrive in the laboratory for testing. It is to this department that the health unit coordinator delivers specimens.

Labeling

All specimens delivered must be correctly identified with the correct patient information and the test being requested. A label must be affixed to the specimen with the patient information (Figure 24-5). The label is generated from the computer system or is hand written by the health unit coordinator. No specimens will be accepted into

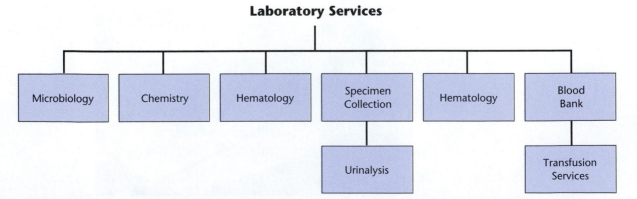

Figure 24-4 • *The laboratory departments are defined by the testing they perform.*

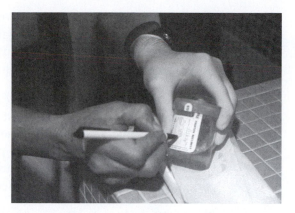

Figure 24-5 • *Laboratory specimens must be labeled correctly.*

the laboratory without proper identification. It is important to label correctly. The laboratory may have a policy stating that unlabeled specimens must be discarded. Some specimens, such as spinal tap fluid or a tissue sample, may not be able to be recollected. The responsibility of this department within the laboratory is to correctly route all properly identified specimens to the correct department for processing. It is very important that all specimens be handled correctly to reduce the risk of biohazard contamination to health system employees.

MICROBIOLOGY

The microbiology department within the laboratory is responsible for identifying organisms. **Microbiology** is the study of microscopic organisms. The microbiology department performs testing on a variety of specimens including blood, stool, urine, sputum, vaginal smears, drainage from wounds, and nose and throat specimens. The following are some common tests that are performed in the microbiology department.

Culture and sensitivity (C&S). A culture can be performed on any specimen placed in a **culture medium** to check for bacterial growth. A culture medium is a special substance that the specimen is placed upon or in to allow bacteria to grow and multiply. The growth takes about 24 hours, after which the species of bacteria is then identified. The identification test takes from 24 hours to 10 days before the final results are completed and able to be reported. Preliminary reports can be provided in 24 hours. If bacteria grow, a sensitivity test is performed to identify what antibiotics are effective in treating the bacteria. A sensitivity is also known as an antibiotic susceptibility test. This test allows the physician to prescribe the correct treatment for the infection. The nursing staff or physician collects the specimen needed for the culture and sensitivity test. The health unit coordinator may order the test, create the label for the specimen, and deliver the specimen to the laboratory. It is important to get the specimen to the laboratory as soon after collection as possible. Although culture tests are ordered to be collected stat, the results will take at least 24 hours. Cultures are also performed on fungi, viruses, and parasites.

AFB culture. This culture is performed on a sputum specimen collected by the nursing or respiratory care staff. This test is performed to identify acid-fast bacilli (AFB), which may cause tuberculosis.

Gram stain. This test may be performed on many types of specimens. This test classifies bacteria as gram negative or gram positive. Gram stain results are available before culture and sensitivity results, giving the physician an early opportunity to order the appropriate gram-negative or gram-positive antibiotic.

Urine for colony count (CC). This test is performed on a urine sample to measure the amount of bacteria present. The urine sample collected must be a clean catch or midstream specimen. The patient collects the specimen if able, otherwise the nursing staff assists the patient in the collection. If needed, the patient may be catheterized to collect the specimen for this test.

Blood cultures. Blood cultures are often ordered on patients when the physician suspects that the patient may have septicemia. Septicemia is a bacterial infection in the bloodstream. The blood culture order usually is written as "Blood cultures 10 minutes apart from 2 different sites." It is important to draw at two different times and from different sites to identify the organism. The phlebotomist, nurse, or physician may draw the blood cultures. The specimen may be drawn by venipuncture or from an arterial line.

The microbiology department may be divided into divisions in large laboratories. Table 24-2 identifies some of the divisions that could be within the microbiology department and test that they perform.

SEROLOGY

The **serology department** is responsible for the testing of specimens that produce a recordable reaction between an antibody and an antigen. An antigen is any substance that triggers an immune response. An antibody is the body's response to a foreign substance. Most antibodies that are produced are produced to fight the specific foreign substance. These tests alone are not able to provide the health care provider with enough information to make a diagnosis, but they do provide supporting information. Serology tests are especially useful in detecting a previous infection as well as exposure to an organism. Testing in this department is performed on patients who have had a transplant or are preparing to have a transplant, patients who are being tested for

TABLE 24-2   Microbiology Department Divisions

Division	Definition	Test
Bacteriology	The study of bacteria that cause diseases	Gram stain
Parasitology	The study of parasites that cause diseases	Stool specimen for O&P (ova and parasites)
Mycology	The study of fungi that cause diseases	Test to determine if fungi present
Virology	The study of viruses that cause diseases	Virus cultures

rheumatoid arthritis (RA), human immunodeficiency virus (HIV), and some types of influenza. Often, the testing is ordered on patients whose antibody production can help identify the foreign substance in the patient's body. Serology specimens can be body fluids or tissue samples, but the most frequent specimen is blood. The results may be ordered as a titer. A titer is the measurement of the antibody level. Titers are often ordered more than once, separated by a specific time interval. Titer results show a rise or fall in the titer. This could show the presence of an infection. Table 24-3 lists common serology tests.

Researchers continue to explore the relationships between antibody-antigen reactions and the autoimmune diseases. These tests provide health care providers with important information.

CYTOLOGY

Cytology is the study of cells. These cells can be from body fluids or body tissues. They are studied in the cytology department to determine the cell type and if a pre-cancer or cancer exists in the cells. The health unit coordinator may not request many laboratory tests from this department. There are two common tests that are ordered from the cytology department; the Pap smear and the biopsy exams. The Pap smear test can be performed on any cells for the presence of cancer, but it is performed most often as a screening tool for cervical cancer. It is a common screening test ordered on women. It is a test that uses a staining method on the cells from the cervix (cervical smear), which are collected during a pelvic exam by the physician, physician's assistant, or nurse practitioner. The other common test ordered is a biopsy. Specimens are collected

TABLE 24-3 Common Serology Tests

Test	Abbreviation	Purpose
Antinuclear antibody	ANA	Determines presence of autoimmune diseases
Antistreptolysin O titer	ASO titer	Elevated titer indicates presence of streptococcal infection
Carcinoembryonic antigen	CEA	Elevated titer indicates liver, colon, or pancreas cancer
Rheumatoid arthritis factor	RA factor	Specific test for rheumatoid arthritis
Human immunodeficiency virus	HIV	Specific test to test for the virus that causes AIDS
Venereal Disease Research Laboratories	VDRL	Screening test for syphilis
Hepatitis B surface antigen	HBsAG	Test used to determine hepatitis B

by the physician and then sent to the cytology department by the health unit coordinator. These specimens may have to be hand delivered or sent by the delivery system after the order has been entered into the laboratory system by the health unit coordinator. The health unit coordinator makes sure these specimens are correctly labeled before being sent to the cytology department.

CHEMISTRY

The **chemistry department** performs tests to determine chemical changes in body fluids. The chemistry testing can be done on a blood or urine specimen. The physician will indicate which specimen type is needed. The tests performed are tests that involve a chemical reaction. When a disease process is occurring in the body, a chemical reaction occurs that varies from the normal range. Chemistry testing can require that the patient fast—that is, not eat or drink anything for a specific amount of time. Usually, patients are asked to fast for 8 to 10 hours. The health unit coordinator requests that no nourishment be delivered to the patient until after the laboratory specimen has been collected. The health unit coordinator notifies the nursing staff and dietary department of this request. Each health care facility has a process for notifying these departments and staff of this request. Table 24-4 contains chemistry tests that are often ordered, including the abbreviation that the doctor may use to request the testing.

The chemistry department is an important area in the laboratory, performing testing that assists in diagnosing heart disease, diabetes, infections, and hypertension. Some chemistry tests that require special setups and processing may be ordered from a department called nuclear chemistry or special chemistry. Tests that may be ordered from this department may include:

- ACTH, adrenocorticotropic hormone
- Cortisol
- Folate
- FSH, follicle-stimulating hormone
- LH, luteinizing hormone
- Schilling test
- TBG, thyroid binding globulin
- TSH, thyroid-stimulating hormone
- T3, triiodothyronine resin uptake
- T4, thyroxine

Most chemistry tests ordered require a serum (blood) specimen; there are some tests that require a urine specimen. If a urine specimen is required, the following tests may be ordered.

Urine glucose. A test used to determine the amount of glucose in the urine. Often ordered in addition to serum glucose.

TABLE 24-4   Chemistry Tests

Test	Abbreviation	Purpose
Acid phosphatase	Acid Phos	To diagnose metastatic cancers
Alkaline phosphatase	Alk Phos	To evaluate bone and liver disease
Ammonia	NH_3	To measure liver function
Amylase		To evaluate acute pancreatitis
Bilirubin	Bili	To measure liver function
Blood sugar	BS	To measure the amount of sugar in the blood
Blood urea nitrogen	BUN	To evaluate kidney function
Calcium	Ca	To measure the amount of calcium in the blood
Cardiac enzymes	AST, SGOT, CPK*, CK*, LDH, troponin	To evaluate whether a heart attack has occurred
Cholesterol	Chol	To measure the function of the liver
Creatine kinase	CK*	To measure the release of an enzyme
Creatine phosphokinase	CPK*	To measure the release of an enzyme
Creatinine clearance		To study kidney function *This test requires a blood specimen and a 24-hour urine specimen.
Electrolytes	Lytes	Includes Na (sodium), K (potassium), Cl (chloride), and HCO_3 (bicarbonate). These elements help maintain the body balance of water and acid.
Fasting blood sugar	FBS	A fasting test to determine the amount of sugar in the blood
Glucose tolerance test	GTT	To determine the amount of sugar in the blood drawn at timed intervals. The patient is required to drink a specific amount of glucose solution. This test looks for changes in the glucose metabolism.
Glycosylated hemoglobin	HbA_{1C}, $HgbA_1C$	Provides a picture of the glucose on the red blood cells for the past 3 months
High-density lipoprotein	HDL	To measure the "good" cholesterol in the blood
Iron	Fe	To measure the amount of iron in the blood

(continues)

TABLE 24-4 *(continued)*

Test	Abbreviation	Purpose
Isoenzymes	Iso's	Determines the variations in the enzymes responsible for an elevation in enzymes such as LDH, CK, and CPK
Magnesium	Mg	To measure the amount of magnesium in the blood
Prostatic specific antigen	PSA	Determines the level of PSA in the body, which is used to diagnose prostate cancer and measure its growth
Serum creatinine	Creat	A serum or urine test to diagnose renal disfunction
Total iron binding capacity	TIBC	To determine the blood's iron-binding capacity, which can be helpful in diagnosing anemia, cirrhosis of the liver, and some infections
Triglycerides	Trig	To identity some types of hyperlipidemia; also is one factor used to determine LDL (low-density lipoprotein) cholesterol
Uric acid		To diagnose gout

Urine creatinine. A test used to determine the amount of creatinine in the urine. May be ordered alone or with a serum creatinine. Elevated creatinine may indicate kidney problems.

Urine protein. A test ordered to determine the amount of protein in the urine. Elevated protein in the urine may indicate urinary system problems including the prostate gland.

Urine osmolality. A test ordered to determine the kidney's ability to dilute and concentrate.

Each health care facility may have a group of chemistry tests that can be ordered as one test (Table 24-5). These test groupings allow the health unit coordinator to order many tests with one request. The groupings, or lab panels, as they may be called, may be built to meet the insurance provider's requirements. These requirements may be nationwide and may have been created to provide needed results at the best possible price.

HEMATOLOGY

Hematology is the study of blood cells, coagulation, and bleeding disorders. Testing is usually performed on serum specimens but can be performed on spinal fluid and bone marrow. Routine hematology tests are now performed by automatic counters (hematology analyzers) instead of by the previous method of counting under the microscope. The counters are more accurate and can perform more tests in a given time. There are many tests performed in the hematology department, but there are some common tests with which the health unit coordinator should be familiar. Table 24-6 lists tests that are performed on a nonfasting serum specimen.

TABLE 24-5 Lab Panels

Panel Name	Abbreviation	Tests Included
Hepatic function (liver function)	HEPF	Albumin, Alk Phos, ALT, AST
Basic metabolic	BMP	Carbon dioxide (CO_2), Cl, Creat, glucose, Ca, BUN, K, Na, Anion gap
Electrolytes	Lytes	CO_2, Cl, Na, K
Comprehensive metabolic	CMP	Albumin, bili total, Ca, Na, Alk Phos, K, protein total, BUN/Creat, AST, CO_2, ALT, Cl, glucose
Renal function (kidney profile)	RFP	Albumin, BUN, Cl, phosphorus, Ca, Creat, CO_2, K, glucose, Na
Coronary risk (lipid profile)	COR	Chol, LDL, Trig, HDL (Ca), Chol/HDL Ratio
Acute hepatitis (hepatitis profile)	AHEPP	Hepatitis A antigen, HBA, hepatitis B core antibody, hepatitis C antibody

TABLE 24-6 Common Hematology Tests

Test	Abbreviation	Purpose
Hematocrit	Hct	To assess blood loss
Hemoglobin	Hgb	To assess the amount of iron in the blood; diagnose anemia
White blood count	WBC	Counts white blood cells; often used to diagnose infections
Red blood count	RBC	Decreasing red blood cells may indicate anemia; increasing may indicate hypoxia due to a chronic condition
Differential	Diff	To test which of the five types of white blood cells is increasing or decreasing
Complete blood count	CBC	Includes Hgb, Hct, WBC, RBC, Diff

Coagulation tests (studies) are performed in the hematology department. These studies provide important information on the clotting ability of the blood. Twelve factors are involved in the clotting process, but not all are necessary for the clotting process to take place. Patients who have these studies ordered by the physician may be at risk for a bleeding problem or for a thrombus to form or may be currently taking medications to thin the blood. Regardless of which of the three conditions is present, it is important that the laboratory test results are reported to the health care team so that the patient's condition can be monitored and the medication adjusted as needed. Table 24-7 lists tests that are commonly ordered.

PT and PTT results are usually reported as time in seconds. The seconds report how long it takes the blood to clot when certain chemicals are added to the serum specimen. There are factors in the environment that can affect this result, so it is important that control values be established. Control values are determined by using a serum sample that is considered normal or as near to normal as possible. Results may also be reported in percentages, or as the INR (international normalized ratio).

URINALYSIS

The function of the **urinalysis department** is to process the tests requested on urine specimens. Urine is generally tested for:

◆ *Color.* How dark it appears, based on a specific color wheel

◆ *Clarity.* How clear or cloudy the specimen appears

◆ *pH.* The acidity or alkalinity

◆ *Specify gravity.* The concentration level

TABLE 24-7   Common Coagulation Studies

Test	Abbreviation	What Is Measured
Prothrombin time	PT	The clotting ability of the blood; also monitors oral anticoagulating therapy
Partial thromboplastin time	PTT	Demonstrates lack of any of the clotting factors except factor VIII; detects many bleeding disorders; also monitors heparin therapy
Fibrinogen level	Fib	The fibrinogen level of the blood; low levels may indicate rare genetic disorders or severe liver disease
Platelet count	PLT CT	The number of platelets; a certain number of platelets are needed for the coagulation process
Clotting time		The length of time it takes for blood to clot
Thrombin clotting time	TCT	To monitor heparin therapy

◆ *Protein.* The amount of protein (albumin) in the urine

◆ *Glucose.* The amount of sugar in the urine

◆ *Blood.* The amount of blood in the urine

◆ *Bilirubin.* The amount of bilirubin in the urine

◆ *Urobilinogen.* The amount of urobilinogen in the urine

◆ *Sediment.* Evaluating the sediment in the urine to detect organisms, intact cells, and crystals

The urine specimen is usually collected by the patient and given to the nursing staff to be sent to the laboratory. If the patient is unable to collect the specimen, the nursing staff assists the patient in the collection process. Before the urine specimen is sent, the test needs to be requested by the health unit coordinator. The test on the urine specimen is not requested until the specimen has been collected and given to the health unit coordinator. The specimen must be labeled correctly with the information that identifies the type of specimen as well as whom the specimen came from (patient name, account number, and any other identifying information required by the health care system) (see Figure 24-5). If this information is not included, the specimen will be discarded and must be recollected. Urine specimens need to arrive in the laboratory within 2 hours of being collected. If the specimen does not arrive in the laboratory within that time, it may become alkaline, providing incorrect results.

Some urine tests require that the specimen be collected in a certain way. The collection process may be stated as follows:

◆ *Random specimen.* No specific time or collection type requested

◆ *Voided specimen.* No specific time, voided specimen requested

◆ *Clean catch midstream specimen.* No specific time, midstream specimen requested; following defined cleaning procedure, specimen is collected in the middle of the voiding process

◆ *Catheterized urine specimen.* No specific time; urine specimen is collected using a catheter (a plastic tube that is inserted into the bladder to obtain urine)

The common abbreviation used for urinalysis is U/A. This test is often ordered because the results provide the health care provider with information to assist in determining health care treatments. Urine specimens may be collected and tests performed in other departments within the laboratory as ordered by the physician.

BLOOD BANK

The function of the **Blood Bank** department (transfusion services) is to provide the blood and blood products to the patient for transfusion. The physician will write an order to transfuse blood products to the patient. The health unit coordinator will send a request to the blood bank for the blood products ordered by the physician. The physician order may be written to type and cross-match the patient. A type and cross-match request requires the lab personnel to draw a sample of the patient's blood to check the patient's blood type. There are four blood types: A, B, AB, and O. Blood types are also classified as positive or negative on the basis of whether the Rh antigen is present (positive) or absent (negative). Patients who require blood during hospitalization must be typed so that they receive blood of a type that is compatible with their blood. The patient's blood must also be cross-matched. Cross-match means that the patient's blood sample is tested to make sure it is compatible with the blood that will be transfused. A sample of the patient's blood is mixed with a sample of the blood unit to be transfused to see if any clumping occurs. If clumping occurs, the blood is not compatible and can not be transfused to the patient. A type and cross-match order does not request that the blood to given to the patient. This process is good for only a set amount of time and, if the time has expired, it must be repeated before blood is sent to be transfused. This request can be sent by paper requisition or by electronic requisition.

If the physician has requested that the patient be transfused, the following would occur when the request is sent to the laboratory. When the laboratory receives the request, they will check to see if the patient has been typed and cross-matched within a certain amount of time. If this process has taken place in the required time frame, the blood bank will then prepare the blood product to be infused. The blood bank will send the blood product to the patient care unit. These products may be brought in person by the lab staff to the nursing unit; they may be sent using the pneumatic tube system or the automated delivery system in the health care facility; or the nursing staff may go to the blood bank department to pick up the blood products. When the blood products arrive, the health unit coordinator notifies the nurse responsible for transfusing the products to the patient. It is important that the nurse be notified immediately. If blood products are not kept at a certain cool temperature they start to warm and bacteria start to grow quickly.

The order written by the physician might say, "T and C, give two units blood." The health unit coordinator would send a request to the laboratory for a type and cross-match to be done as well as a request to prepare two units of blood to be given to the patient. After receiving the request, the laboratory will send a phlebotomist to the patient to draw the blood sample used to perform the type and cross-match tests. After the type and cross-match have been completed, transfusion services will prepare the units of blood to be infused to the patient. Blood products are prepared following strict guidelines to provide the safest products available. Blood consists of different components. A patient's health condition may require a specific component rather than whole blood. Table 24-8 lists blood components that may be ordered for patients.

DONOR SERVICES

Donor Services is a department of the laboratory that collects blood from donors. Usually the department is easily accessible by the public so that potential donors can get in and out in a short amount of time (Figure 24-6). This department conducts blood drives off-site, encouraging people to donate blood without having to come to the blood donor site. At these events, donors can donate blood and blood products. The collected blood is sent to the transfusion services department, where it is processed to be provided to patients when ordered by their physician. Donor services is an important part of the health system because it recruits donations that enable the health system to provide blood products for patients. Patients may donate their own

TABLE 24-8 Blood Components for Transfusions

Blood Component	Reason ordered
Albumin	Shock, low blood volume, electrolyte imbalance, low protein
Whole blood	To restore blood volume, could be decreased because of hemorrhage or trauma
Erythrocytes	To restore red blood cell count
Immunoglobulin	To provide globulin when there is a deficiency
Leukocytes	To aid in treating infections; restore cells damaged by chemotherapy
Plasma	Increases blood volume; used to treat blood-clotting deficiency; may be used to treat hepatitis
Platelets	Used to treat blood-clotting deficiency

blood at these departments if they are having a planned surgery that will require a transfusion. This type of donation is called autologous blood and will be provided to the patient when needed. Before donating, the potential donor must fill out a questionnaire and may be required to have a health physical. These steps are taken to ensure that the donor and donation will be safe. Some health care facilities may purchase their needed blood products from private donor service businesses.

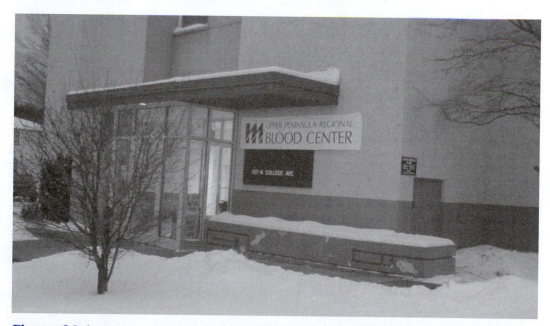

Figure 24-6 • *Donor services may be located in a building outside of the main hospital for easy access by the public to donate blood products. (Courtesy of Marquette General Health System, Marquette, MI)*

PATHOLOGY

The pathology department of the health system is often included as a department within the laboratory. **Pathology** is the study of disease. Medical doctors called pathologists staff the pathology department of the laboratory. The function of the pathology department is to interpret the results of the laboratory tests for the attending physicians. The pathologists use highly specialized tools to aid in their interpretation of the laboratory tests.

ORDERING PRIORITIES FOR LABORATORY TESTS

The physician must order all tests that are to be completed in the laboratory setting. The physician or the physician's assistant writes orders to request the specific tests. The laboratory tests requested may be completed while the patient is in the health care facility, or the patient may need to return to have the testing completed after being discharged. The health unit coordinator will process the physician's laboratory orders. The health unit coordinator completes the processing of physician laboratory orders according to the health care system's procedures. Transcription of orders is explained in detail in Chapter 23. The physician's order specifies the time the specimen is to be drawn from the patient. Each health care system and laboratory define the ordering time frame. Table 24-9 lists examples of physician orders, which reflect different time requests.

TABLE 24-9   Examples of Physicians' Orders for Lab Tests

Physician's Order	Time Requested	What It Means
CBC today	Routine time request	Next time the laboratory makes a routine run to the unit they will draw the specimen for the test requested. The laboratory makes a run every 2 hours to the surgical unit.
CBC in AM	AM time request	The test needs to be ordered for the morning of the next day. The laboratory draws the AM lab specimens on the surgical unit at 6 A.M.
CBC now	Stat	The lab would go to the surgical unit and draw the specimen as soon as possible after the request is received.
CBC at 11 am	Specimen to be drawn at 11 A.M.	The laboratory would draw the specimen at the time requested (11 A.M.)
CBC	Unknown time	The health unit coordinator would ask the physician at what time the test should be ordered.

MICROBIOLOGY

MARQUETTE GENERAL HOSPITAL, INC. MARQUETTE, MICHIGAN

☐ STAT TODAY ☐ SPECIAL INST. **B 21937**

TIME COLLECTED	DATE COLLECTED	REQ. COMP BY	SPECIMEN SOURCE

☐ SMEAR - GRAM STAIN
☐ CULTURE - AEROBIC ROUTINE (INCLUDE SENS)
☐ CULTURE - ANAEROBIC
☐ CULTURE - BLOOD
☐ CULTURE - GC SCREEN (GONORRHOEA)
☐ CULTURE - HOSPITAL
☐ CULTURE - LEGIONELLA
☐ CULTURE - RESP (SPUTUM OR EYE OR EAR)
☐ CULTURE - STOOL (SAL, SHIG, CAMPY, HEM E. COLI, YER SC.
☐ CULTURE - THROAT ROUTINE
☐ CULTURE - THROAT BETA STREP A ONLY
☐ CULTURE - URINE
☐ CULTURE - VIRUS (HSV, CMV, VZ ONLY)
☐ CULTURE - YERSINIA
☐ TB-AFB - SMEAR
☐ TB-AFB - SMEAR
☐ DARKIELD ☐ MINIMAL BACT. CONC.
☐ MISCELLANEOUS ____________________

☐ THROAT SCREEN - RAPID BETA STREP A ANTIGEN
☐ CLOST DIFFICILE PROTOCOL (RAPID & TOXIN ON (+) RAPIDS)
☐ CLOST DIFFICILE CULTURE
☐ CLOST DIFFICILE RAPID ANTIGEN
☐ CLOST DIFFICILE TOXIN ASSAY
☐ DNA PROBE - CHLAMYDIA
☐ DNA PROBE - GC
☐ FUNGUS - CULTURE
☐ FUNGUS - INDIA INK PREP
☐ FUNGUS - KOH PREP
☐ FUNGUS - SILVER STAIN SMEAR
☐ FUNGUS - WET PREP
☐ PARASITE - AMOEBA SMEAR (TRICHROME)
☐ PARASITE - SMEAR CRYPTOSPORIDIUM/GIARDA
☐ PARASITE - KOH PREP
☐ PARASITE - O & P CONC.
☐ PARASITE - PINWORM PREP
☐ PARASITE - WET PREP AMOEBA/GIARDIA
☐ SERUM BACT. TITER ☐ SMEAR LEGIONELLA

DATE
NAME
RT. NO / DOCTOR
ADDRESS
SEX/ AGE

REQN RECD
SPEC RECD
TEST COMP

CHART FINAL

Figure 24-7 • *A paper request form is used to order a microbiology test. (Courtesy of Marquette General Health System, Marquette, MI)*

Ordering priorities, or the times the specimens are collected, are determined by the health care system and the laboratory facility that provides the services.

Laboratory requests are processed either by using a computerized ordering system or with a paper ordering system. In some health care systems a combination of computer and paper requests may be used (Figures 24-7 and 24-8).

```
                --- Enter/Edit Demographics & Orders ---
                         Privacy Act of 1974
ID:                    Name:                              LOC:  MDM    -
ëëëëëëëëëëëëëëëëëëëëëëëëëëëëëëëëëëëëëëëëëëëëëëëëëëëëëëëëëëëëëëëëëëëëëëëëëëë
Ø GENERAL LAB                  Accession Number:  3352-GL0922              Ø
Ø  Charge Type: BILL FACILITY/DR  Ordered: 12/18/2003  14:26   By: MDUMOU  Ø
Ø                       To Be Collected: 12/18/2003            By:         Ø
Ø                              Received:                       By:         Ø
Ø  Comment:                                                                Ø
áááááááááááááááááááááááááááááááááááááááááááááááááááááááááááááááááááááááááááá
Ø  # ° Procedure                              ° Doctor ° Loc    ° Priority Ø
áááááááááááááááááááááááááááááááááááááááááááááááááááááááááááááááááááááááááááá
Ø 01 ° [CBC   ] ____________________________ ° ______ ° ______ ° ________ Ø
Ø 02 ° [______] ____________________________ ° ______ ° ______ ° ________ Ø
Ø 03 ° [______] ____________________________ ° ______ ° ______ ° ________ Ø
Ø 04 ° [______] ____________________________ ° ______ ° ______ ° ________ Ø
Ø 05 ° [______] ____________________________ ° ______ ° ______ ° ________ Ø
Ø 06 ° [______] ____________________________ ° ______ ° ______ ° ________ Ø
Ø 07 ° [______] ____________________________ ° ______ ° ______ ° ________ Ø
Ø 08 ° [______] ____________________________ ° ______ ° ______ ° ________ Ø
ëëëëëëëëëëëëëëëëëëëëëëëëëëëëëëëëëëëëëëëëëëëëëëëëëëëëëëëëëëëëëëëëëëëëëëëëëë
```

Figure 24-8 • *A computer request is used to order a CBC. (Courtesy of Marquette General Health System, Marquette, MI)*

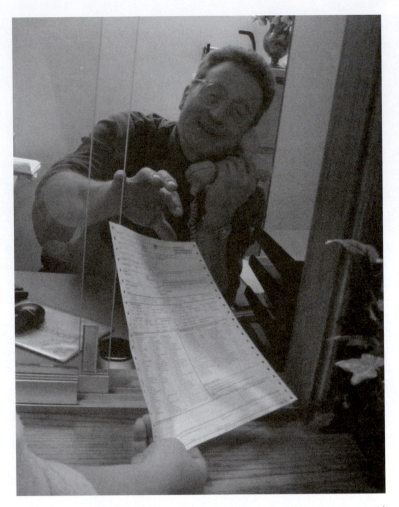

Figure 24-9 • *An outpatient laboratory request is given to a patient for tests to be completed after discharge.*
(Courtesy of Marquette General Health System, Marquette, MI)

If the patient is discharged and must return for laboratory testing, a requisition must be provided to the patient to bring to the laboratory where the test is scheduled (Figure 24-9).

It is important to remember that not all requested laboratory testing can be done on-site. Some tests must be sent out. If a test is to be sent to another laboratory the process for requesting that testing may be unchanged from an in-house test, or the request may be different. The results from an off-site laboratory will not be returned to the patient chart as quickly as will the results from an in-facility test. In fact, the results will have a different look and may be filed in a specially identified location in the patient record.

RECEIVING LABORATORY RESULTS

It is the responsibility of the laboratory department to complete all testing requested and return the verified results to the patient chart. All laboratory reports must be attached to the correct patient chart (Figure 24-10). The health care team uses this

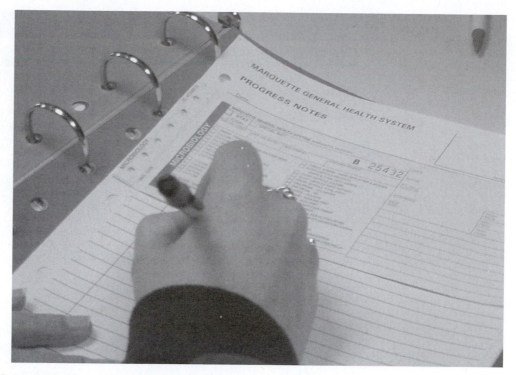

Figure 24-10 • *Lab reports filed in the patient chart are cumulative from the date of admission.*
(Courtesy of Marquette General Health System, Marquette, MI)

information in making decisions regarding patient care. The results may be paper reports or electronic reports (Figure 24-11). How and where the reports are filed are defined by the health care system's procedures. Table 24-10 lists examples of reports and where they are placed.

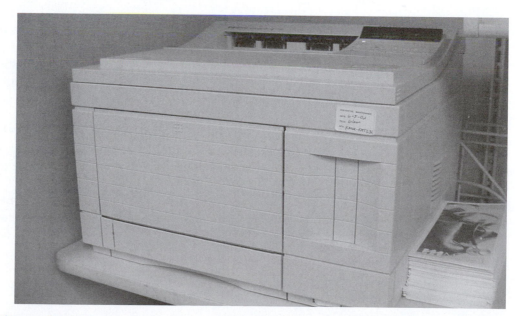

Figure 24-11 • *Stat lab reports print at the workstation printer upon lab staff verification.*
(Courtesy of Marquette General Health System, Marquette, MI)

TABLE 24-10	Lab Reports	
Lab Order	**When Report Available**	**Where It Is Found**
CBC today	After enough specimens are collected to run a batch. No report sent to unit.	◆ On the computer ◆ On daily lab reports that are sent at 8:30 A.M. and 4:30 P.M. ◆ On the patient chart tomorrow
CBC in AM	After all A.M. labs are drawn and run	◆ On the computer ◆ On daily lab reports that are sent at 8:30 A.M. and 4:30 P.M. ◆ On the patient chart tomorrow
CBC now	As soon as specimen is drawn, test is immediately run	◆ On the computer ◆ Report prints on the printer on the unit as soon as it is verified ◆ On daily lab reports that are sent at 8:30 A.M. and 4:30 P.M. ◆ On the patient chart tomorrow
CBC at 11 am	As soon as it is run after being drawn at 11 A.M.	◆ On the computer ◆ Report prints on the printer on the unit as soon as it is verified ◆ On daily lab reports that are sent at 8:30 A.M. and 4:30 P.M. ◆ On the patient chart tomorrow
CBC	After test is verified, not run until enough for a batch. No report sent to unit.	◆ On the computer ◆ On daily lab reports that are sent at 8:30 A.M. and 4:30 P.M. ◆ On the patient chart tomorrow

TRANSCRIPTION STEPS

Table 24-11 lists the steps that should be taken when transcribing laboratory orders.

TABLE 24-11   Transcription Steps

Transcription Step	Key Points
1. Read the entire order set thoroughly.	Careful reading of the orders allows the health unit coordinator to review, prioritize, and check for incomplete or illegible orders.
2. Prioritize orders.	Determine the urgency of the orders within all the charts needing transcription. Decide what orders in the order set need to be transcribed first. A patient who has laboratory orders stat and in the A.M. should have the stat orders transcribed right away.
3. If medications are included in the order set, send the order carbon or a copy to the pharmacy.	This step may be omitted for lab orders. However, IV fluids are needed to transfuse certain blood products; these fluids may be stocked in the pharmacy.
4. Communicate the order to the individual or department that will be performing the order.	The health unit coordinator will communicate laboratory orders to the laboratory department and to the patient care staff responsible for the patient.
5. Record the orders on the patient Kardex or care plan.	Record the lab order as written from the physician's order form to the patient Kardex, care plan, and/or lab board.
6. Record medication orders on the medication administration record (MAR).	This step may be omitted for lab orders, except for transfusion orders. Transfusion orders are usually recorded on the MAR.
7. Check off each order in the set as completed.	Placing a check mark by each order as it is transcribed can help the health unit coordinator track orders even when interrupted.
8. Re-read and check all work for accuracy.	Because of multiple requests received by the health unit coordinator, re-reading and checking work is a necessity.
9. Sign off the order with name, title, date, and time.	The health unit coordinator is accountable for the orders transcribed.

SUMMARY

Ordering of laboratory tests is an important responsibility of the health unit coordinator. For every laboratory test that is ordered, the health unit coordinator needs to know the type of specimen that is needed, who will collect the specimen, if a consent form is required, and in what type of container the specimen will be transported. There are many different laboratory tests done within specific departments located within the laboratory. The health unit coordinator must know which department within the laboratory performs the testing ordered. The health care team must know where the results can be located and when the results are completed. The health unit coordinator provides that information to the health care team. Each health care facility has a defined set of ordering priorities and procedure for filing reports. The health unit coordinator assists the health care team in locating laboratory results. It is important to remember that not all testing requested can be performed at the health care laboratory facility and that tests may be sent out to other laboratories.

REVIEW QUESTIONS

1. List two different methods to obtain a urine specimen for laboratory testing.

2. Describe the purpose of the blood bank.

3. List four different divisions within the laboratory and the main purpose of each.

4. Describe a send-out test and explain why tests are sent out.

5. List five chemistry tests that might be ordered.

TRANSCRIPTION PRACTICE

Go to the CD-ROM for transcription exercises that support the content in this chapter.

NAHUC CERTIFICATION EXAM

CONTENT AREAS

I. A. 2   Interpret medical symbols, abbreviations, and terminology

I. A. 6   Enter orders on a Kardex

I. A. 9   Schedule diagnostic tests and procedures

I. A. 10   Initiate and follow test preparation procedures

I. A. 13   Process orders for diagnostic and therapeutic tests and procedures

I. B. 1   Notify staff of new orders

II. B. 2   Notify physicians of diagnostic test results

II. E. 11   Retrieve test results

III. B. 2   Retrieve diagnostic result from computers

III. B. 4   Enter orders via computers

THROUGH THE EYES

OF A HEALTH CARE PROFESSIONAL

A laboratory technician shares her thoughts.

The health unit coordinator is a key health care team member who provides the lab personnel with important information. The health unit coordinator is knowledgeable as to the patient location, which nurse is responsible for which patients, if the patient has been NPO, where the patient is scheduled to be at each hour of the day, and what laboratory tests have been ordered on each patient on the patient care unit. Health unit coordinators are truly a valuable resource for the laboratory technician.

REFERENCES

Corbett, J. V. (2004). *Laboratory tests and diagnostic procedures with nursing diagnoses* (6th ed.). Stanford, CT: Appleton and Lange.

Kerschner, V. (1992). *Health unit coordinating principles and practices*. Clifton Park, NY: Thomson Delmar Learning.

CHAPTER 25

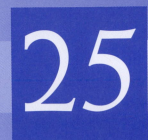

Diagnostic Exam Orders

Learning Objectives

Upon completion of this chapter and review questions, the learner should be able to:

1. Define the ordering process for diagnostic examinations.

2. Describe the importance of communicating and documenting test results.

3. Define contrast medium.

4. List seven examples of clinical data.

5. Name two justifications for the reason of the examination to be included when ordering diagnostic exams.

6. List three examinations completed by the cardiology department.

7. List the nine steps to the transcription process for all diagnostic exams.

8. Describe the seven divisions of radiology.

9. Recognize abbreviations for tests done in computer tomography.

10. Describe the difference between an electrocardiogram and an echocardiogram.

11. Differentiate a cardiac catheterization procedure from an angiogram.

12. Differentiate between a KUB and an IVP.

13. List two abbreviations for magnetic resonance imaging tests.

14. Explain the parts of the body being examined when an EGD and ERCP are performed.

Key Terms

contrast medium Dye or iodine-containing substance that is injected into the body to illuminate inner structures that are hard to see.

electrode A conductor used to establish electrical contact with a nonmetallic part of a circuit.

fluoroscopy A procedure for observing the internal structure of the body.

Holter monitor A device that monitors heart activity throughout the course of the day.

invasive Procedure in which a part of the body is entered, such as an incision or cutting.

telemetry The process of measuring and transmitting heart activity.

Abbreviations

ABD Abdomen

AP Anterior to Posterior

BaE Barium Enema

BAER Brainstem Auditory Evoked Response

BE Barium Enema

CAT Computed Axial Tomography

CT Computed Tomography

CXR Chest x-ray

DSA Digital Subtraction Angiogram

DVI Digital Vascular Imaging

ECG Electrocardiogram

Echo Echocardiogram

EEG Electroencephalogram

EGD Esophagogastroduodenoscopy

GB Gallbladder

GI Gastrointestinal

EKG Electrocardiogram

ERCP Endoscopic Retrograde Cholangiopancreatography

HOH Hard of Hearing

IV Intravenous

IVP Intravenous Pyelogram

KUB Kidneys, Ureters, and Bladder

L Left

Lat Lateral

MAR Medication Administration Record

MBO Monitored Bed Orders

MRA Magnetic Resonance Angiography

MRI Magnetic Resonance Imaging

OCG Oral Cholecystogram

PA Posterior to Anterior

Preps Preparation for an Examination

PROCTO Proctopscopy

Sigmoid Sigmoidoscopy

SONO Sonogram

UGI Upper Gastrointestinal

VER Visual Evoked Response

W/C Wheelchair

PROCESSING DIAGNOSTIC EXAM ORDERS

Chapter 6 introduced some of the many diagnostic departments that are part of health care facilities. The emphasis in this chapter will be the *ordering* of tests and examinations from the diagnostic departments, with the exception of laboratory tests, which were covered in Chapter 24. Abbreviations are often used in writing orders in a patient chart. The health unit coordinator must be able to recognize these abbreviations and have an understanding of the exams requested in order to communicate with the diagnostic departments for the correct test and their needed services. When transcribing a diagnostic exam order, the health unit coordinator must be prepared to find the answers to the following questions:

◆ When is the exam performed?

◆ How is the patient prepared?

◆ How is the patient transported?

◆ Why is the exam ordered?

◆ What department performs the exam?

SCHEDULING

To answer the question "when is the exam performed?" the health unit coordinator needs to understand scheduling protocols. To schedule a test properly, the health unit coordinator needs to know which tests can be done right away and needs to become familiar with the hours of service of each department at the health care facility. These times will range from being open 24 hours a day to 8 hours a day.

The health unit coordinator must also know in what sequence the exams should be ordered. Physicians may determine that several diagnostic exams are needed and write orders for multiple exams on one patient. The health unit coordinator should know which exam should be scheduled first. For example, a barium enema, which is a test using a contrast medium, will affect another exam such as a nuclear scan of the intestines. Most health care facilities have sequencing policies and procedures available at the workstation. When in doubt, the health unit coordinator should contact the department that is responsible for performing the exam.

PREPARATION

The health unit coordinator must also answer the question, "how is the patient to be prepared?" Preparation may include a diet change or a meal to be held before the exam. The process of a patient's receiving preparation for an exam is often referred to as being "prepped." It is the health unit coordinator who initiates many of the preps for the exams. If an exam requires a contrast medium, there will probably be an accompanying prep. In order for some contrast media to be effective, the patient must have empty or clean intestines. That is why many preps involve changing or limiting the patient's food intake and administering laxatives or enemas. Examples of steps the health unit coordinator may take include communicating with the dietary department of the meal prep or pulling and completing a procedure form. Preps to be followed are found in a reference manual, in a Rolodex file, or even printed as part of the requisition from the workstation computer. Some tests will require consent forms to be signed before the procedure. Other tests will require that some type of preparation be completed before the exam. Scheduling may be affected by the requirement that the patient be prepped with some type of contrast medium before the exam or procedure. The health unit coordinator must have and use knowledge about all these factors before scheduling exams.

Consent Forms

Part of the preparation process includes explaining the exam to the patient. A patient will be asked to sign a consent form or procedure form before the procedure is started, in order to ensure that the patient and physician have thoroughly discussed the procedure technique, the risks as well as the benefits. Many of the consent forms for the examinations in this chapter are completed by the department that will be conducting the test. Any **invasive** procedure in which a part of the body is entered, such as an incision or cutting, will require a consent form. Often it is the health unit coordinator who pulls a consent form from a file, completes parts of it, and places it in the patient's chart.

Contrast Medium

A **contrast medium** is a substance that is opaque to x-rays or a substance that will appear solid on an x-ray. A contrast medium illuminates inner structures that are hard to see. It is used to differentiate between body tissues and organs. There are different types of contrast media. Examples of contrast media include air, barium, and iodine dyes. The contrast medium may be swallowed, injected into a patient's vein, or introduced into the rectum. Some contrast media will be given *before* an exam. For example, for a gallbladder series the patient takes tablets the night before. Some contrast media are given *during* the test, such as a barium enema (BE) or upper gastrointestinal (UGI) series.

CLINICAL DATA

The health unit coordinator must also be able to answer the question "how is the patient transported?" The health unit coordinator will be responsible for sharing clinical data. Data that must be shared include diabetes, allergy, and isolation information; mode of transportation; and oxygen and intravenous information. Other examples of clinical information include whether the patient is on telemetry or has special needs such an interpreter or if the patient is visually or hearing impaired or confused. Communicating all of this information assists the diagnostic department in scheduling, transporting, preparing the room, and performing the exam for each individual's needs.

If the patient is a diabetic, the performing location will schedule exams before meal times to allow the nursing staff and the patient to follow the insulin and eating routines. If the patient has an allergy to something, a check will be made to see if it conflicts with the contrast medium to be given to the patient. For example, shellfish contain iodine, which may be the substance that causes a patient's allergic reaction to shellfish. Because iodine is a common contrast medium, the performing department must be aware of the shellfish allergy. If the patient is in airborne isolation, health care workers need to wear masks within three feet of the patient. Patients moving about the hospital away from the isolation room should wear a mask.

The mode of transportation may change quickly depending on the patient's condition. The three most common types of transportation are wheelchair (w/c), cart, and portable. A wheelchair can be ordered for patients who are able to sit or stand. A cart is used for patients who are able to leave the room but are not able to sit or stand. Portable in a true sense is not a mode of transportation because the patient is not transported anywhere. Instead, the department comes to the patient's room with a machine to complete the test in the room. These portable exams are also known as bedside exams.

It is very important to communicate the most current mode of transportation so a transporter does not arrive on the unit with a wheelchair when the patient can be transported only via a cart.

When the patient requires oxygen and intravenous (IV) fluids, supplying this information again assists the transporters so they know to bring the right equipment to hold an oxygen tank and an IV bag.

For patients whose heart rhythm is being monitored via telemetry, the transporter needs to notify someone at the workstation that the patient is going off the unit.

When a patient has special needs, the diagnostic department must be notified. For example, if the patient is hard of hearing (HOH) in the left ear and they are aware of this condition, the department will know to speak to the patient from the right side. Also, if a patient does not speak English, the diagnostic department will need to schedule an interpreter for the department at the same time the patient is scheduled for the exam.

REASON FOR EXAM

The health unit coordinator must also be able to answer "why is the exam ordered?" The reason for the exam is often a required component of the computer order entry screen or the exam requisition.

Stating the reason, such as signs and symptoms the patient is having, gives the physicians and technicians guidance when performing tests and reading the test results. Many tests can be ordered for very different reasons. For example, one left knee x-ray may be ordered for a patient to see the severity of arthritis, while another left knee x-ray may be ordered to determine and view a fracture.

Another reason for stating why an exam is needed is to control costs. Hospitals, long-term health care facilities, physicians, and insurance companies are all working to contain or cut the cost of health care. One way to control costs is to make sure that unnecessary exams are not ordered or completed. Therefore, if a physician orders an electrocardiogram (ECG) on a patient who is hospitalized for a broken arm, there has to be a valid reason why the ECG was ordered. Health care facilities are very conscious of what insurance companies will and will not pay for. A reason of "rule out," such as rule out pneumonia or rule out fracture, is not recognized as a reimbursable reason for an exam.

DIAGNOSTIC DEPARTMENTS

The health unit coordinator must also be able to answer the question, "what department performs the exam?" The following sections discuss various diagnostic testing departments and their commonly performed exams.

CARDIOLOGY

The cardiology department performs procedures and exams related to the heart. Table 25-1 shows common cardiology tests along with their abbreviation, whether a consent is typically required, prep information, and definition.

A common mistake by new health unit coordinators is to confuse an "**echo**" with an "ECG." One way to differentiate the two is to keep in mind that an electrocardiogram records electrical impulses; it is a very quick process, and a complete ecg exam takes only a minute to perform. An echocardiogram uses sound waves that bounce off the heart to create a picture of the position, size, and movement of the valves and chamber walls. It is a longer process; an echo takes 30–45 minutes to complete.

Table 25-2 describes the steps for transcribing cardiac orders.

TABLE 25-1 Common Cardiology Ordering Information

Test	Abbreviation	Written Consent	Prep Needed	Definition/Reason
Cardiac catheterization	Cardiac cath	Yes	Yes	An invasive procedure in which a long catheter is passed into the heart through a large blood vessel in an arm or leg to diagnose heart disease. X-ray allows the physician to view the catheter as it is inserted. This exam is performed by a radiologist or qualified physician. Some large health care facilities have a separate cardiac catheterization lab department.
Echocardiogram	Echo	No	No	A noninvasive exam performed by a technician using sound frequencies to study the function of the heart.
Electrocardiogram	ECG, EKG	No	No	A noninvasive exam that records electrical impulses of the heart, performed by a technician. Often performed with portable equipment at the patient's bedside.
Holter monitor	24-hour Holter	No	No	A device that monitors heart activity throughout the course of the day. A patient wears **electrodes**, and the heart activity is recorded on a small tape recorder that the patient wears around the waist or chest. The patient records in a diary his or her physical activity throughout the day. The nursing staff places the electrodes on the patient and observes the telemetry monitors.
Telemetry; monitored bed orders	Tele; MBOs	No	No	The process of measuring and transmitting heart activity during hospitalization. The patient wears electrodes, and the heart activity is transmitted to monitors normally kept at the nursing workstation.

DIAGNOSTIC IMAGING

In many health care facilities, the diagnostic imaging, or radiology, department has seven divisions: angiography, computer tomography, diagnostic x-ray, magnetic resonance imaging, mammography, nuclear medicine, and ultrasound. These divisions are defined in Chapter 6; in this chapter, we will focus on the tests performed in these departments.

TABLE 25-2	Transcription Steps for Cardiac Orders
Transcription Step	**Key Points**
1. Read the entire order set thoroughly.	Careful reading of the orders allows the health unit coordinator to review, prioritize, and check for incomplete or illegible orders.
2. Prioritize orders.	Determine the urgency of the orders in all the charts needing transcription. Decide what orders in the order set need to be transcribed first.
3. If medications are included in the order set, send the order carbon or a copy to the pharmacy.	It is crucial that the pharmacy receive the physician's medication orders.
4. Communicate the order to the individual or department that will be performing the order.	The health unit coordinator enters the order for the exam on a paper requisition and sends the requisition to the department. In some facilities, the order is entered into the computer to notify the department of the order. Be sure to send clinical data.
5. Record the orders on the patient Kardex or care plan.	Most health care facilities have a form used to keep track of current orders and the plan of care for a patient. Documentation on the Kardex is usually done in pencil and updated as orders are changed, discontinued, and added.
6. Record medication orders on the medication administration record (MAR).	If the order contains preprocedure medications, the health unit coordinator may be responsible for writing the medications on the MAR. Check your facility's policies and procedures.
7. Check off each order in the set as completed.	Placing a check mark by each order as it is transcribed can help the health unit coordinator track orders even when interrupted.
8. Re-read and check all work for accuracy.	Because of multiple requests received by the health unit coordinator, re-reading and checking work is a necessity.
9. Sign off the order with name, title, date, and time.	The health unit coordinator is accountable for the orders transcribed.

Position of Patient

The physician may order the patient to be positioned in a specific way during a diagnostic procedure in order to get the best view of the body structure. One such order may be "chest x-ray PA & lat." When the physician writes the position with the order, it is extremely important to include that information when transcribing the order. The most common position orders are:

> AP—anterior to posterior, or front to back
>
> Decubitus—a position assumed when lying down
>
> PA—posterior to anterior, or back to front
>
> Lat—lateral or side
>
> Oblique view—a slanting angle

Angiography

Table 25-3 consists of information the health unit coordinator needs to transcribe tests performed in the angiography department.

Magnetic resonance angiography (MRA) and computed tomography (CT) angiography are replacing conventional angiography in many situations because these tests are less invasive and easier to perform than conventional angiography.

Computed Tomography

Computed tomography (CT), sometimes called a CAT (computed axial tomography) scan, is a diagnostic procedure in which cross-sectional pictures of the body are made by special x-ray equipment. Doctors use a CT scan to study internal parts of the body. Computed tomography has advantages over other x-ray techniques in diagnosing dis-

TABLE 25-3 Common Angiography Ordering Information

Test	Abbreviation	Written Consent	Prep Needed	Definition/Reason
Digital subtraction angiogram	DSA	Yes	Yes	Two x-ray pictures are taken: one before the contrast material is injected into a blood vessel and a second one after the contrast material is injected. A computer then subtracts images of bone, tissues, and other interfering structures that appear in the first picture from the second picture. The resulting x-ray image, displayed on a video monitor, shows only the blood vessels.
Digital vascular imaging	DVI	Yes	Yes	An exam that allows for the visualization of arteries by a special technique using **fluoroscopy** and computer enhancements.

TABLE 25-4 Common CT Ordering Information

Test	Abbreviations	Written Consent	Prep Needed
Computed tomography of the abdomen	CT scan of the abdomen, CT of the abdomen, CAT scan of abdomen	No	Yes
Computed tomography of the head	CT scan of the head, CT of the head, CAT scan of head	No	No
Computed tomography of the pelvis	CT scan of the pelvis, CT of the pelvis, CAT scan of pelvis	No	Yes
Computed tomography of the spine	CT scan of C1–L5, CT of C1–L5, CAT scan of C1–L5	No	No

eases, particularly because it clearly shows the shape and exact location of organs, soft tissues, and bones. Computed tomography may be ordered with or without contrast media. Here again, it is important for the health unit coordinator to order the test exactly how the physician wrote the order. Table 25-4 lists some of the common tests ordered from the CT department.

See Figure 25-1 for a picture of the abdomen obtained via computed tomography.

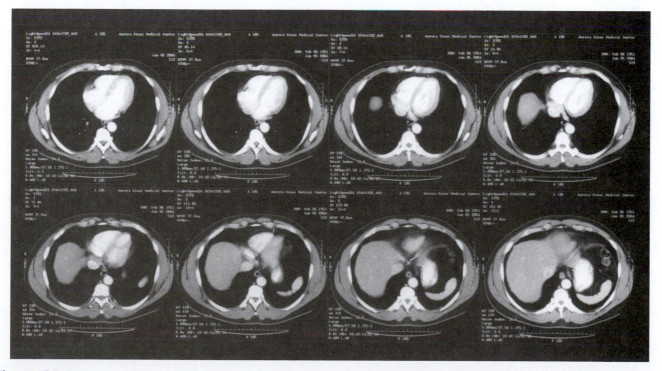

Figure 25-1 • *CT image of the abdomen (Courtesy of Aurora Health Care)*

Diagnostic X-ray

X-rays, also known as radiographs, are used to examine soft and bony tissues of the body. Images are made on photographic film, displayed on video screen, or recorded on digital media. The basic principle of radiography is that differences in density among various body structures produce images of varying light or dark intensity, like the negative print of a photograph. Dense structures appear light, whereas air-filled areas are black. Some common diagnostic x-ray orders that need to be transcribed are listed in Table 25-5.

TABLE 25-5 Common Diagnostic X-ray Ordering Information

Test	Abbreviations	Written Consent	Prep Needed	Definition/Reason
GI barium enema, lower gastrointestinal	BaE, BE, lower air contrast BaE	No	Yes	A test to view the large intestine. There are two types of this test. In the single-contrast technique, barium sulfate is injected into the rectum to view the large intestine. In the double-contrast (or "air contrast") technique, air is inserted into the rectum.
Chest x-ray	AP & Lat CXR	No	No	Front-to-back and side view x-rays of the chest.
X-rays of the extremities		No	No	X-rays of the left, right, or both arms, hands, and wrists and x-rays of the left, right, or both feet and ankles.
Gallbladder, oral cholecystogram	GB, OCG	No	Yes	An x-ray exam of the gallbladder (GB), a saclike organ that stores bile that is located under the liver. The study involves taking tablets containing dye (contrast), which outlines any abnormalities when x rays are taken the following day.
Intravenous pyelogram	IVP	No	Yes	Contrast medium is injected into a vein and the kidneys, ureters, bladder, and urethra are viewed.
Kidneys, Ureters, Bladder	KUB	No	No	An x-ray showing the size and location of the kidneys in relation to other organs in the abdominal region.
Spine x-rays	X-ray of C1–C7, X-ray of T1–T12, X-ray of L1–L5, X-ray of C1–L5	No	No	X-ray of the cervical spine, x-ray of thoracic spine, x-ray of the lumbar spine, x-ray of the spine all the way from the cervical to the lumbar spine.
Upper gastrointestinal series	UGI	No	Yes	X-ray using barium to view the upper digestive tract, including the esophagus, stomach, and part of the small intestine.

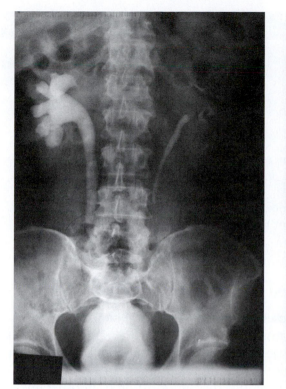

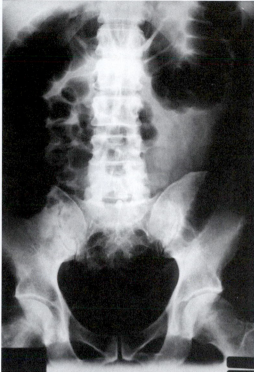

Figure 25-2 • *X-ray image of an intravenous pyelogram (Courtesy of Aurora Health Care)*

Figure 25-3 • *X-ray image of the kidneys, ureters, and bladder (KUB) (Courtesy of Aurora Health Care)*

Figures 25-2 and 25-3 show the difference between IVP and KUB images.

Magnetic Resonance Imaging

Magnetic resonance imaging (MRI) is a diagnostic technique that produces images of organs and structures. The MRI scanner uses strong magnetic fields, not x-rays, to create these images. Hydrogen atoms in the patient react to the magnetic fields, and a computer analyzes the results to produce a picture. An MRI provides highly detailed information without exposing the body to radiation. At times, an MRI provides more detailed and useful images than CT scans or ultrasound.

Because of the strong magnetic fields used, it is important for the patient to complete a questionnaire inquiring about any metal that may be in the patient's body. Internal metals could be a surgical pin, aneurysm clip, ear implant, or pacemaker. Table 25-6 gives information regarding MRI exams.

Figure 25-4 shows the how the abdomen looks on an a MRI scan.

Mammography

A mammogram is an x-ray image of the soft tissues of the breast. Mammograms are used to detect breast cancer at its earliest stage. Ordering a mammogram is usually a straightforward procedure. The reason for the exam, such as "lump in left breast," is included as part of the order.

TABLE 25-6   Common MRI Exam Ordering Information

Test	Abbreviations	Written Consent	Prep Needed
Magnetic resonance imaging of the head	MRI of the head, MRI scan of the head	No	No
Magnetic resonance imaging of the abdomen	MRI of abd, MRI scan of the abd	No	No
Magnetic resonance imaging of the left knee	MRI of L knee, MRI scan of L knee	No	No

Nuclear Medicine

Nuclear medicine uses very small amounts of radioactive materials that are introduced into the body. Because the radioactive materials are attracted to specific organs, bones, or tissues, the emissions they produce can provide crucial information about a particular type of cancer or disease. Information gathered during a nuclear medicine procedure is more comprehensive than information from other imaging procedures because it describes organ function, not just structure. Because nuclear medicine procedures use very small doses of short-lived isotopes (ones that stay radioactive for only a few

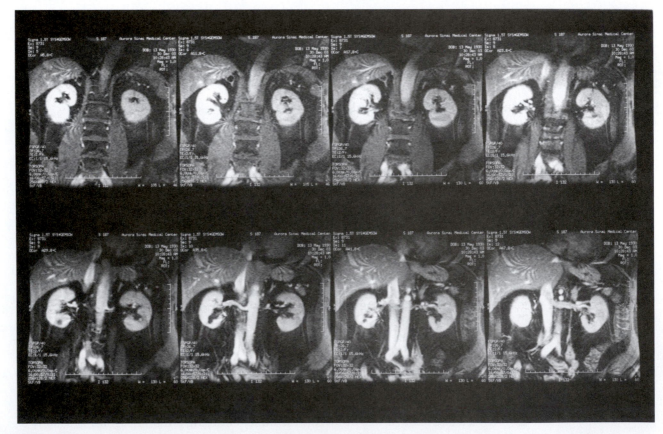

Figure 25-4 • *MRI image of the abdomen (Courtesy of Aurora Health Care)*

TABLE 25-7   Common Nuclear Medicine Ordering Information

Test	Written Consent	Prep Needed
Brain scan	No	No
Bone scan	No	No
Liver/spleen scan	No	No
Lung scan	No	No
Thyroid scan	No	Yes

hours or days), the amount of radiation received is generally less than or equal to that of an x-ray. Table 25-7 is a list of common nuclear medicine tests.

Figure 25-5 shows a nuclear medicine bone scan.

Although this chapter deals with diagnostic tests, because of the advancement of technology, some of the means used for diagnosing may also be used for treatment in nuclear medicine. During the last decade, major progress has been made in the treatment of disease with radioisotopes. Treatments involving the use of medical isotopes are increasing in the race against many types of cancer. Currently, the most common therapeutic uses of medical isotopes are for treatment of thyroid and prostate cancer, hyperthyroidism, cancer bone pain, and polycythemia (abnormal red blood cell and blood increase).

Ultrasound

The use of high-frequency sound to image internal structures is the procedure used in ultrasounds. Ultrasound diagnosis differs from radiological diagnosis in that there is

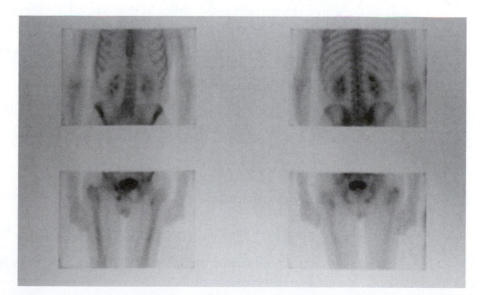

Figure 25-5 • *Nuclear medicine bone scan (Courtesy of Aurora Health Care)*

TABLE 25-8   Common Ultrasound Ordering Information

Test	Abbreviations	Written Consent	Prep Needed
Ultrasound of the abdomen	US abd, echo of the abd, sono of the abd	No	Yes
Ultrasound of the liver	US of liver, echo of the liver, sono of the liver	No	Yes
Ultrasound of the pancreas	US of pancreas, echo of the pancreas, sono of the pancreas	No	Yes

no ionizing radiation involved. Echography and sonography are synonymous with ultrasound. So the physician may order an ultrasound using the terms *ultrasound*, *echo*, or *sono*. A word of caution here: If the physician orders an echo of the liver or an echo of the pancreas, these tests will be ordered from the ultrasound division of radiology. If the physician just orders an "echo" and does not specify what part of the body, an echocardiogram would be ordered from the cardiology department. Table 25-8 lists common ultrasound orders.

Transcription Steps for Diagnostic Imaging Orders

When ordering any tests from the radiology department, follow the steps in Table 25-9.

DIGESTIVE DISORDERS EXAMS

Tests or examinations related to the digestive system may be ordered from the imaging department or from the gastroinstestinal laboratory (GI lab). Orders from the imaging department were addressed earlier in this chapter. Orders from the GI lab are invasive procedures and most often are completed by the physician who ordered them. For this reason, GI tests are scheduled by the physician or the physician's office, not by the health unit coordinator. Some common tests and ordering data for tests completed in the GI lab are listed in Table 25-10.

Figure 25-6 shows the special room used for GI studies. Table 25-11 describes the transcription steps to be followed when ordering tests from the GI lab.

NEUROLOGY EXAMS

The neurology department studies the nervous system, especially in respect to its structure, functions, and abnormalities. Some of the most common neurology tests, along with their abbreviations and other information, are listed in Table 25-12.

Health unit coordinators should follow the steps for transcription in Table 25-13 for neurology department examinations.

TABLE 25-9 Transcription Steps for Radiology Orders

Transcription Step	Key Points
1. Read the entire order set thoroughly.	Careful reading of the orders allows the health unit coordinator to review, prioritize, and check for incomplete or illegible orders.
2. Prioritize orders.	Determine the urgency of the orders in all the charts needing transcription. Decide which orders in the order set need to be transcribed first.
3. If medications are included in the order set, send the order carbon or a copy to the pharmacy.	It is crucial that the pharmacy receive the physician's medication orders.
4. Communicate the order to the individual or department that will be performing the order.	The health unit coordinator enters the order for the exam on a paper requisition and sends the requisition to the department. In some facilities, the order is entered into the computer to notify the department of the order. Be sure to send clinical data.
5. Record the orders on the patient Kardex or care plan.	Most health care facilities have a form used to keep track of current orders and the plan of care for a patient. Documentation on the Kardex is usually done in pencil and updated as orders are changed, discontinued, and added.
6. Record medication orders on the medication administration record (MAR).	If the order contains preprocedure medications, the health unit coordinator may be responsible for writing the medications on the MAR. Check your facility's policies and procedures.
7. Check off each order in the set as completed.	Placing a check mark by each order as it is transcribed can help the health unit coordinator track orders even when interrupted.
8. Re-read and check all work for accuracy.	Because of multiple requests received by the health unit coordinator, re-reading and checking work is a necessity.
9. Sign off the order with name, title, date, and time.	The health unit coordinator is accountable for the orders transcribed.

TABLE 25-10 Common Ordering Information for GI Lab Tests

Test	Abbreviations	Written Consent	Prep Needed	Definition/Reason
Colonoscopy		Yes	Yes	Visualization of the lining of the large intestine using a colonoscope.
Esophagogastro-duodenoscopy	EGD	Yes	Yes	Visualization of the inside of the esophagus, stomach, and duodenum by a flexible fiber-optic tube placed in the mouth.
Endoscopic retrograde cholangio-pancreatography	ERCP	Yes	Yes	Combines the use of x rays and an endoscope. The physician can see the inside of the stomach and duodenum and inject dyes into the ducts in the biliary tree and pancreas so they can be seen on x rays.
Esophageal motility		Yes	Yes	Endoscopy: First. the physician passes a small, flexible fiber-optic tube through the mouth, down the esophagus and into the stomach, providing an opportunity to assess the lining and muscular activity of the esophagus and stomach. Then an x-ray of the esophagus is done while the patient swallows a thick liquid that is visible under x-rays, creating a picture of the lining of the esophagus and stomach.
Gastroscopy		Yes	Yes	Visualization of the inside of the stomach by a gastroscope inserted through the esophagus.
Proctoscopy	Procto	Yes	Yes	Visualization of the rectum and lower end of the colon using a proctoscope.
Sigmoidoscopy	Sigmoid	Yes	Yes	Examination of the rectum and sigmoid colon with the aid of a special instrument called a sigmoidoscope.

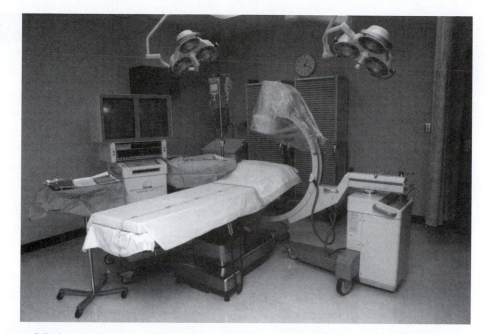

Figure 25-6 • *GI procedure room (Courtesy of Aurora Health Care)*

TABLE 25-11 Transcription Steps for GI Lab Orders

Transcription Step	Key Points
1. Read the entire order set thoroughly.	Careful reading of the orders allows the health unit coordinator to review, prioritize, and check for incomplete or illegible orders.
2. Prioritize orders.	Determine the urgency of the orders in all the charts needing transcription. Decide what orders in the order set need to be transcribed first.
3. If medications are included in the order set, send the order carbon or a copy to the pharmacy.	It is crucial that the pharmacy receive the physician's medication orders. Medications are often a part of the preprocedure preparation.
4. Communicate the order to the individual or department that will be performing the order.	Most often the physician who orders the GI test will schedule the test to coincide with his or her work schedule.
5. Record the orders on the patient Kardex or care plan.	Most health care facilities have a form used to keep track of current orders and the plan of care for a patient. Documentation on the Kardex is usually done in pencil and updated as orders are changed, discontinued, and added.

(continues)

TABLE 25-11   *(continued)*

Transcription Step	Key Points
6. Record medication orders on the medication administration record (MAR).	If the order contains preprocedure medications, the health unit coordinator may be responsible for writing the medications on the MAR. Check your facility's policies and procedures.
7. Check off each order in the set as completed.	Placing a check mark by each order as it is transcribed can help the health unit coordinator track orders even when interrupted.
8. Re-read and check all work for accuracy.	Because of multiple requests received by the health unit coordinator, re-reading and checking work is a necessity.
9. Sign off the order with name, title, date, and time.	The health unit coordinator is accountable for the orders transcribed.

TABLE 25-12   Common Neurology Exam Ordering Information

Test	Abbreviations	Written Consent	Prep Needed	Definition/Reason
Brainstem auditory evoked response	BAER	No	No	Evaluates the function of nerve pathways in the brain that are needed to hear. Clicking noises or tones are sent through earphones to the person being tested, and each response is recorded from brain waves by using electrodes taped to the head. The electrical response in the brain is called a brainstem auditory evoked response or potential.
Electroencephalo- gram	EEG	No	Yes	Records the electrical activity of the brain. Sensors are attached with adhesive to the head and connected by wires to a computer. The computer records the brain's electrical activity on paper as wavy lines. Certain brain abnormalities can be detected by observing changes in the normal pattern of the brain's electrical activity.
Visual evoked response	VER	No	No	When the eyes are stimulated by looking at a test pattern, the response is called a visual evoked response or potential.

TABLE 25-13 Transcription Steps for Neurology Department Orders

Transcription Step	Key Points
1. Read the entire order set thoroughly.	Careful reading of the orders allows the health unit coordinator to review, prioritize, and check for incomplete or illegible orders.
2. Prioritize orders.	Determine the urgency of the orders in all the charts needing transcription. Decide what orders in the order set need to be transcribed first.
3. If medications are included in the order set, send the order carbon or a copy to the pharmacy.	It is crucial that the pharmacy receive the physician's medication orders.
4. Communicate the order to the individual or department that will be performing the order.	The health unit coordinator enters the order for the exam on a paper requisition and sends the requisition to the department. In some facilities, the order is entered into the computer to notify the department of the order. Be sure to send clinical data.
5. Record the orders on the patient Kardex or care plan.	Most health care facilities have a form used to keep track of current orders and the plan of care for a patient. Documentation on the Kardex is usually done in pencil and updated as orders are changed, discontinued, and added.
6. Record medication orders on the medication administration record (MAR).	If the order contains preprocedure medications, the health unit coordinator may be responsible for writing the medications on the MAR. Check your facility's policies and procedures.
7. Check off each order in the set as completed.	Placing a check mark by each order as it is transcribed can help the health unit coordinator track orders even when interrupted.
8. Re-read and check all work for accuracy.	Because of multiple requests received by the health unit coordinator, re-reading and checking work is a necessity.
9. Sign off the order with name, title, date, and time.	The health unit coordinator is accountable for the orders transcribed.

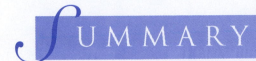

SUMMARY

Understanding abbreviations is the first step in reading physicians' orders. Reading and understanding the orders thoroughly will assist in prioritizing and ordering all the patients' exams needed to be transcribed throughout the day. Knowledge of preprocedure requirements and communicating the orders to ancillary departments such as pharmacy and dietary will ensure timely scheduling. The health unit coordinator must document the tests by writing the tests on the Kardex in order to notify the nurses. Signing the orders off at the end of the set should never done without double-checking for completeness and accuracy. Signing off the orders with the current date and time makes tracking the order easier and tells everyone that the set of orders is complete. Although these are the generic rules for the transcription of orders, each health care facility will have its own exact policy. Always know and follow your individual health care facility's policies and procedures.

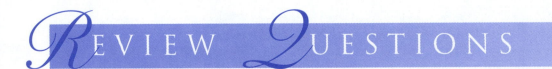

REVIEW QUESTIONS

1. List three exams completed by the cardiac services department.

2. Explain the parts of the body being examined when an EGD and ERCP are performed.

3. Differentiate cardiac catheterization from angiography.

4. List the nine steps to the transcription process for all diagnostic exams.

5. Define contrast medium.

6. Name two justifications for the reason of the exam to be included when ordering diagnostic exams.

7. Recognize abbreviations for tests done in computed tomography.

8. List two abbreviations for magnetic resonance imaging tests.

9. List the seven divisions of radiology.

10. Describe the importance of communicating and documenting test results.

11. List seven examples of clinical data.

12. Differentiate between a KUB and an IVP.

TRANSCRIPTION PRACTICE

Go to the CD-ROM for transcription exercises that support the content in this chapter.

NAHUC CERTIFICATION EXAM

CONTENT AREAS

I. A. 2   Interpret medical symbols, abbreviations, and terminology

I. A. 6   Enter orders on a Kardex

I. A. 9   Schedule diagnostic tests and procedures

I. A. 10   Initiate and follow test preparation procedures

I. A. 13   Process orders for diagnostic and therapeutic tests and procedures

I. B. 1   Notify staff of new orders

II. H. 4   Demonstrate knowledge of informed consent

III. B. 4   Enter orders via computers

THROUGH THE EYES

OF A HEALTH CARE PROFESSIONAL

The radiology department staff shares their thoughts.

Scheduling the right test at the right time and having the patient prepped properly helps to make the radiology department run more smoothly. When the complete and correct information is provided to the department, we can complete our jobs in an organized and timely fashion. Proper communication from the health unit coordinators helps us serve our patients in a kind and professional manner.

REFERENCES

http://www.cbvcp.com/nmrc Accessed October 2003.

http://www.healthatoz.com Accessed October 2003.

http://www.radiologymalaysia.org Accessed October 2003.

Fischbach, F. (2000). *A manual of laboratory and diagnostic tests* (6th ed.). Philadelphia: Lippincott

Greathouse, J. S. (1998). *Radiographic positioning and procedures* (Vol. 1). Clifton Park, NY: Thomson/Delmar Learning.

Nutrition Orders

Learning Objectives

Upon completion of this chapter and review questions, the learner should be able to:

1. Define vocabulary and abbreviations related to diets.

2. Explain the functions of the food management and nutritional support services within the dietary department.

3. List the diets that progress in consistency.

4. List special or therapeutic diets.

5. Identify supplements.

6. Identify different administration routes and types of tube feedings.

7. Explain how the health unit coordinator communicates orders to the dietary department.

8. Interpret and transcribe physicians' orders.

Key Terms

bolus   A single amount given all at once.

diet board   A list of all of the department's patients and the nutrition and meals that have been ordered for them.

enteral   By way of the intestine or gastrointestinal tract.

gastostomy tube A small plastic hose inserted into a cut or incision in the skin directly to the stomach or small intestine.

nasogastric tube A tube inserted in the patient's nose and routed directly into the stomach.

nutrients The substances that provide the body with energy and the materials necessary for growth and the maintenance of body tissues and proper cell functioning.

nutrition The process by which the body absorbs food and uses it for growth and maintenance.

parenteral Apart from or away from the intestine.

therapeutic diet A diet that is modified to improve or treat specific conditions.

tube feeding Food in liquid form is given to a patient through a tube that is inserted into the stomach.

Abbreviations

ADA American Dietetic Association

As tol As Tolerated

Cal Calorie

cc Cubic Centimeters

CDR Commission on Dietetic Registration

Chol Cholesterol

Cl liq Clear Liquids

DAT Diet As Tolerated

G-tube Gastostomy Tube

Gen General

Gen liq General Liquids

gm Gram

Hi protein High Protein

I/O Intake and Output

K potassium

Lo chol or low chol Low Cholesterol

Lo Na or Low Na Low Sodium

Lo NaCl or Low NaCl Low Salt

Lo protein Low Protein

Lo res or low res Low Residue

Mech soft Mechanical Soft

ml Milliliters

Na Sodium

NaCl Sodium Chloride (salt)

NAS No Added Salt

NG Nasogastric

NPO Nothing by Mouth

P or Phos Phosphorus

Reg Regular

DIETARY DEPARTMENT

In Chapter 6, the dietary department was defined. Another name for the dietary department is food management and nutrition services. The responsibilities of food management and nutrition services may be divided. The food management division may be responsible for ordering and preparing food for patients or residents and staff and visitors. This division is staffed with chefs and dietary assistants who assemble food trays as well as deliver and collect meal trays. They may deliver meal trays to the patients and collect trays after mealtime.

Nutrition services employs registered dietitians and registered dietetic technicians. Registered dietitians are food and nutrition experts who have met the criteria to earn the registered dietitian credential from the American Dietetic Association (ADA). In addition to meeting the educational requirement of a minimum of a baccalaureate degree, they must also pass a national examination administered by the Commission on Dietetic Registration (CDR). Registered dietetic technicians are also trained in food and nutrition and must have an approved associate's degree and pass an examination administered by the CDR.

Dietitians assess the patient's needs and assist the patient and, often, family members with hospital menu selections. Patients are often required to follow a restricted diet both while in the hospital and when they return home. Dietitians teach and recommend food choices and guidelines for patients on restricted diets. They also recommend food choices based on patient allergies or likes and dislikes.

DIET AND NUTRITION

A person cannot live long without food and water. **Nutrition** is defined as the process by which the body absorbs food and uses it for growth and maintenance. Food supplies **nutrients**, the substances that provide the body with energy and the materials necessary for growth and the maintenance of body tissues and proper cell functioning.

There are six major nutrients:

- Water
- Lipids
- Proteins
- Carbohydrates
- Vitamins
- Minerals

Diet is an important factor in one's health. Therefore, diet orders are an important factor in the plan of care the physician orders for the patient. Physicians must write an order for special food and liquids, just as they do for laboratory and diagnostic imaging tests.

REGULAR DIETS

The term *regular diet* is given to a balanced, nutritional diet with no restrictions. A regular diet has all the essential nutrients. It will consist of breakfast, lunch, and dinner. A patient receiving a regular diet may also have snacks and beverages as desired. A regular diet may also be referred to as a general or house diet. The diet order may be abbreviated as:

Gen diet—general diet

Reg diet—regular diet

A physician may write a diet order as "diet as tolerated," "DAT, "Diet as tol," or "advance diet as tolerated." *Diet as tolerated* can be defined as a regular diet that progresses or changes in consistency or texture. A diet as tolerated will progress from ice chips and water to clear liquids (Cl liq) to general liquids (Gen liq) or full liquids to soft foods to a regular general diet.

The DAT diet order requires a nurse to assess what consistency of food the patient may tolerate. The dietary department will call for clarification if a diet is entered as diet as tolerated. The dietary department needs to know specifically if the diet tray should contain clear liquid, general or full liquid, soft foods, or general diet. May be abbreviated as:

DAT or Diet as tol—diet as tolerated

Cl liq—clear liquids

Gen liq—general liquid

THERAPEUTIC OR SPECIAL DIETS

Therapeutic means tending to improve or restore health. A **therapeutic diet** is a diet that is modified to improve or treat specific conditions. It may also be called a special diet. The therapeutic diet may have specific nutrients that are restricted or controlled or specific nutrients that are increased. The dietary department in each health care facility has a list of available diets that can be ordered for the patient (Figure 26-1). Examples of therapeutic diets follow. This list does not include all of the therapeutic diets that are available.

		SPECIAL DIETS	
Diet	**General Use**	**Foods Allowed**	**Foods to Limit/or Avoid**
Low-calorie	Overweight	Skim milk, fresh fruits, lean meat or fish, vegetables, 1–2 servings of cereal per day	Fried foods, rich gravies and sauces, jams, jellies, rich desserts
High-calorie	Undeweight	Peanut butter, eggnog, jellies, ice cream, desserts, frequent snacks, milk shakes	None
Bland	Stomach or intestinal precaution; ulcers	Eat three well-balanced meals.	Highly seasoned, fried foods, raw vegetables and fruit, whole grains and cereals, spices such as chili peppers or powder, black pepper, red pepper, caffeinated and alcoholic beverages. Decaffeinated coffee or tea will be served according to individual tolerance.
Diabetic	Diabetes	Canned fruits in natural juices, fresh fruits, regular meat, vegetables, bread, sugarless gelatin, custards	Foods containing sugar, alcoholic beverages, gravy, sauces, chocolate; sweetened carbonated beverages
Low-sodium	Fluid retention; heart problems; high blood pressure	Foods cooked without salt, regular meat, vegetables, fruits, salt substitutes (are not recommended in renal conditions)	Smoked, cured, canned fish and meats; cold cuts; cheese; potato chips; pretzels; pickles; bouillon; prepared mustard; catsup; commercial salad dressings; soy sauce
Low-fat, low-cholesterol	Heart disease; liver disease; gallbladder	Veal, poultry, fish, skim milk, buttermilk, yogurt, low-fat cottage cheese, fat-free soup broth, fresh fruits and vegetables, cereals, gelatin, angel cake, ices, carbonated beverages, coffee, tea, jams, jellies	Fatty meats, bacon, butter, whole milk, cheese, kidney, liver, heart, fried foods, rich desserts, sauces

(continues)

Figure 26-1 • *Special diets table*

Diet	General Use	Foods Allowed	Foods to Limit/or Avoid
Clear-liquid	Preoperative or postoperative	Tea or black coffee with sugar, apple juice, plain gelatin (no fruit), clear broth or bouillon	Solid foods
Full-liquid	Gastrointestinal problems; chewing problems	All foods in clear-liquid diet; strained juices, milk, cream, buttermilk, eggnog, strained cream soups, strained cereal, cocoa, carbonated beverages, ices, ice cream, gelatin, custard puddings, sherbets, milk shakes, bouillon, yogurt	Solid foods
Soft, mild	Gastrointestinal conditions; chewing problems	Milk, cream, butter, mild cheeses (cottage, cream cheeses), eggs (not fried), soup, broth, strained cream soups, tender cooked vegetables, fruit juices, cooked fruits, bananas, grapefruit and oranges peeled with all section skins removed, white bread, cereals, cooked cereals, spaghetti, noodles, macaroni, pasta, tea, coffee, carbonated beverages, sherbets, ices, sponge cake, tender chicken, fish, ground beef or lamb, only small amounts of salt and spices	Fibrous meat, coarse cereals, fried foods, raw fruits and vegetables, rich pastries
Pureed	Difficulty or discomfort in swallowing	All semisolid foods, foods put through a blender, and liquids of a viscous nature such as nectars	Sticky foods such as peanut butter or melted cheese, thin liquids such as water
Low-residue	Postoperative; colitis; diverticulitis	Milk, buttermilk, butter, mild cheeses, tender chicken, fish, ground beef, ground lamb, soup broths, fruit juices, breads and cereals, macaroni, noodles, custards, sherbet, vanilla ice cream, sponge cake, plain cookies, strained and cooked vegetables	Fried foods, fresh fruits and vegetables, fibrous meats, nuts, seeds
High-fiber	Constipation	Whole grain breads and cereals, raw and cooked vegetables, fruit juices, dried beans, bran or bran flakes, nuts, seeds, and dried fruits	
High-potassium	Potassium loss due to medication	Fresh fruits and vegetables, especially bananas and raisins	Canned tomato juice, raw clams, sardines, frozen lima beans, frozen peas, canned spinach, canned carrots

NOTE: This chart is a general guide to special diets. Always follow the dietitian's prescribed diet plan.

Figure 26-1 • *continued*

Diabetic or American Dietetic Association (ADA) diet. A diet intended to decrease the need for diabetic medication and to control weight by managing calories and carbohydrates.

Bland. A diet of easily digested foods and foods that do not irritate the digestive tract.

Calorie controlled. May be ordered as a high-calorie (high-cal) or a low-calorie (low-cal) diet, or the specific number of calories may be indicated, for example, a 1200-calorie diet. May be abbreviated as:

High cal—high calorie

Low cal—low calorie

1800 cal diet—1800 calorie diet

Consistent carbohydrate or carbohydrate controlled. A diet intended to decrease the need for diabetic medication and/or to control weight by managing carbohydrates.

Fluid restricted. A diet that controls or monitors liquids. This type of diet limits the amount of liquids in cubic centimeters or milliliters. For example, "Restrict fluids to 1200 cc per day." The health unit coordinator may use the facility's guidelines for dividing the fluids among meals. A fluid restriction order may be written as "350 cc at breakfast, 350 cc at lunch, 350 cc at dinner, and 150 cc in evening."

Low cholesterol. A diet restricted in cholesterol. May be abbreviated as low chol or lo chol.

Low fat. A diet restricted in fat.

Low fiber or low residue. A diet restricted in bulk or fiber. May be abbreviated as low res or lo res.

Low sodium or low salt. A diet that restricts sodium. May be abbreviated as:

Lo Na or low Na—low sodium

Lo NaCl or low NaCl—low salt

NAS—no added salt

2 gm Na—two grams sodium

3.5 gm Na—three point five grams sodium

Mechanical soft. A diet that is easy to chew. This type of diet would be ordered for a patient who has difficulty chewing. It may also be ordered as a regular diet with ground meat. May be abbreviated as mech soft.

Potassium restricted. A diet that restricts potassium. The potassium-restricted diet usually specifies in milliequivalents the amount of potassium the patient may have. For example, "30 mEq K."

Pureed or blenderized. A diet that breaks down the solid foods into a liquid form for ease of chewing and swallowing.

Protein. May be written as high-protein or low-protein. May be abbreviated as: hi protein, lo protein.

Renal. A diet for the patient with kidney disease. A renal diet will likely restrict protein, sodium (Na), potassium (K), and phosphorus (P or Phos).

Small feedings. A diet for the patient who would benefit from smaller, more frequent meals. A physician may write an order for six small meals instead of the standard three of breakfast, lunch, and dinner.

RELIGIOUS OR CULTURAL DIETS

Therapeutic or special diets do not just address health conditions. Special diets may address the religious or cultural needs of the patient. For example, the patient may not eat meat on certain days of the week, or may not eat specific types of meat, or may not eat meat at all. Some religions and cultures require that one's food be prepared a specific way. Examples of these diets may be written as kosher, vegetarian, or no pork. It is important for the health unit coordinator to contact the dietary department when a patient has special dietary needs.

HOLDING DIETS

Sometimes, the diet order is that the patient is not to have anything to eat or drink. The abbreviation for nothing by mouth is NPO. For example, a patient going to surgery may be ordered to not eat or drink anything after midnight before surgery. Another example would be when a patient has breakfast held in order to fast for a blood test. The order may be written as "Hold breakfast." When a patient is NPO, the dietary department is informed so that no meal trays are delivered for the patient until further notification. However, if only breakfast is to be held before laboratory testing, the dietary department is not usually notified to hold delivery of the meal tray. Instead, the breakfast meal tray is held on the unit or department until the patient's tests are completed. The meal is held on the unit to ensure that the patient receives breakfast as soon as possible after the tests.

MONITORING DIETS

A physician may order that a patient's food or liquids, or both, be monitored. If food intake is to be monitored, an order for a calorie count will be written. After a patient is served a meal, a patient care staff member will record the amount of food that was eaten. This information is usually sent back to the dietary department so they can calculate the amount of calories consumed.

If fluids are to be monitored, an order for I/O will be written. I/O is the abbreviation for intake and output. The patient care staff will record all liquids the patient consumes, both orally and intravenously. The patient care staff will also record the amount when the patient voids. Usually an I/O form is placed close to the patient for ease of recording or charting.

VISITOR MEALS

Many patients come to health care facilities with family or friends, and a visitor or family member may be at the health care facility during mealtime. Most health care facilities have vending machines, coffee shops, or cafeterias that provide food for visitors. In rare cases, a visitor may not be able to eat the vending machine food or go to the coffee shop or cafeteria. In this case, a guest tray may be ordered for the visitor to be delivered along with the patient's meal.

PATIENT SELECTION AND SATISFACTION

Because diet is important for the restoration of health, the health team strives to interest the patient in maintaining a good diet. Whether the patient is on a regular or a therapeutic diet, individual choice is important. Many health care facilities offer a menu of meal choices for general diets and commonly ordered therapeutic diets. It is also important that food be served as appetizingly as possible. If a patient's meals are held or delayed for diagnostic testing, it is important that the health unit coordinator resume the meal as soon as possible. It is important for a health unit coordinator to communicate the correct diet to the dietary department because this is one area over which the patient has some control while hospitalized; the patient can choose from a variety of food selections on the menu (Figure 26-2).

DIETITIAN CONSULTATION

As stated earlier, dietitians teach and recommend food choices and guidelines for patients on restricted diets. An order may be written for a dietitian to consult with the patient. The dietitian is specially trained to make nutritional assessments and recommendations.

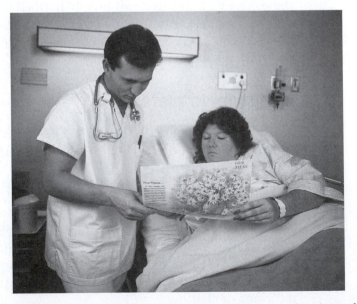

Figure 26-2 • *Patients may choose a variety of food selections from a menu*

SUPPLEMENTS, TUBE FEEDINGS, AND PARENTERAL NUTRITION

A patient may need more nutrients than diet alone can provide. A patient who is a poor eater or who is malnourished may not be able to eat enough food to obtain all the necessary nutrients to heal and build strength. In this case, a dietary supplement or a tube feeding may be ordered for the patient.

SUPPLEMENTS

A dietary supplement is a type of food or drink that is fortified with additional nutrients and vitamins. Most supplements are in the form of a canned liquid, but supplements may also be served in the form of puddings or candy-type bars. Common examples of a supplement are Sustacal and Ensure.

TUBE FEEDINGS

The diets that have been discussed so far have been diets that are taken into the body by mouth. Sometimes, a patient's condition may prohibit him or her from taking food in by mouth. For example, a patient who has had a stroke may have difficulty swallowing or sucking. When a patient is unable to eat, a feeding tube may be inserted. A **tube feeding** is food in liquid form that is given to a patient through a tube that is inserted into the stomach. A tube feeding may also be referred to as an **enteral** feeding. *Enteral* means by way of the intestine or gastrointestinal tract. Enteral nutrition is sometimes used when the patient is able to eat small amounts by mouth but cannot obtain enough food that way. The patient may continue to eat or drink as able, and the tube feeding provides the balance of calories and nutrients that are needed.

There are two common routes used for tube feedings. A tube can be inserted into the patient's nose and routed directly into the stomach. This type of tube is called a **nasogastric tube**, or NG, tube. *Naso* is the word root meaning nose, and *gastro* is the word root meaning stomach. A small plastic hollow hose may also be inserted into a cut or incision in the skin directly to the stomach or small intestine. This procedure is done under x-ray guidance. This is called a **gastrostomy** tube or a g-tube (Figure 26-3). The word root *gastro* means belly or stomach, and the suffix *stomy* means artificial or surgical opening.

Food in liquid form is given to the patient through the tube. Different tube feeding formulas are available. Some provide complete nutrition, and others provide certain nutrients. Formulas that meet the patient's specific needs are selected. For example, some formulas may be suited for diabetic patients, and other formulas for patients who are on a ventilator. Examples of formulas include Ensure, Isocal, Jevity, Osmolite, Pediasure, and Pulmocare.

Food may be given through the tube in prescribed amounts several times a day or continuously. The term **bolus** may be used for feedings that are not continuous. *Bolus* means a single amount given all at once. The order may include the type of formula, the amount of formula, and the number of times per day it is to be administered. For example, "Isocal 200 cc tid." Isocal is the formula; 200 cc is the amount; and tid is the frequency. The patient care staff would prepare a tube feeding of 200 cc of the formula and administer it to the patient three times a day.

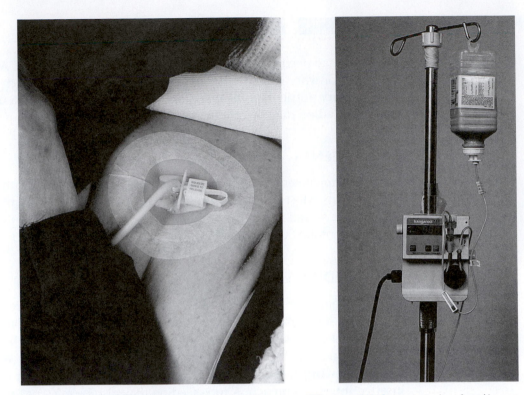

Figure 26-3 • *A gastrostomy tube*   **Figure 26-4** • *A tube feeding pump*

In a continuous tube feeding, the liquid is going through the tube all of the time at a specific flow rate. The order may include the type of formula and a flow rate expressed as cubic centimeters or milliliters (ml) per hour. For example "Pulmocare 50 cc/hr." The type of formula is Pulmocare, and the flow rate is 50 cc per hour. The patient care staff would prepare a tube feeding to drip continuously through the feeding tube at a rate of 50 cc per hour.

The health unit coordinator may be responsible for ordering the equipment that the patient care staff needs to administer the tube feeding. A tube feeding bag and tubing will be required. Depending on the way the feeding is ordered, a tube feeding pump may also be needed. A tube feeding bag and tubing can be connected to an electronic pump that will regulate the flow of the formula through the tubing (Figure 26-4).

PARENTERAL NUTRITION

Some patients cannot get the necessary nutrients by mouth or by enteral feeding. In such cases, the patient will receive **parenteral** nutrition. The term parenteral comes from the prefix *para*, which means apart from, and the word root *enteral*, which means by way of the intestine or gastrointestinal tract. Therefore, *parenteral* means apart from or away from the intestine. In health care, parenteral usually refers to administering fluids or medications by injection. Parenteral nutrition is delivered to the patient directly into the blood, through a catheter (thin tube) inserted into a vein. Parenteral nutrition is discussed in more detail in Chapter 28.

COMMUNICATING DIETARY ORDERS

The health unit coordinator communicates diet orders to the dietary department. Dietary services and diet orders may be requested via the computer order entry system or by paper requisition. Once the service or diet is ordered, the information is also communicated to the patient care staff responsible for the patient. The health unit coordinator may also need to contact central supply if tube feeding supplies are needed. The health unit coordinator may need to add additional chart forms for calorie count or I/O orders.

DIET BOARD

Some facilities use a **diet board** to record patient diets. A diet board is a list of all of the department's patients and the nutrition and meals that have been ordered for them. The diet board serves as a centralized list of the patients and their diets. The diet board may be used for cross-checking the patient meal trays against the physician's order (Figures 26-5 and 26-6). The health unit coordinator may generate the diet board

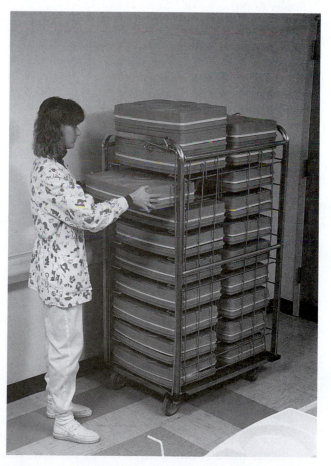

Figure 26-5 • *Meal trays should be checked carefully with the physician's diet order as indicated on the diet board.*

The Best Care Hospital
Diet Report

Room #	Patient Name	Breakfast	Lunch	Dinner	Snacks
Room 101	Hammers, Harry	General			
Room 102	Nails, Nancy	Hold	NAS		
Room 103	Pliers, Peter	General			
Room 104					
Room 105	Tape, Thomas	Clear Liquids	Full Liquid	Soft	
Room 106	Saw, Samuel	General			
Room 107	Wire, Wendy	Tube Feeding			
Room 108	Socket, Sally	Soft			
Room 109	Test, Tammy	No Added Salt, Lo Chol			
Room 110	Apple, Annie	General			

Figure 26-6 • *Diet board*

electronically or may manually create a diet board. For a manual diet board, the health unit coordinator would list the patients and record the most recent diet order for the patients from the patient chart or Kardex.

STOCKING NOURISHMENTS

Small kitchens are usually found in health care facility departments that have patients stay for extended periods time. This is a convenience because patients will need and require food and liquids at times other than scheduled mealtimes. The health unit coordinator may be responsible for maintaining the supply of nourishments for the department. A typical list of nourishments is shown in Figure 26-7.

DIET ORDERS

Most diet orders are written as standing orders. Standing orders remain active or in place until orders are written to change or discontinue them. The physician has to write the diet order only once as a standing order, and the patient will receive that diet every meal, every day until the physician writes another order to change or discontinue the diet. If the diet order is a standing order, it will probably be written just as the type of diet. For example, the physician may write "NAS diet." It is implied that the diet

Nourishments

Date of Order: _____

Date to be Delivered: _____

Department: _____

Cost Center No.: _____

Ordered by: _____

Item	Stock Quantity	Quantity Ordered
Sherbet	each	
Popsicles	each	
Jello	each	
2% Milk	8 oz carton	
Skim Milk	8 oz carton	
Chocolate Milk	8 oz carton	
Wheat bread	loaf	
White bread	loaf	
Saltines	packets of two	
Margarine	pats	
Artificial sweetener	packets	
Sugar	packets	
Creamer	packets	

Figure 26-7 • *Nourishment order form*

order is a standing order. The physician probably would not write, "NAS diet breakfast, lunch, dinner, every day of the week."

A diet order can be written as a one-time order. One-time orders are active or in place only once or just for a specified short amount of time. In this case, the physician writes the diet type and when the patient is to receive the diet or the length of time the order will be in effect. Many diagnostic tests require that the patient have an empty intestinal tract. Because of this requirement, the patient may receive a preparation diet before a test. For example, the physician may write the order, "Cl. Liq. today" or "NPO after midnight."

Table 26-1 lists transcription steps as they apply to diet orders.

TABLE 26-1 Transcription Steps for Diet Orders

Transcription Step	Key Points
1. Read the entire order set thoroughly.	Careful reading of the orders allows the health unit coordinator to review, prioritize, and check for incomplete or illegible orders.
2. Prioritize orders.	Determine the urgency of the orders in all the charts needing transcription. Decide what orders in the order set need to be transcribed first. A patient whose meals have been held and may now eat is a priority. The health unit coordinator should promptly resume meals when a "hold" has been lifted.
3. If medications are included in the order set, send the order carbon or a copy to the pharmacy.	This step may be omitted for diet orders. However, in some health care facilities, tube-feeding formulas are stocked in the pharmacy.
4. Communicate the order to the individual or department that will be performing the order.	The health unit coordinator communicates diet orders to the dietary department and to the patient care staff responsible for the patient. The health unit coordinator may also need to contact central supply if tube-feeding supplies are needed. The health unit coordinator may need to add additional chart forms for calorie count or I/O orders.
5. Record the orders on the patient Kardex or care plan.	Record the diet order as written from the physician's order form to the patient Kardex, care plan, and/or diet board.
6. Record medication orders on the medication administration record (MAR).	This step may be omitted for diet orders. Diet orders are not usually recorded on the MAR.
7. Check off each order in the set as completed.	Placing a check mark by each order as it is transcribed can help the health unit coordinator track orders even when interrupted.
8. Re-read and check all work for accuracy.	Because of multiple requests received by the health unit coordinator, re-reading and checking work is a necessity.
9. Sign off the order with name, title, date, and time.	The health unit coordinator is accountable for the orders transcribed.

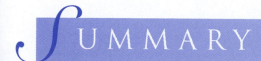

SUMMARY

The patient's physician will determine the diet that gives the patient the most beneficial combination of nutrients. The dietary department supports the patient's plan of care by preparing and providing meals and teaching the patient and the family about diet choices.

REVIEW QUESTIONS

Write out the meanings of the following orders:

1. NPO p 2400

2. 60 mg Na, 40 mEq K diet

3. 1000 cal ADA

4. List five therapeutic or special diets.

5. List the diets that may be selected for a DAT.

6. Explain the difference between a g-tube and an NG tube.

TRANSCRIPTION PRACTICE

Go to the CD-ROM for transcription exercises that support the content in this chapter.

NAHUC CERTIFICATION EXAM

CONTENT AREAS

I. A. 2 Interpret medical symbols, abbreviations, and terminology

I. A. 6 Enter orders on a Kardex

I. B. 1 Notify staff of new orders

III. B. 4 Enter orders via computers

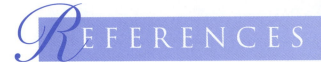

THROUGH THE EYES

OF A HEALTH CARE PROFESSIONAL

A dietitian shares her thoughts.

Someone who is a patient in a hospital usually is subjected to tests and treatments that can be uncomfortable and distressing. The dietary department performs an important service *for* the patient instead of doing something *to* the patient. I like to think that a patient's meal is the highlight of his day. It is my job to make sure that the patient still has as much choice as possible regarding meal choices. It can be a challenge to encourage a patient who has a therapeutic or special diet to make meal choices that are healthy and still taste good. The health unit coordinator can assist me in that challenge by communicating the diet orders promptly and accurately. The health unit coordinator can let me know when a patient and his family are available to discuss the diet the physician has ordered. Good communication between the dietitian and the health unit coordinator can help ensure that mealtime is a bright spot in the patient's stay.

REFERENCES

Hegner, B. R., Caldwell, E., & Needham, J. F. (2004). *Nursing assistant* (9th ed.). Clifton Park, NY: Thomson Delmar Learning.

Huber, H., & Spatz, A. (1998). *Homemaker/home health aide* (5th ed.). Clifton Park, NY: Thomson Delmar Learning.

CHAPTER 27

Nursing Orders

Learning Objectives

Upon completion of this chapter and review questions, the learner should be able to:

1. Describe the nursing interventions that can be provided to the patient.

2. Describe the role of the health unit coordinator in nursing interventions.

3. Define five comfort orders that the health unit coordinator documents on the Kardex.

4. Differentiate nursing orders from activity orders.

5. Explain four different types of activity orders.

6. List two objectives for palliative care.

Key Terms

activity The extent or level of body movement, function, or exercise.

afebrile Refers to body temperature within normal limits.

apical pulse A pulse taken over the chest in the area of the apex of the heart.

axillary Refers to under the arm.

blood pressure The measure of the pressure of the blood against the walls of the blood vessels.

diastolic The bottom value in the blood pressure reading.

febrile Refers to elevated body temperature, not within normal range.

Kardex A communication tool used by health unit coordinators to communicate nursing orders to the nursing staff.

neurological vital signs Signs used to assess the nervous system; include checking the eye pupils for reaction to light and checking the level of consciousness by asking the patient questions relating to time, place, and events.

nursing care The attention and treatment provided to the client by the clinical staff. The physician can order the care, or the nursing staff can provide the care on the basis of nursing judgment.

nursing care orders Orders written by the nurse with specific instructions for implementing the nursing care plan.

nursing judgment The thought process used by the nursing staff to provide care to the patient.

palliative care Comfort care measures given to patients near the end of life. All diagnostic testing is stopped, and most treatments are discontinued. The main objective of the nursing staff is to ensure the patient's comfort.

pulse The rate at which the heart is beating.

radial artery The artery located in the wrist.

respirations The rate at which breathing occurs.

systolic The top value in the blood pressure reading.

tympanically Refers to the ear.

vital signs The measurement of the body's temperature, blood pressure, pulse, and respirations.

Abbreviations

Amb Ambulatory

BP Blood Pressure

BRP Bathroom Privileges

BSC Bedside Commode

C Celsius

CBR Complete Bed Rest

D/c Discontinue

F Fahrenheit

HOB Head of Bed

HR Hours

I & O Intake and Output

I/O Intake and Output

IV Intravenous

LOC Level of Consciousness

MIN Minutes

NG Nasogastric

NVS Neurological Vital Signs

OOB Out of Bed

P Pulse

PRN As necessary

Q Every

R Respirations

RR Respiratory Rate

SOB Shortness of Breath

SSE Soapsuds Enema

Temp Temperature

tol Tolerated

TPR Temperature, Pulse, Respirations

TWE Tap Water Enema

UO Urinary Output

VS Vital Signs

NURSING CARE

Patients are admitted to a health care facility under the specific care of an admitting physician. The nursing care team provides the majority of the hands-on patient care. **Nursing care** is defined as the care provided to patients by the nursing staff. Either the physician can order the care, or the nursing staff can provide the care on the basis of nursing judgment. **Nursing judgment** is the thought process used by the nursing staff to provide care to the patient. Nurses have been educated to assess the patient for potential health issues that can surface because of their current health status. After assessing the patient, the nursing staff often initiates **nursing care orders**, which are orders written by the nurse with specific instructions for implementing the nursing care plan. To provide patients with quality nursing care for their specific health care diagnosis, a plan of care is written by the nursing care team. This plan of care may include the current diagnosis and conditions other than the reason for the hospitalization or an ongoing health issue such as diabetes or congestive heart failure. The health unit coordinator requests the services to be provided or orders the supplies and equipment required. The services provided may be unique to the health care facility. The nursing care orders are communicated to the nursing staff verbally and are documented on the correct form.

The form used in many health care facilities is called a **Kardex**. An example of a Kardex is shown in Figure 27-1. The Kardex can be in paper or electronic format. Another form that may be used is called a nursing care plan. Figure 27-2 is an example of a nursing care plan.

VITAL SIGNS

Vital signs (VS) are the signs that members of the patient care team monitor and measure to diagnose and monitor a patient's health condition. They are requested by physicians, may be part of the health care system standard procedures, and are often done by the patient care team as an assessment of the patient. It is important that they be recorded as soon as possible after being taken. **Vital signs** include the measurement of the patient's temperature, pulse, respirations (TPR), and blood pressure. At times, neurological vital signs are also ordered.

TEMPERATURE

Temperature (temp) is the internal degree of heat of the body. The normal body temperature for each individual varies. This can be measured on the Fahrenheit (F) or Celsius (C) scale. The normal temperature average is 98.6 degrees Fahrenheit, or 37 degrees Celsius. Temperature can be measured in the mouth (oral), by the ear (**tympanic**), or the rectum (rectal), or under the arm (**axillary**). The length of time that is required for an accurate reading depends on the method used to measure the temperature as well as the device used. The temperature device can be an electronic device or a manual thermometer. The health unit coordinator may be required to chart on the graphic sheet for each patient the results and the type of thermometer used. The health care provider may refer to the patient temperature as being **afebrile** (temperature not elevated, within normal range) or **febrile** (temperature elevated). Temperature results are graphed on a temperature graphic chart (Figure 27-3).

An order for a routine temperature would be communicated to the nursing staff. The nursing staff would follow the health system's routine procedure for checking and recording a patient's temperature. The health unit coordinator would document the temeprature on a Kardex or on the nursing care plan.

MARQUETTE GENERAL HOSPITAL —Patient Information Kardex

Diagnosis:	Patient Label	Room #

Code Status:	OR/Procedure Date:

Daily Weights	

Activity:	Isolation:

	Other:

Fluid Restriction:
Diet:

Contrast Allergy: ☐ YES ☐ NO	Social Security #:

Date	To Be Done	Test/Labs	Date	To Be Done	Test/Labs

Daily Labs:

Contact Person:
Place Staying:
Phone #:

D:/IC/PTinfoKARDEX.PM6.5P   Rev. 12/01

Item #: 760428

Figure 27-1 • *Kardexes are used by the patient care staff to review current patient information. (Courtesy of Marquette General Health System, Marquette, MI)*

MARQUETTE GENERAL HOSPITAL
CLINICAL PATHWAY —
Generic Surgical

PATIENT LABEL

Date of Admission:	LOS:	Date:	Surgical Procedures
Diagnosis:			Pertinent PMH:
			D/C Disposition:

Date Ordered:	REFERRALS / CONSULTS	Date Ordered:	REFERRALS / CONSULTS

PATIENT PROBLEM LIST	Discipline	Date	Initials	D/C'd	Initials
☐ Pain					
☐ Activity intolerance					
☐ Alteration in nutrition					
☐ Knowledge deficit					
☐ Financial concerns					
☐ Discharge needs					

	Date/Init.	If Outcome not met document in plan	Expected Date	Met	Revised	Date Goal Met
INDIVIDUAL OUTCOMES				Y N		
				Y N		
				Y N		
				Y N		
				Y N		
INTERMEDIATE OUTCOMES		1. Tolerating activity progression		Y N		
		2. Pain control acceptable to patient		Y N		
		3. Surgery specific education initiated by POD #1		Y N		
				Y N		
				Y N		
DISCHARGE OUTCOMES		1. Pain managed with rest and P.O. meds.		Y N		
		2. Tolerating diet as ordered.		Y N		
		3. No signs/symptoms of infection.		Y N		
		4. Pt./family verbalize understanding of self-care.		Y N		
		5. Independent with ADL's or home help or to rehab or SNF		Y N		

C:/PROJECTS/Surgical/PWGenericSurgical8-1-2x11.pmd 6/01, Rev. 1/22/04

Figure 27-2 • *Nursing care plans are used to provide the nursing care team with patient information.* *(Courtesy of Marquette General Health System, Marquette, MI) (continues)*

**MARQUETTE GENERAL HOSPITAL
PATIENT OUTCOMES CONTINUED**

PATIENT LABEL

	Date/Init.	If outcome not met document in plan	Expected Date	Met		Revised	Date Goal Met
OUTCOMES				Y	N		
				Y	N		
				Y	N		
				Y	N		
				Y	N		
				Y	N		
				Y	N		
OUTCOMES				Y	N		
				Y	N		
				Y	N		
				Y	N		
				Y	N		
				Y	N		
				Y	N		
OUTCOMES				Y	N		
				Y	N		
				Y	N		
				Y	N		
				Y	N		
				Y	N		
				Y	N		
OUTCOMES				Y	N		
				Y	N		
				Y	N		
				Y	N		
				Y	N		

Figure 27-2 • *(continued)*

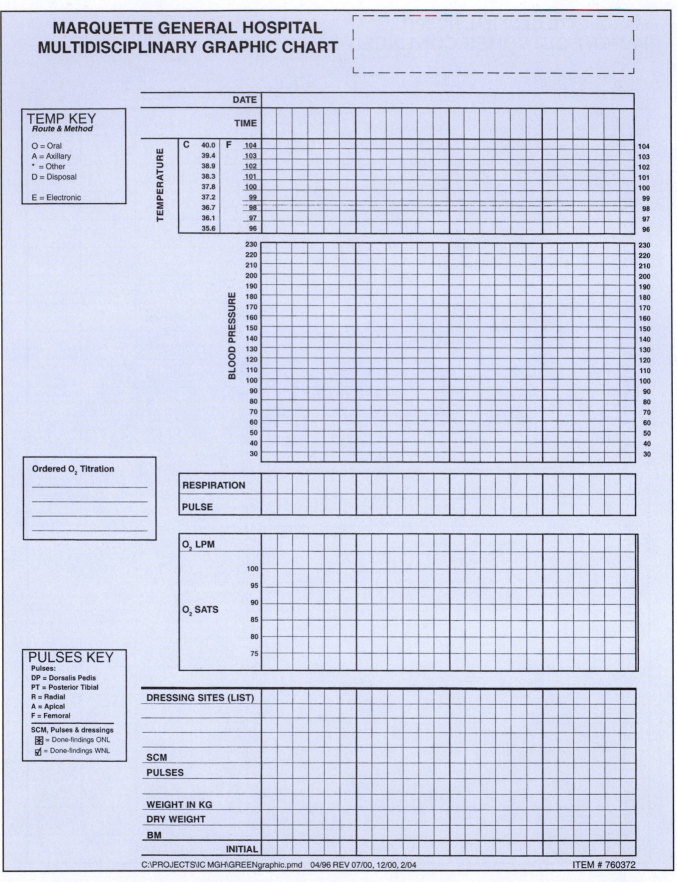

Figure 27-3 • *Temperature results are graphed on the graphic sheet. (Courtesy of Marquette General Health System, Marquette, MI)*

BLOOD PRESSURE

Blood pressure (BP) is the measure of the pressure of the blood against the walls of the blood vessels. The blood pressure measurement has two numbers, usually reported as one number over another number such as 130 over 80. It is written like a fraction, with the first number over the second number, such as 130/80. The top number is the **systolic value**, and the bottom number is the **diastolic value**. Blood pressure readings can vary on a patient throughout the day. The health unit coordinator may be required to graph the patient blood pressure readings on the chart form. The physician may call requesting the blood pressure reading for the patient. The health unit coordinator needs to know how to provide this information to the physician and must be able to locate the information in the patient record.

A physician's order for blood pressure measurements might say, "Check BP in the Right and Left arm Q 30 min. then Q 4 hrs." This order would be communicated to the nursing staff to check the blood pressure in both the left and right arm every 30 minutes four times and then every four hours until the order is changed.

A physician may order that the patient's orthostatic blood pressure reading be taken and recorded. This requires the blood pressure to be taken on the patient in a lying, sitting, and standing position. It is important for the health unit coordinator to clearly communicate this physician order to the patient care staff, because this is not a routine blood pressure procedure.

PULSE

Pulse (P) is the rate at which the heart is beating. The pulse can be located at different places in the body. It is important to record on the patient's record the location from which the pulse reading was taken so that comparisons can be made correctly. Usually, the health care provider takes the pulse reading from the **radial artery**. This site is located on the wrist area. **Apical pulses** are pulses taken over the chest in the area of the apex of the heart using a device called a stethoscope. Pulses may also be taken at the femoral artery or the carotid artery, and can be taken with the fingers, a stethoscope, or an electronic device automatically programmed. Pulse rate is usually recorded and reported as a number of beats per minute.

A nursing order may indicate that the pulse should be taken at two different sites and recorded as such. For example: "Check apical and radial pulse Q4 hours for 24 hours." This order would be communicated to the nursing staff to check the apical and radial pulse every 4 hours for the next 24 hours. A total of 12 values will be provided and charted on a graphic sheet to complete this order (Figure 27-4).

RESPIRATIONS

Respirations (R) are the rate at which breathing occurs. The respiratory rate (RR) is usually recorded and reported as a number of breaths per minute. Respirations are an observed rate. The normal rate varies by the age of the patient and can be decreased by certain medications. Adults' average respiration is 16 breaths a minute, and infants' is 20 breaths a minute.

If the patient is having an episode of SOB, shortness of breath, this would be observed when taking the respiration count. The patient may alert the care provider that he or she is short of breath, at which point the health unit coordinator may be requested to

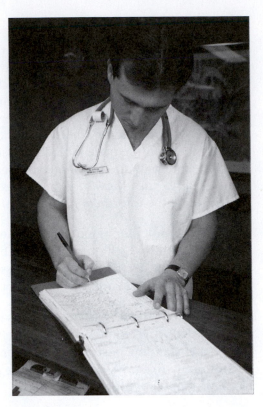

Figure 27-4 • *Graphing of blood pressure and pulse rates is completed after each reading is taken.*

notify the physician. The respirations are charted in the patient's chart and can be requested by the physician at set intervals. For example, "Check respirations Q 8 hours for 3 days and record. If ↑ 32 per minute call me." This order would be communicated to the patient care provider and charted on a graphic sheet (Figure 27-5). If the respirations were greater than 32 breaths per minute, the health unit coordinator would be asked to call the health care professional who wrote the order.

NEUROLOGICAL VITAL SIGNS

Neurological vital signs (NVS) include checking and recording observations of the patient's nervous system. These signs include checking the eye pupils for reaction to light and checking the level of consciousness (LOC) by asking the patient questions relating to time, place, and events. These vital signs may be ordered in addition to vital signs or alone.

ACTIVITY

Activity is the extent or level of body movement, function, or exercise the patient is to participate in during hospitalization. Activity orders change during the patient stay depending on the health condition of the patient. It is important to communicate the activity orders to the nursing care team, because activity is part of the patient care plan. Table 27-1 lists activities that are frequently ordered for patients.

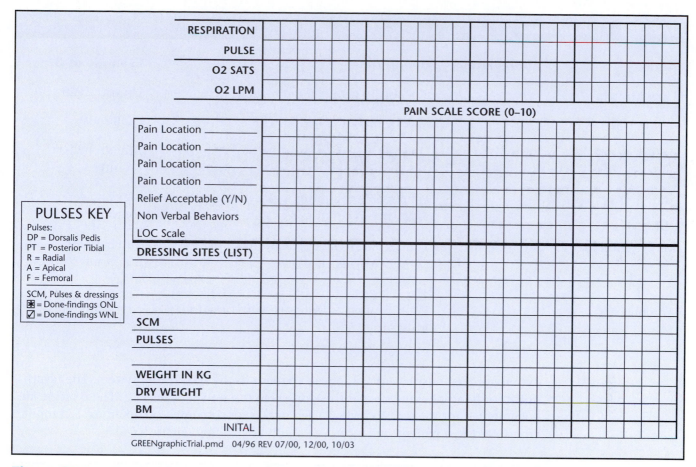

Figure 27-5 • *The health unit coordinator graphs respirations on the graphic sheet in the time frame requested. (Courtesy of Marquette General Health System, Marquette, MI)*

TABLE 27-1 Activities Often Ordered

Activity	Abbreviation	Definition	Example of Order
Complete bed rest	CBR	Must stay in bed at all times	CBR today
Complete bed rest with bathroom privileges	CBR c̄ BRPs	Must stay in bed at all times except able to get up to use the bathroom	CBR with BRPs for 3 days
Dangle		Able to put legs over the side of the bed to "dangle"	Dangle tonight for 10 minutes
Bedside commode only	BSC	May use the bedside commode only, otherwise must stay in bed	BSC only
Up ad lib		Up at will, no restrictions	Up ad lib
Activity as tolerated	Up as tol	Up as able to be, as tolerated without problems	Up as tol

(continues)

TABLE 1-1 *continued*

Activity	Abbreviation	Definition	Example of Order
Up with help		Not able to get up alone without help	Up with help only
Out of bed	OOB	May be up out of bed	OOB today
Ambulatory	Amb	Up with no restrictions	Amb in halls Q shift
May shower		Patient able to shower with or without assistance as condition warrants	May shower tomorrow
May take tub bath		Patient able to take tub bath with or without assistance	Tub bath for 20 minutes twice a day
Ambulate		Walk as often as requested with or without assistance	Ambulate prn

Activity orders must be written for each patient in the health care system. The health unit coordinator communicates these orders to the nursing care staff. These orders are documented for the staff to review. They may be documented on a Kardex, a computerized Kardex, a patient care record, or a unit activity log (Figure 27-6).

Unit Activity Log
ORTHO UNIT

DATE: 5/9
SHIFT: EVENINGS

Room Number	Transport	Room Number	Transport
804D	w/c	814D	empty
805D	cart	815D	w/c
806D	w/c	816D	empty
808D	BED	817D	cart
809D	w/c	818D	BED
810D	cart	819D	cart
811D	cart	820D	w/c
812D	BED	821D	empty
813D	w/c	822D	w/c

Total w/c = 7
Total carts = 5
Total BEDS = 3

Figure 27-6 • *The unit activity log states the mode of activity for each patient.*

POSITIONING

Physicians write patient positioning orders when a position is required for healing. The patient care staff writes positioning orders for patient comfort. All positioning orders need to be communicated to the nursing care staff by the health unit coordinator. Table 27-2 lists some common positioning orders.

OBSERVATION

The nursing care staff assesses and observes the patient frequently during hospitalization. Every time the staff enters the patient room, the patient is observed. The physician may order that the nursing staff perform tasks more often than they are usually done on normal rounds. Normal rounds are defined by each health care facility. The nursing staff documents these rounds and their observations on the patient care record. The health unit coordinator needs to be familiar with the documentation process to access requested information quickly. The nursing care staff observes the patient for signs and symptoms of normal behavior; anything that is not normal is reported to the physician. A patient who is confused and must be restrained for safety

TABLE 27-2   Common Positioning Orders

Position	Abbreviation	Definition
Elevate head of bed 45 degrees	↑ HOB 45°	Put the head of the bed up 45 degrees to facilitate the patient's ability to breathe
Elevate right leg on two pillows	↑ R leg on 2 pillows	Put two pillows under the patient's right leg to elevate it off the bed. Often this is used to reduce pressure on the leg.
Semi-Fowler's position		This position is accomplished by elevating the head of the bed 30 degrees and slightly elevating the knees.
Fowler's position		This position is accomplished by elevating the head of the bed 45 degrees and slightly elevating the knees.
Log roll		This is a roll used when turning the patient from side to side. The body is kept straight, like a log, with a pillow placed between the knees to roll the patient.
Turn every 3 hours	Turn Q3 hr	Turning can be ordered for a specific time frame. Usually, turning is ordered so that the patient changes position and skin breakdown is prevented.

is observed more often than normal, and the observations are recorded in the patient record. Health care facilities have programs that alert all employees of patients who are at risk to fall and need to be closely observed and assisted so that they do not have an accident. Some facilities have a form alerting staff to a patient's risk for falls and other risks (Figure 27-7).

When a patient is admitted to the nursing unit, a data base is completed. During this process, the health care team evaluates the patient for risk to fall. If the patient meets the criteria to be at risk to fall, a colored armband is placed on the patient. The patient chart is identified with a colored dot, and one is placed on the outer side of the patient's room door. All employees are educated regarding the meaning of a colored armband or dot. These practices reduce the number of patient falls in health care facilities.

INTAKE AND OUTPUT

Often patients need to be encouraged to take fluids during hospitalization. It is important to record the amount of fluids taken in as well as the patient output. This record is called intake and output (I & O or I/O). The record used to record this information is the I & O form (Figure 27-8). The physician may order that I & O be recorded for a set amount of time, or the nurse may order I & O. The nurse may be concerned that the patient is not voiding in amounts equal to the fluids being taken in. If the patient is unable to take in nutrition orally, an alternative way of providing nutrition may be ordered. The method used most frequently for short-term nutrition is to provide fluids intravenously (IV). Physicians who are concerned about a patient's output may write an order to be called if the urinary output (UO) is less than a specific amount in a specific time frame. For example, "Call Dr. Brown if the UO is <250cc in 2 hours."

SUPPORT SERVICES

Support services provided by outside agencies are also coordinated by the nursing care staff. These support services can be described as any service that offers support to the patient and family. Care providers are aware of support services both within the health care system and within the community. Businesses, churches, social organizations, and neighbors provide these services. Support services are requested by the health care team, the family, or the patient. The health unit coordinator is responsible for contacting these support service providers. The support services may vary from community to community. One community may have a strong system of support groups for patients with Parkinson's disease and their family members, and another community may have a strong cancer support group. The health unit coordinator will be requested to provide the contact information either directly to the patient or to the nursing staff, who will provide the information to the patient. In some health care systems, patients with selected diagnoses are routinely referred to support services. For example, if a patient is diagnosed with breast cancer, the health unit coordinator would notify the American Cancer Society, provided the patient has given permission.

These support systems are in place throughout communities. An awareness of these groups and how and when to contact the groups is a responsibility of the health unit coordinator. Other support services include clergy support, home health care, and other organizations that offer various services or educational support in the community.

MARQUETTE GENERAL HEALTH SYSTEM
PATIENT CARE RECORD

PATIENT LABEL

RISK FOR FALLS	N	D	E
☐ **Initiate Spot the Dot if ≥ 3 shaded/ History of Previous Falls/Lower Extremity Amputee**	O	O	O
24-48 hours post-op	O	O	O
> 70<5 years of age or behavior outside of developmental milestones	O	O	O
Postural Hypotension	O	O	O
Nocturia	O	O	O
Sensory Deficit, Hearing or Speech Impaired	O	O	O
Uses ambulatory aids / unsteady gait / weakness	O	O	O
Meds (hypnotics, psychotropics, diuretics, laxatives, sedatives, narcotics, bowel prep, antihypertensives)	O	O	O
Impaired memory / judgment / confusion / altered mentality	O	O	O
"Spot the Dot" Maintained	O	O	O
RISK FOR IMPAIRED SKIN INTEGRITY	N	D	E
☐ **Initiate skin care measures and/or ET referral if: > 2 SHADED**	O	O	O
Cannot Verbalize Discomfort	O	O	O
Poor Nutrition	O	O	O
Diabetic	O	O	O
Skin Always Moist/Incontinence	O	O	O
Complete Bed Rest	O	O	O
Mobility Severely Limited	O	O	O
↑ Friction/Red Skin	O	O	O
Ulcers	O	O	O
SKIN CARE MEASURES	N	D	E
Position changes & avoid prone position & suspend heels off mattress	O	O	O
Keep Pt. off pressure points	O	O	O
Specialty mattress if needed	O	O	O
Orthotics/positioning device	O	O	O
ET REFERRAL	O	O	O
SAFETY INTERVENTIONS	N	D	E
Call light within reach	O	O	O
Side rails ↑	O	O	O
Bed low / locked	O	O	O
Crib Bubble / Bed Check	O	O	O
NUTRITION	N	D	E
NPO	O	O	O
Fluids: Controlled sips / chips / force / limit	O	O	O
Serve Meals – Routine Setup	O	O	O
Assist Feed / Breast Feed	O	O	O
Total Feed / Infant/Bottle	O	O	O
• Tube Feed	O	O	O
• Dysphagia	O	O	O
PLAN OF CARE REVIEWED WITH PATIENT	O	O	O
ISOLATION PROCEDURES MAINTAINED	O	O	O

Time	24	01	02	03	04	05	06	07	08	09	10	11	12	13	14	15	16	17	18	19	20	21	22	23
C & DB																								
Incentive Spirometry																								
Position Changes (L R S P)																								
Rounds																								
Initials																								

Awake = A   S = Sleeping   R = Resting   L = Left   R = Right   S = Supine   P = Prone

D:\MGH IC\PCR&I&O.pmd   Rev. 11/30/00, 1/04

Item # 760495

Figure 27-7 • *Some facilities use a patient care record to alert staff to a patient's risk for falls and other risks. (Courtesy of Marquette General Health System, Marquette, MI)*

MARQUETTE GENERAL HEALTH SYSTEM | *I & O RECORD*

EQUIPMENT BEING UTILIZED BY PATIENT

IVAC Controller		Bili Light	
IVAC Pump		Auto Syringe	
Dinamap BP Monitor		Mini-Med	
Food Pump		Isolation Cart	
Aquamatic Heat Pad		Hypothermia Blanket	
Egg Crate Mattress		Bear Hugger	
PCA		Sequential Teds	
IABP		Camino	
Specialty Bed		Blood Warmer	
Bumper Pads		Continuous Sx	
Apnea Monitor		Intermittent Sx	
Floatation Pad			

PATIENT LABEL

DATE: _____

DIET		APPETITE	B	L	D
		G-ATE 75-100%			
NOURISHMENTS		F-ATE 50-75%			
		•P-UNDER 50%			

	Intake ORAL/NG	TUBE FDS	IV.	1	2	3	4	5	6	7	8	9	PRESSURE FLUSH LINE	Output URINE	N/G	CT		
Credit																		
Hour 2300																	po/FT_____	
2400																	IV_____	
0100																	8°I_____	
0200																	U_____	
0300																	O_____	
0400																		
0500																	8°O_____	
0600																		
8° TOTAL																		
Credit																		
Hour 0700																	po/FT_____	
0800																	IV_____	
0900																	8°I_____	
1000																	U_____	
1100																	O_____	
1200																		
1300																	8°O_____	
1400																		
8° TOTAL																		
Credit																		
Hour 1500																	po/FT_____	
1600																	IV_____	
1700																	8°I_____	
1800																	U_____	
1900																	O_____	
2000																		
2100																	8°O_____	
2200																		
8° TOTAL																		

24° TOTAL PO/TF _____ IV _____ 24° INTAKE _____ URINE _____ OTHER _____ 24° OUTPUT _____

Cumulative Total Since Surgery: _____

Figure 27-8 • *The I & O form is used to document what a patient takes in and puts out. (Courtesy of Marquette General Health System, Marquette, MI)*

COMFORT

It is important to provide comfort to the patient during hospitalization. Comfort is provided in a variety of ways. The attending or consulting physician may order the comfort measures. The members of the patient care team may request comfort measures, as may members of the nursing care staff. Depending on the measures requested, there may or may not need to be a written order by the physician. The nursing care team members usually provide the majority of patient comfort measures. One such comfort measure may be to provide the patient with a back rub each evening.

BOWEL ELIMINATION ORDERS

During hospitalization, the bowel elimination patterns of the patients are often altered. They may be altered because of the patient's condition, medications, lack of activity, nutritional intake, or required preps for ordered exams or procedures. If the patient requires an enema, the nursing staff would give this treatment.

Enemas are given to patients to relieve gas (flatus), to remove stool due to constipation, or as a preparation for surgery or an exam. The most common types of enemas are:

Tap water enema (TWE)

Soapsuds enema (SSE)

Oil retention enema

Fleets enema

CATHERTIZATION ORDERS

Urinary retention (inability to pass urine) or collection of a urine specimen may require that a urinary catheter be placed to drain the urine from the bladder. The catheter may be inserted, the urine drained, and the catheter removed; or the catheter may be left in the bladder until the physician orders that it be removed. The equipment required for this treatment is packaged together and will be disposed of after the patient has had the catheter inserted. The health unit coordinator needs to be familiar with the name of the equipment and where the equipment is located so that it can be found when requested. There are many sizes and kinds of catheters that may be requested. Each health care facility has standard sizes in stock.

INTRAVENOUS THERAPY ORDERS

Intravenous therapy (IV) is administered by the clinical patient care provider. The therapy is used to provide the patient with nutrition, blood products, fluids, and medications. The intravenous therapy may be flowing continuously or intermittently. It may flow through a peripheral line or through a central line. The type of IV line used to supply the solution to the patient is selected on the basis of the length of time the line will be used as well as the solution that the patient will have infusing. IV orders are discussed in detail in Chapter 28.

SUCTION ORDERS

At times, patients are unable to clear the secretions in their throat and must be assisted with suctioning. The inability to clear the throat may be due to an ineffective cough, a decreased level of consciousness, thick secretions, or anesthesia administered for surgery. Suctioning is done through the nose or the mouth. The suctioning device is connected to a wall-mounted suction machine or a portable suction machine. The suctioning may be continuous or intermittent.

Another type of suctioning is the NG (nasogastric) tube. This may be inserted if the patient needs to have the stomach emptied. Sometimes, the patient's stomach needs to be emptied continually for several days. If this is the case, the patient will have the NG tube connected to a suction machine that will keep the stomach empty. The order may read, "Insert NG tube. Connect to suction continuously." The health unit coordinator would document this order on the form used to communicate orders to the nursing staff and order a suction machine for the patient from the area that houses these machines.

Another example may read, "Insert NG tube and send contents to the lab for analysis." The health unit coordinator would alert the nurse of this request, document the request, and prepare the lab request for the gastric contents when the nurse alerts the health unit coordinator that the specimen is ready to be sent to the laboratory.

HEAT AND COLD THERAPY ORDERS

Patients may require heat and cold treatments as part of their therapy during hospitalization. The physical therapy department or the nursing staff, depending on the practice of the health care facility, may provide these treatments. Both heat and cold treatments may be provided for comfort. It is important that the health unit coordinator be familiar with the practices at the facility and know whom to alert regarding these requests. If the therapy is to be provided by the physical therapy department, the health unit coordinator sends the order to the department. If the treatment is to be provided by the nursing staff, the health unit coordinator documents the order for nursing, usually on the Kardex or patient care plan. Table 27-3 provides some examples of these treatments.

THE PATIENT BED

If the patient is restricted to bed, the nursing staff will often need to provide some of the equipment listed in Table 27-4 for comfort. The patient, the patient's family, or the patient care team may request this equipment. This equipment may be equipment that the patient takes home upon discharge or uses only while in the hospital.

PALLIATIVE CARE

Palliative care may also be referred to as comfort care orders. Palliative care is a multidisciplinary approach to providing care for patients near the end of life. This care may include providing pain relief medications and nutritional supplements, while at the same time discontinuing all diagnostic tests and treatments. Spiritual assistance is offered. Nursing staff are available only to supply comfort care, and usually no vital signs or other assessment or observation orders are carried out.

TABLE 27-3   Heat and Cold Therapy Orders

Treatment	Abbreviation	Order
Dry heat to an area using an electronic heating device	K-pad	K-pad to knee three times per day for 15 minutes
Warm wet compress	H. comp	H. comp to R wrist for 10 min twice a day
Soaking in a warm solution	H_2O soak	H_2O soak to L foot for 20 min four times per day
Cold compress	Ice pack	Ice pack to L elbow 20 min four times a day prn
Cooling blanket	Cool blanket	Cooling blanket if temp over 101, d/c when temp 99

TABLE 27-4   Comfort Equipment

Item	Reason for Use
Air bed	A bed that allows for air flow even though the patient does not move. Decreases the breakdown of skin.
Foot cradle	Keeps the bedclothes off the feet and legs.
Overhead trapeze	Allows the patient to move in the bed by lifting, using the arms on the device overhead.
Pressure mattress	Reduces skin breakdown (called alternating pressure mattress or Gaymar mattress).
Sheepskin	Adds a barrier between the bedclothes and the patient. Reduces skin breakdown.

TRANSCRIPTION STEPS

Table 27-5 lists the steps that should be taken when transcribing nursing orders.

TABLE 27-5 Transcription Steps for Nursing Orders

Transcription Step	Key Points
1. Read the entire order set thoroughly.	Careful reading of the orders allows the health unit coordinator to review, prioritize, and check for incomplete or illegible orders.
2. Prioritize orders.	Determine the urgency of the orders in all the charts needing transcription. Decide what orders in the order set need to be transcribed first.
3. If medications are included in the order set, send the order carbon or a copy to the pharmacy.	The pharmacy requires a copy of a signed order.
4. Communicate the order to the individual or department that will be performing the order.	The health unit coordinator may schedule appointments, notify ancillary departments of needs, order equipment necessary to perform the order, and contact the nursing personnel responsible for the patient.
5. Record the orders on the patient Kardex or care plan.	Most health care facilities have a form used to keep track of current orders and the plan of care for a patient.
6. Record medication orders on the medication administration record (MAR).	Most health care facilities automatically generate medication administration records every 24 hours based on orders entered into a computer. Orders that are received after the record has been generated may require that the order be added or handwritten on the MAR. Some facilities document on the medication records items from the pharmacy such as enemas.
7. Check off each order in the set as completed.	Placing a check mark by each order as it is transcribed can help the health unit coordinator track orders even when interrupted.
8. Re-read and check all work for accuracy.	Because of multiple requests received by the health unit coordinator, re-reading and checking work is a necessity.
9. Sign off the order with name, title, date, and time.	The health unit coordinator is accountable for the orders transcribed.

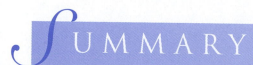

SUMMARY

Patients are provided with the majority of their care during hospitalization on the patient care unit. It is important that the patient be provided with this care by the nursing staff with as much comfort as possible. With this in mind, the nursing care staff strive to provide the patient with comfort based on the physician's requests and the patient's requests. It is very important that the requests be processed as soon as possible to provide the care as comfortably as possible. The health unit coordinator, by promptly communicating these requests to the correct staff members, is a pivotal staff member in having patient comfort needs correctly attended.

REVIEW QUESTIONS

Match the term in the left column to the abbreviation in the right column.

1. Pulse	a. VS
2. Tap water enema	b. CBR
3. Temperature	c. Amb
4. Bed rest	d. Temp
5. Complete bed rest	e. BR
6. Soapsuds enema	f. HOB
7. Head of bed	g. TWE
8. Celsius	h. C
9. Ambulatory	i. P
10. Vital signs	j. SSE

TRANSCRIPTION PRACTICE

Go to the CD-ROM for transcription exercises that support the content in this chapter.

NAHUC CERTIFICATION EXAM

CONTENT AREAS

I. A. 2   Interpret medical symbols, abbreviations, and terminology

I. A. 6   Enter orders on a Kardex

I. A. 14   Process nursing treatment orders

I. B. 1   Notify staff of new orders

III. B. 4   Enter orders via computers

THROUGH THE EYES

OF A HEALTH CARE PROFESSIONAL

The nursing staff share their thoughts.

Health unit coordinators are the eyes and ears of the workstation. They read the orders of the physicians, hear the conversations at the workstations, and provide the needed requests and information to the staff providing the hands-on care to the patients. They often greet the patient's family members, receiving not only the questions but also the concerns and requests of the family members for their loved ones. The health unit coordinators truly are the ones who direct the requests to the patient care providers.

REFERENCES

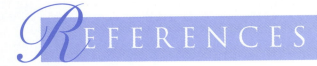

Smith, S. (2004). *Clinical nursing skills* (6th ed.). Upper Saddle River, NJ: Prentice Hall.

Wilkinson, J. M. (1996). *Nursing process: A critical thinking approach* (2nd ed.). Menlo Park, CA: Addison-Wesley Nursing.

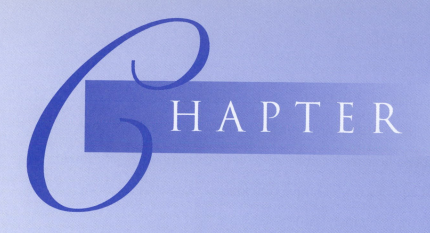
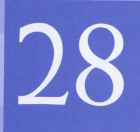

CHAPTER 28

Medication and Intravenous Therapy Orders

Learning Objectives

Upon completion of this chapter and review questions, the learner should be able to:

1. Define vocabulary and abbreviations related to medications and intravenous therapy (IV).

2. Explain the role of the pharmacy and pharmacist in the health care setting.

3. List and describe the components of a medication order.

4. Explain chemical, generic, and trade medication names.

5. List the common forms of medications.

6. Name two weight and measure systems used in medication orders and identify the symbols used in each.

7. List routes by which medications are administered.

8. List and describe the parenteral routes of administration.

9. Explain the use of an intermittent IV line and list two other names given to this device.

10. Demonstrate knowledge of military time.

11. List the standard medication times.

12. Calculate start and stop times for medications.

13. List the classifications of medications.

14. Explain how medications are dispensed, transported, and stored.

15. List and describe the three components of an IV order.

16. List the commonly used IV solutions.

17. Explain the use of supplemental forms related to medication and IV orders.

18. Demonstrate knowledge of drug resource materials.

19. Interpret and transcribe medication and IV orders.

Key Terms

apothecary   An old European term given to a druggist, meaning one who prepares or sells drugs.

chemical name   The chemical and molecular formula of a drug.

generic name   The common name given to the drug by the developer.

metric   A modern measurement system based on the meter, kilogram, and decimal system.

sliding scale   The medication dose is written to be dependent on a laboratory result.

trade or brand name   The name given to the drug by the manufacturer or seller.

Abbreviations

ac   Before Meals

ASA   Aspirin

Aer   Aerosol

Bid   Twice a Day

cap   Capsule

cc   Cubic Centimeter

chew   Chewable

CNS   Central Nervous System

Conc   Concentrate

CSA Controlled Substance Act

CVC Central Venous Catheter

D5 Dextrose 5%

D5W Dextrose 5% Water

DEA Drug Enforcement Administration

dr Delayed Release

dr Dram

Drsg Dressing

effrv Effervescent

elcon Electronically Controlled

er Extended Release

g Gram

gm Gram

gr Grain

gran Granule

gtt Drop

h Hour

H Hypodermic

HA Hyperalimentation

Hep loc Heparin lock

hr Hours

hs Hour of sleep, or bedtime

Hyperal Hyperalimentation

ID Intradermal

IM Intramuscular

imp Implant

inj Injection

INT Intermittent IV needle

IV Intravenous

IVP Intravenous push

IVPB Intravenous piggyback

L Liter

l Liter

liq Liquid

loz Lozenge

LR Lactated Ringer's

MAR Medication Administration Record

mcg Microgram

mEq Milliequivalent

met Metered

mg Milligram

ml, **mL** Milliliter

MOM Milk of Magnesia

NaCl Sodium Chloride (Saline)

NF *National Formulary*

NS Normal Saline

NSAID Nonsteroidal Anti-inflammatory Drug

oz Ounce

pc After Meals

PCA Patient-controlled analgesia

PDR *Physician's Desk Reference*

PICC Peripherpherally Inserted Central Catheter

po oral, or by mouth

prn As Necessary

pwd Powder

q day Every Day

qid Four Times a Day

RL Ringer's Lactated

sc Subcutaneous

sol Solution

sq Subcutaneous

subl sublingual

subling sublingual

subq subcutaneous

supp Suppository

susp Suspension

tab Tablet

tid Three Times a Day

TPN Total Parenteral Nutrition

USP *United States Pharmacopeia*

VAD Vascular Access Device

PHARMACY DEPARTMENT

In Chapter 6, the pharmacy department was defined. Patients who are seeking care from a health care facility may be offered some type of medication. Medication orders are often included as part of the physician order set written for the patient. The responsibilities of health unit coordinators will vary from facility to facility. The health unit coordinator needs to be able to recognize orders that need to be communicated to the pharmacy department. Knowledge of the components of medication orders will make recognizing medication orders and communicating with the pharmacy department easier.

COMPONENTS OF A MEDICATION ORDER

A physician will write an order for medications. As must all orders, medication orders must be carefully transcribed. Because of the many problems medication errors can cause, special precautions and practices should be followed. There is a structure to medication orders that helps in transcribing. The structure is that medication orders have specific identifiable components, or parts. Medication orders can be divided into four parts: name, dose, route, and frequency.

MEDICATION NAME

The name component of the medication order answers the question "What?" This part of the order lists what drug the physician wants to give to the patient.

Every medication can be referred to by three different names:

Chemical name. The chemical and molecular formula of the drug. The chemical name could also be described as the recipe of the drug.

Generic name. The common name given to the drug by the developer. Generally, the generic name is not capitalized.

Trade, or brand, name. The name given to the drug by the manufacturer or seller. Generally, the brand name is capitalized. A drug may have more than one trade or brand name.

Table 28-1 gives the three names for two familiar drugs.

DRUG FORMS

In addition to the name, the physician's order may also include the way the drug is prepared, such as syrup, tablet, or capsule. The form or way the drug is prepared is not always included in medication orders. Knowing the different forms in which medications are prepared is helpful when transcribing the order. The drug form is often a clue as to the means of administering the drug (Table 28-2).

MEDICATION DOSE

The dose component of the medication order answers the question; "how much?" The dose is the measured amount of the medication that is to be given. There are two main systems of measurement for medications, apothecary and metric.

Apothecary Doses

Apothecary is an old European term given to a druggist meaning one who prepares or sells drugs. The apothecary system of weights and measures is an older system that was formerly used to measure medications. This system of measurement is based on the ounce, which is divided into 8 drams or 480 grains. In this system of measurement, the drug is written in lower case Roman numerals following the measurement unit symbol. For example if a drug were to be measured for 15 grains, it would be written as grain (gr) xv. Apothecary symbols that are still used include:

Grain (gr)

Dram (dr)

Ounce (oz)

TABLE 28-1   Medication Names

Chemical Name	Generic Name	Brand Name
Acetylsalicylic acid	aspirin	Anacin
(+) –2- (p-isobutylphenyl)	ibuprofen	Motrin or Advil

TABLE 28-2 Drug Forms

Name	Definition	Short Name/Abbreviation
Aerosol	A product that is packaged under pressure and contains therapeutically active ingredients that are released upon activation of an appropriate valve system; it is intended for topical application to the skin as well as local application into the nose (nasal aerosols), mouth (lingual aerosols), or lungs (inhalation aerosols).	Aer
Aerosol, metered	A pressurized dosage form consisting of metered dose valves, which allow for the delivery of a uniform quantity of spray upon each activation.	Aer met
Capsule	A solid dosage form in which the drug is enclosed within either a hard or soft soluble container or "shell" made from a suitable form of gelatin.	cap
Capsule, delayed release	A solid dosage form in which the drug is enclosed within either a hard or soft soluble container made from a suitable form of gelatin, and which releases a drug (or drugs) at a time other than promptly after administration. Enteric-coated articles are delayed-release dosage forms.	cap dr
Capsule, extended release	A solid dosage form in which the drug is enclosed within either a hard or soft soluble container made from a suitable form of gelatin, and which releases a drug (or drugs) in such a manner to allow a reduction in dosing frequency as compared to that drug (or drugs) presented as a conventional dosage form.	cap er
Capsule, liquid filled	A solid dosage form in which the drug is enclosed within a soluble, gelatin shell which is plasticized by the addition of a polyol, such as sorbitol or glycerin, and is therefore of a somewhat thicker consistency than that of a hard-shell capsule; typically, the active ingredients are dissolved or suspended in a liquid vehicle.	cap liq filled
Core, extended release	An ocular system placed in the eye from which the drug diffuses through a membrane at a constant rate over a specified period.	Core er
Cream	A semisolid dosage form containing one or more drug substances dissolved or dispersed in a suitable base; more recently, the term has been restricted to products consisting of oil-in-water emulsions or aqueous microcrystalline dispersions of long-chain fatty acids or alcohols that are water washable and more cosmetically and aesthetically acceptable.	Cream
Disc	A circular platelike structure.	Disc

(continues)

TABLE 28-2 *(continued)*

Name	Definition	Short Name/Abbreviation
Douche	A liquid preparation, intended for the irrigative cleansing of the vagina, that is prepared from powders, liquid solutions, or liquid concentrates and contains one or more chemical substances dissolved in a suitable solvent or mutually miscible solvents.	Douche
Dressing	The application of various materials for protecting a wound.	Drsg
Elixir	A clear, pleasantly flavored, sweetened hydroalcoholic liquid containing dissolved medicinal agents; it is intended for oral use.	Elixir
Emulsion	A two-phase system in which one liquid is dispersed throughout another liquid in the form of small droplets.	Emulsion
Enema	A rectal preparation for therapeutic, diagnostic, or nutritive purposes.	Enema
Extract	A concentrated preparation of vegetable or animal drugs obtained by removal of the active constituents of the respective drugs with a suitable menstrua, evaporation of all or nearly all of the solvent, and adjustment of the residual masses or powders to the prescribed standards.	Extract
Film	A thin layer or coating.	Film
Gel	A semisolid system consisting of either suspensions made up of small inorganic particles or large organic molecules interpenetrated by a liquid.	Gel
Gel, jelly	A class of gels—semisolid systems that consist of suspensions made up of either small inorganic particles or large organic molecules interpenetrated by a liquid—in which the structural coherent matrix contains a high portion of liquid, usually water.	Gel, jelly
Granule	A small particle or grain.	gran
Granule, effervescent	A small particle or grain containing a medicinal agent in a dry mixture usually composed of sodium bicarbonate, citric acid, and tartaric acid which, when in contact with water, has the capability to release gas, resulting in effervescence.	gran effrv
Gum	A mucilaginous excretion from various plants.	Gum
Implant	A material containing a drug intended to be inserted securely or deeply in a living site for growth, slow release, or formation of an organic union.	Imp

(continues)

TABLE 28-2 *(continued)*

Name	Definition	Short Name/ Abbreviation
Inhalant	A special class of inhalations consisting of a drug, or combination of drugs, that by virtue of their high vapor pressure, can be carried by an air current into the nasal passage where they exert their effect; the container from which the inhalant generally is administered is known as an inhaler.	Inhalant
Injection	A sterile preparation intended for parenteral use; five distinct classes of injections exist as defined by the U.S. Pharmocopeia.	inj
Injection, solution	A liquid preparation containing one or more drug substances dissolved in a suitable solvent or a mixture of mutually miscible solvents that is suitable for injection.	inj sol
Injection, suspension	A liquid preparation, suitable for injection, which consists of solid particles dispersed throughout a liquid phase in which the particles are not soluble. It can also consist of an oil phase dispersed throughout an aqueous phase, or vice-versa.	inj susp
Insert, extended release	A specially formulated and shaped solid preparation (e.g., ring, tablet, or stick) intended to be placed in the vagina by special inserters, where the medication is released, generally for localized effects; the extended-release preparation is designed to allow a reduction in dosing frequency.	Insert er
Irrigant	A sterile solution intended to bathe or flush open wounds or body cavities; they are used topically, never parenterally.	Irrigant
Liniment	A solution or mixture of various substances in oil, alcoholic solutions of soap, or emulsions intended for external application.	Liniment
Liquid	A state of a substance that is an intermediate one entered into as matter goes from solid to gas; liquids are also intermediate in that they have neither the orderliness of a crystal nor the randomness of a gas. (Note: This term should not be used to describe solutions, only pure chemicals in their liquid state.)	liq
Lotion	The term *lotion* has been used to categorize many topical suspensions, solutions, and emulsions intended for application to the skin.	Lotion
Lozenge	A solid preparation containing one or more medicaments, usually in a flavored, sweetened base, which is intended to dissolve or disintegrate slowly in the mouth. A lollipop is a lozenge on a stick.	loz

(continues)

TABLE 28-2 *(continued)*

Name	Definition	Short Name/ Abbreviation
Oil	An unctuous, combustible substance, which is liquid, or easily liquefiable, on warming, and is soluble in ether but insoluble in water. Such substances, depending on their origin, are classified as animal, mineral, or vegetable oils.	Oil
Ointment	A semisolid preparation intended for external application to the skin or mucous membranes.	Ointment
Paste	A semisolid dosage form that contains one or more drug substances intended for topical application.	Paste
Patch	A drug delivery system that contains an adhesive backing and that permits its ingredients to diffuse from some portion of it (e.g., the backing itself, a reservoir, the adhesive, or some other component) into the body from the external site where it is applied.	Patch
Patch, extended release	A drug delivery system in the form of a patch that releases the drug in such a manner that dosing frequency is reduced compared to that drug presented as a conventional dosage form (e.g., a solution or a prompt drug-releasing, conventional solid dosage form).	Patch er
Patch, extended release, electrically controlled	A drug delivery system in the form of a patch which is controlled by an electric current that releases the drug in such a manner that dosing frequency is reduced compared to that drug presented as a conventional dosage form (e.g., a solution or a prompt drug-releasing, conventional solid dosage form).	Patch er elcon
Pill	A small, round solid dosage form containing a medicinal agent intended for oral administration.	Pill
Poultice	A soft, moist mass of meal, herbs, seed, etc., usually applied hot in cloth that consists of gruel-like consistency.	Poultice
Powder	An intimate mixture of dry, finely divided drugs and/or chemicals that may be intended for internal or external use.	Pwd
Rinse	A liquid used to cleanse by flushing.	Rinse
Salve	A thick ointment or cerate (a fat- or wax-based preparation with a consistency between an ointment and a plaster).	Salve
Shampoo	A liquid soap or detergent used to clean the hair and scalp and often used as a vehicle for dermatologic agents.	Shampoo

(continues)

TABLE 28-2 *(continued)*

Name	Definition	Short Name/ Abbreviation
Solution	A liquid preparation that contains one or more chemical substances dissolved, i.e., molecularly dispersed, in a suitable solvent or mixture of mutually miscible solvents.	sol
Solution, concentrate	A liquid preparation (i.e., a substance that flows readily in its natural state) that contains a drug dissolved in a suitable solvent or mixture of mutually miscible solvents; the drug has been strengthened by the evaporation of its nonactive parts.	Sol conc
Spray	A liquid minutely divided as by a jet of air or steam.	Spray
Stick	A dosage form prepared in a relatively long and slender often cylindrical form.	Stick
Suppository	A solid body of various weights and shapes, adapted for introduction into the rectal, vaginal, or urethral orifice of the human body; they usually melt, soften, or dissolve at body temperature.	Supp
Suspension	A liquid preparation which consists of solid particles dispersed throughout a liquid phase in which the particles are not soluble.	Susp
Syrup	An oral solution containing high concentrations of sucrose or other sugars; the term has also been used to include any other liquid dosage form prepared in a sweet and viscid vehicle, including oral suspensions.	Syrup
Tablet	A solid dosage form containing medicinal substances with or without suitable diluents.	tab
Tablet, chewable	A solid dosage form containing medicinal substances with or without suitable diluents that is intended to be chewed, producing a pleasant-tasting residue in the oral cavity that is easily swallowed and does not leave a bitter or unpleasant aftertaste.	tab chew
Tablet, coated	A solid dosage form that contains medicinal substances with or without suitable diluents and is covered with a designated coating.	tab coated
Tablet, delayed release	A solid dosage form, which releases a drug (or drugs) at a time other than promptly after administration. Enteric-coated articles are delayed release dosage forms.	tab dr
Tablet, effervescent	A solid dosage form containing, in addition to active ingredients, mixtures of acids (citric acid, tartaric acid) and sodium bicarbonate, which release carbon dioxide when dissolved in water; it is intended to be dissolved or dispersed in water before administration.	tab effrv

(continues)

	TABLE 28-2 *(continued)*	
Name	**Definition**	**Short Name/ Abbreviation**
Tablet, extended release	A solid dosage form containing a drug which allows at least a reduction in dosing frequency as compared to that drug presented in conventional dosage form.	tab er
Tincture	An alcoholic or hydroalcoholic solution prepared from vegetable materials or from chemical substances.	Tincture
Troche	A discoid-shaped solid containing the medicinal agent in a suitably flavored base; troches are placed in the mouth where they slowly dissolve, liberating the active ingredients.	Troche
Wafer	A thin slice of material containing a medicinal agent.	Wafer

Source: U.S. Food and Drug Administration, Center for Drug Evaluation and Research. *http://www.fda.gov/cder/* Accessed January 2004.

Metric Doses

Metric is a modern decimal measurement system of weights and measures based on the meter as a unit length and the kilogram as a unit of mass. In health care, the common unit of measurement for weight is the gram and the unit for volume is the liter, or cubic centimeter. The prefix of the gram and the liter reflect either fractions or multiples of the measurement. Metric system prefixes are:

Deci: 1/10 or 0.1

Centi: 1/100 or 0.01

Milli: 1/1000 or 0.001

Micro: 1/1,000,000

Kilo: 1000 times

The amount of the drug is written in Arabic numerals before the measurement unit symbol. For example, if a drug were to be measured for 50 milligrams, it would be written as 50 milligrams (or 50 mg). Metric symbols used are:

Gram (g or gm)

Liter (L or l)

Microgram (mcg)

Milligram (mg)

Milliliter (mL or ml)

Cubic centimeter (cc)

There are other units of measurement that are used in medication orders that are not part of either system. Examples of those units of measurements include:

Drop (gtt)

Unit

Milliequivalent (mEq)

Sliding Scale Doses

Often the dose of the medication is indicated by a specific condition or diagnostic examination result. If the medication dose is written to be dependent on a laboratory result, it is called a **sliding scale** dose. The most common medication ordered as a sliding scale dose is insulin. Insulin doses are often determined by the patient's blood glucose. A sliding scale insulin dose will be written as a range of doses dependent on blood glucose values. For example:

Sliding Scale Insulin QID ac and hs

For blood glucose of 70–150 = no insulin

For blood glucose of 151–250 = 2 units regular insulin

For blood glucose of 251–300 = 4 units regular insulin

For blood glucose of 301–350 = 6 units regular insulin

For blood glucose of 351–400 = 8 units regular insulin

For blood glucose greater than 400, call physician

MEDICATION ROUTE

The route answers the question "How will the patient take the drug or how will it get into the patient's system?" (See Table 28-3.) The most common medication routes are topical, oral or enteral, and parenteral. Topical medications have a local effect and are applied directly where the action is desired. Oral medications enter the patient's system through the digestive tract either by mouth or through a feeding tube. In medication orders, a parenteral route refers to an injection (Figure 28-1).

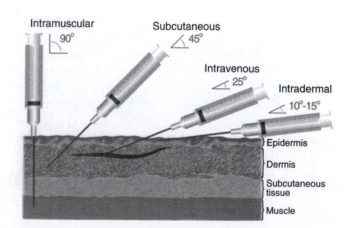

Figure 28-1 • *Angle of injection*

TABLE 28-3 Medication Routes

Route	Abbreviation	Definition
Oral	po	By mouth, orally
Sublingual or buccal	subling or subl	Dissolved under the tongue or inside the cheek
Aerosol inhalation		Directly inhaled into the lungs
Topical or transdermal		Applied directly to the skin
Instillation		Dropped into the ear, eye, or nose
Intraocular		A disk similar to a contact lens
Insertion		Introduced into body openings, such as a suppository
Intradermal hypodermic	ID or H	Injected into the upper layer of the skin
Subcutaneous	subq, sc, or sq	Under the skin into fat or connective tissue
Intramuscular	IM	Injected into deep muscle
Intravenous	IV	Injected into the vein
IV push or bolus	IVP	Given directly into a vein by a syringe and needle or an injection port of IV tubing, used for relatively large volumes of fluid or dose of a drug given rapidly to hasten or magnify a response
Intermittent IV	INT	Needle connected to a small length of tubing with a resealable cap used for intermittent infusions of small amounts
Heparin lock or flush, saline lock or flush	Hep loc	Needle connected to a small length of tubing with a resealable cap used for intermittent infusions of small amounts
IV piggyback	IVPB	Used when a patient has an established continuous IV; a bag is connected to a side arm of an existing IV
Admixture		For a continuous even drip of a med, a drug is added to a commercially prepared IV solution

(continues)

TABLE 28-3	*(continued)*

Route	Abbreviation	Definition
Patient-controlled analgesia	PCA	Allows patient to administer his or her own IV med via a special pump and IV tubing
Central venous catheter	CVC	IV line inserted through the subclavian vein. A consent may be needed for the insertion procedure. Used for total parenteral nutrition (TPN), hyperalimentation (HA or hyperal), or IV solutions with a dextrose concentration greater than 10%
Epidural		Injected into epidural space of spinal cord
Intrathecal		Injected into subarachnoid space for the purpose of instilling a medication for diffusion throughout the spinal fluid

Parenteral Routes of Administration

IV medication can be injected into the port of an existing IV line or through an IV catheter (Figure 28-2). This direct route is referred to as IV push or bolus. When an IV catheter is used to administer IV medications, it is also referred to as an intermittent IV line. The intermittent, or INT line, is an IV needle or catheter connected to a small length of tubing with a resealable cap. It is used for medication infusions when needed, or intermittently. The INT line may also be referred to as a heparin, or saline, lock or a capped IV. Those names evolved from the need for the INT line to be flushed with saline or heparin and then capped.

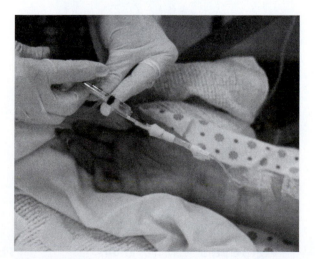

Figure 28-2 • *Intravenous push*

One way to administer medications intravenously is to use an already existing IV line. The term IV piggyback (IVPB) is given to the method of adding a medication to a small amount of fluid and joining the small bag of fluid to the primary or existing IV line (Figure 28-3).

Patient-controlled analgesia (PCA) allows the patient to administer his or her own medication for pain. A special programmable pump is connected to a subcutaneous, intravenous, or epidural catheter. The pump is carefully programmed to control the correct dose and the dose limit. Once a patient has been connected to the PCA pump, he or she presses a button to administer the programmed dose (Figure 28-4). This device allows a patient to have control over pain because there is no time waiting for the medication to be prepared and administered.

Vascular Access Devices

"Vascular access devices (VAD) include various catheters, cannulas, and infusion ports that allow for long-term IV therapy or repeated access to the central venous system" (DeLaune & Ladner, 2002, p. 1106). Types of vascular access devices are listed in Table 28-4.

FREQUENCY

The frequency component of the medication order answers the question, "When or how often will the medication be given?" Health care facilities have a standard medication schedule that includes the frequency and the time of day (Table 28-5). The time of day is usually given in military time, which is discussed later in the chapter. The frequency may be written as every A.M. and the standard administration time as 9:00 A.M. The physician will designate the frequency, but the health unit coordinator may assign the times or hours the medication is to be given according to the facility's medication time schedule. In addition to the facility's standard administration time,

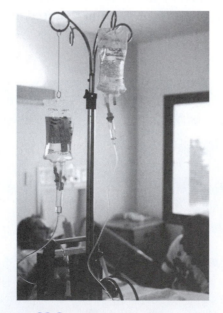

Figure 28-3 • *Intravenous piggyback*

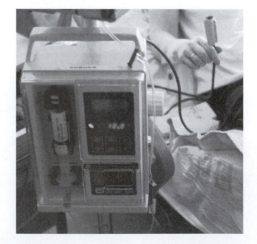

Figure 28-4 • *Patient-controlled analgesia pump*

TABLE 28-4 Vascular Access Devices

Type	Brand Name	Use
Nontunneled central venous catheter (triple-lumen)	Hohn, Deseret	Short-term fluid or blood administration, obtaining blood specimens, and administering medications
Tunneled central venous catheter (single or double lumen)	Hickman, Broviac, Groshong	Long-term (months to years) fluid replacement therapy, medication administration, nutritional supplement, and blood specimen withdrawal
Implanted infusion port	Chemo-Port, Infuse-a-Port, Mediport, Port-a-Cath	Long-term (months to years) fluid replacement therapy, medication administration (espcially chemotherapy), blood or blood product administration, and blood specimen withdrawal
Peripherally inserted central catheter (PICC)	C-PICC, Groshong PICC, SoloPICC	Long-term fluid replacement therapy, medication administration (chemotherapy, antibiotics, controlled narcotics), blood or blood product administration, and blood specimen withdrawal

TABLE 28-5 Standard Medication Administration Schedule

Frequency	Abbreviation	Time
Every day	Q day	0900
Twice a day	bid	0900-1700
Three times a day	tid	0900-1300-1700
Four times a day	qid	0900-1300-1700-2100
Before meals	ac	1000-1400-1800
After meals	pc	0730-1130-1630
Bedtime, or hour of sleep	hs	2100
Every 12 hours	Q 12 hr	0900-2100
Every 8 hours	Q 8 hr	0800-1600-2400
Every 6 hours	Q 6 hr	0600-1200-1800-2400
Every 4 hours	Q 4 hr	0900-1300-1700-2100-0100-0500

circumstances that affect the administration times include how the medication interacts with food, side effects, who administers the medication, the purpose of the medication, and the duration of the medication. Most medications are given between meals and during waking hours if possible.

Order Duration

As covered in Chapter 23, physician orders can be categorized by the time frame or duration of the order. Medication order categories include stat, standing, standing prn, and one-time or short-series orders.

> *Stat.* Orders that are activated immediately. For example, "Heparin 5000 units subq stat."
>
> *Standing.* Orders that remain active or in place until further orders are written to discontinue or change. This means the physician has to write the order only once as a standing order and the patient will receive that medication every day as ordered until the physician writes another order to change or discontinue the medication. For example, "Verapamil 80 mg po tid."
>
> *Standing prn.* Orders that remain active or in place until further orders are written to discontinue or change but for which the medication is administered only as necessary. For example, "Dalmane 15 mg po qhs prn for sleep."
>
> *One-time or short-series.* Orders that are active or in place only once or just for the specified amount of time. For example, the physician may order the medication to be given for 4 days or for 10 doses. The health unit coordinator may have to indicate the times for the short-term frequency order.

For example, on August 12 at 4:00 P.M., the physician writes, "Keflex 500 mg bid for 6 doses." The health unit coordinator may calculate the start and stop times. The medication would first be given on August 12 at 1700, and five doses would follow, with the last dose given on August 15 at 0900.

> August 12 1700 (first dose)
>
> August 13 0900-1700 (second and third dose)
>
> August 14 0900-1700 (fourth and fifth dose)
>
> August 15 0900 (sixth dose)

PRN Frequencies

Often, when a medication is ordered as necessary, or prn, the physician will write a qualifying phrase. A qualifying phrase answers the question "Why is the medication being given or under what condition should the medication be given?" Examples of qualifying phrases are:

- ◆ While awake
- ◆ For nausea

◆ For pain

◆ If unable to sleep

Military Time

Most health care facilities use military time. Military time is the term given to the 24-hour clock (Figure 28-5). Military time is used to reduce errors than can occur when trying to decipher if one has written A.M. or P.M. Military time, or the 24-hour clock, eliminates the use of A.M. and P.M. To convert time to the 24-hour format, use the "add 12" concept. Time conversion between the hours of midnight and noon is the easiest. Basically, there is no conversion. One would write 0100 and say "O one hundred," instead of 1 A.M. Time conversions between noon and midnight are done by adding 12. To convert time between noon and midnight, add 12 hours to whatever hour it happens to be. For example, to convert 1 P.M. to the 24-hour format, add 12 + 1 to get 13.

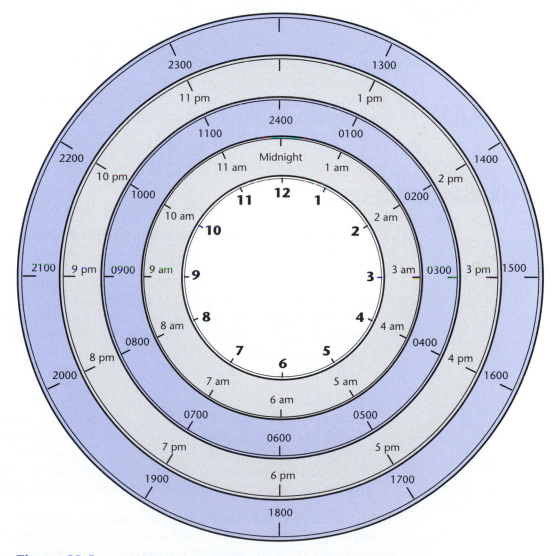

Figure 28-5 • *24-hour clock*

One would write 1300 and say "13 hundred." Likewise, if the time is 5 P.M., add 5 + 12 to get 17, or 1700 hours. The colon between the hours and the minutes is optional.

Automatic Stop Dates and Renewals

Medication orders may have automatic stop dates. Even if the physician writes the medication order as a standing order, the health care facility may have a policy in place that gives the maximum duration of medication orders. For example, an order for a controlled substance may expire automatically after 4 days, or an antibiotic may expire after 2 weeks. If the health care facility has an automatic stop date policy, it will also have a notification procedure in place. There will be some process to notify the physician that the medications will be automatically expiring and will need to be renewed if the administration is to continue.

CLASSIFICATIONS

Medications are usually classified or grouped according to the disease or body system they affect. A health unit coordinator's exposure to the different types of medications will depend on the area in which he or she works. It may be helpful to ask for a list of medications commonly used and prescribed in the department. Table 28-6 lists common medication classifications and examples of each.

CONTROLLED SUBSTANCES

The U.S. Drug Enforcement Administration (DEA) Web site explains the Controlled Substance Act.

> The Controlled Substance Act (CSA) places all substances that are regulated under existing federal law into one of five schedules. This placement is based upon the substance's medicinal value, harmfulness, and potential for abuse or addiction. Schedule I is reserved for the most dangerous drugs that have no recognized medical use, while Schedule V is the classification used for the least dangerous drugs.

> The CSA also creates a closed system of distribution for those authorized to handle controlled substances. The cornerstone of this system is the registration of all those authorized by the DEA to handle controlled substances. All individuals and firms that are registered are required to maintain complete and accurate inventories and records of all transactions involving controlled substances, as well as security for the storage of controlled substances.

Health care facilities have specific rules for controlled substances. Controlled substances are locked up. Each time a controlled substance is administered, it is recorded on a special form. Controlled substances are counted frequently and compared with the administration forms.

TABLE 28-6 Drug Classifications

Classification	Action/Uses	Medication Generic and Brand Name
CARDIOVASCULAR SYSTEM		
Antianginal	Treat angina (chest pain)	isosorbide (Isordil), nitroglycerine
Antiarrhythmic	Treat cardiac arrythmias	atropine (Atropair), digoxin (Lanoxin), lidocaine, procainamide (Pronestyl), propranolol (Inderal)
Blood modifiers and anticoagulants	To form or thin blood	clopidogrel bisulfate (Plavix), dipyridemole (Persantine), enoxaparin (Lovenox), epoetin alfa recombinant (Procrit), heparin, warfarin (Coumadin)
Antihypertensive	Treat hypertension (high blood pressure)	atenolol (Tenormin), captopril (Capoten), clonidine (Catapres), quinapril hydrochloride (Acupril), verapamil (Isoptin)
Antihyperlipidemic	Treat high cholesterol	atorvastatin (Lipitor), clopidogrel (Plavix), lovastatin (Mevacor), pravastatin (Pravachol)
Diuretics	Treat hypertension, fluid retention	Hydrocholorthiazide (Hydro-diuril)
Potassium supplements	Replaces potassium—often lost because of the use of diuretics	potassium bicarbonate (K+care), potassium chloride (Kaochlor, Klor-con, Klorvess, Slow-K), potassium gluconate (Kaon)
ANTI-INFECTIVE		
Antibiotics	Treat bacterial infections	amoxicillin (Amoxil), ceflacor (Ceclor), gentamicin (Garamycin), tetracycline (Panmycin), tobramycin (Nebcin)
Antiviral	Treat viral infections	acyclovir (Zovirax)
CENTRAL NERVOUS SYSTEM (CNS)		
Amphetamine	CNS stimulant	dextroamphetamine sulfate (Dexadrine)
Anti-anxiety drug	Treat anxiety	diazepam (Valium), hydroxyzine (Atarax), lorazepam (Ativan), ranitidine (Zantac)

(continues)

TABLE 28-6 *(continued)*

Classification	Action/Uses	Medication Generic and Brand Name
Anticonvulsants	Treat seizures	carbamazepine (Tegretol), divalproex (Depakote), phenytoin (Dilantin)
Antidepressants	Treat depression	amitriptyline (Elavil), bupropion hydrochloride (Wellbutrin), sertraline hydrochloride (Zoloft)
Antiparkinson agents	Treat Parkinson's disease	amantadine (Symmetrel), entacapone (Comtan), levodopa (L-dopa)
Antipsychotic	Treat mental illness	haloperidol (Haldol), quetiapine (Seroquel)
Analgesics—narcotic	Treat pain	codeine, fentanyl (Sublimaze), hydrocodone and acetaminophen (Vicodan), hydromorphone (Dilaudid), meperidine (Demerol), morphine sulfate
Analgesics—non-narcotic	Treat pain	acetaminophen (Tylenol), aspirin (abbreviated ASA)
Tranquilizers/hypnotics	Induce rest	flurazepam (Dalmane), temazepam (Restoril), zolpiden tartrate (Ambien)
ENDOCRINE SYSTEM		
Antidiabetic agents—hypoglycemics	Treat diabetes	glipizide (Glucotrol), metformin (Glucophage), tolbutamide (Orinase)
Antidiabetic agents—insulin	Treat diabetes	lente insulin, NPH insulin, regular insulin
Corticosteroids	Treat diseases of metabolism, anti-inflammatory or immunosuppressant therapy	betamethasone, hydrocortisone, methylprednisone (Solu-Medrol), prednisone
Thyroid drugs	Treat hypothyroidism	levothyroxin (Levothroid)
GASTROINTESTINAL SYSTEM		
Antidiarrheal	Treat diarrhea	diphenoxylate hydrochloride (Lomotil), loperamide (Imodium)
Anitemetics	Treat nausea and vomiting	prochlorperazine (Compazine), thiethylperazine (Torecan)
Laxatives	Treat constipation	bisacodyl (Dulcolax), docusate sodium (Colace), magnesium hydroxide (Milk of Magnesia, abbreviated MOM)

(continues)

TABLE 28-6	*(continued)*	
Classification	**Action/Uses**	**Medication Generic and Brand Name**
RESPIRATORY SYSTEM		
Antihistamines	Treat allergies	diphenhydramine (Benadryl), fexofenadine (Allegra), hydroxyzine hydrochloride (Atarax)
Histamine antagonists	Treat allergies	cimetidine (Tagamet), Prochlorperazine (Compazine)
Bronchodilators	Open bronchial tubes	albuterol (Proventil), bitolterol (Tornalate), metaproterenol sulfate (Alupent), terbulatine (Brethine), theophylline (Theolair, Theo-bid)
MUSCOSKELETEL SYSTEM		
Nonsteroidal anti-inflammatory drugs (NSAIDs)	Treat inflammatory disease and pain	etodolac (Lodine), ibuprofen (Motrin), indomethacin (Indocin), naproxen (Naprosyn)
Skeletal muscle relaxants	Treat musculoskeletal and neurological disorders	methocabamol (Robaxin)
Antineoplastic	Chemotherapeutic, treat cancer	carmustine (BICNU), cyclophosphamide (Cytoxan), cytarabine (Cytosar-U), melphalan (Alkeran), tamoxifen (Tamofen Nolvadex)

DISPENSING, STORING, AND TRANSPORTING MEDICATIONS

Medications are dispensed or distributed from the pharmacy to the patient care department. The methods for dispensing vary. Once the medication has been delivered, it is the responsibility of the receiving department to store it safely. In the inpatient health care facility, the two most common ways to dispense medications are unit dose and automated dispensing.

UNIT DOSE

In the Agency for Healthcare Research and Quality Web site, Murray and Shojania state,

Unit-dose carts are prepared daily, often manually, by technicians and then checked by pharmacists. These carts, containing thousands of patient-specific dosages of drugs, are sent to the wards (or departments) daily, for nurses to administer medications to patients. Dosing frequencies vary widely, ranging from regular intervals around the clock to "stat" doses given to control acute pain or other symptoms.

In unit-dose dispensing, medication is dispensed in a package that is ready for administration to the patient. For example, when a physician orders one ibuprofen four times a day, four individually wrapped ibuprofen tablets are wrapped and sent to the unit. Unit-dose dispensing can be used for medications administered by any route; however, oral, parenteral, and respiratory routes are especially common. When unit-dose dispensing first began, hospital pharmacies equipped themselves with machines that packaged and labeled tablets and capsules, one pill per package. They also purchased equipment for packaging liquids in unit doses. As the popularity of this packaging increased, the pharmaceutical industry began prepackaging pills in unit-of-use form. Many hospitals now purchase prepackaged unit-dose medications. However, it is still common for hospital pharmacies to purchase bulk supplies of tablets and capsules from manufacturers and repackage them in the central pharmacy into unit-dose packages.

There are many variations of unit-dose dispensing. As just one example, when physicians write orders for inpatients, these orders are sent to the central pharmacy (by pharmacists, nurses, other personnel, or computer). Pharmacists verify these orders and technicians place drugs in unit-dose carts. The carts have drawers in which each patient's medications are placed by pharmacy technicians—one drawer for each patient [Figure 28-6]. The drawers are labeled with the patient's name, ward (unit), room, and bed number. Before the carts are transported to the wards, pharmacists check each drawer's medications for accuracy. Sections of each cart containing all medication drawers for an entire nursing unit often slide out and can be inserted into wheeled medication carts used by nurses during their medication administration cycles. A medication administration recording form sits on top of the cart and is used by the nurse to check off and initial the time of each administration of each medication. The next day, the carts are retrieved from the wards (units) and replaced by a fresh and updated medication

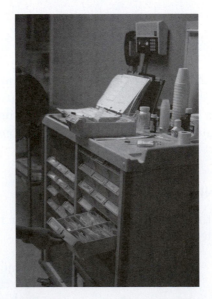

Figure 28-6 • *Unit dose cart*

supply. Medications that have been returned to the central pharmacy are credited to the patient's account.

Murray and Shojania go on to state,

> Studies often compare unit-dose dispensing to a ward (unit) stock system. In this system, nurses order drugs in bulk supplies from the pharmacy; the drugs are stored in a medication room on the ward (unit). Nurses prepare medication cups for each patient during medication administration cycles. The correct number of pills must be taken out of the correct medication container for each cycle and taken to the patient for administration. Liquids must be poured by the nurse from the appropriate bottle and each dose carefully measured. Nurses are responsible for any necessary labeling. Any medications taken from stock bottles and not administered to patients are generally disposed of.

AUTOMATED DISPENSING

In his explanation of the automated dispensing system (Figure 28-7), Murray states:

> In the 1980s, automated dispensing devices appeared on the scene, a generation after the advent of unit-dose dispensing. The invention and production

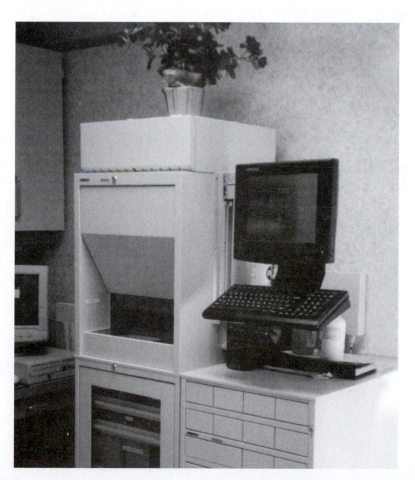

Figure 28-7 • *Automated medication dispensing the via Pyxis automated dispensing devise (Courtesy of All Saints Health Care, Racine, WI)*

of these devices brought hopes of reduced rates of medication errors, increased efficiency for pharmacy and nursing staff, ready availability of medications where they are most often used (the nursing unit or inpatient ward), and improved pharmacy inventory and billing functions.

Automated dispensing systems are drug storage devices or cabinets that electronically dispense medications in a controlled fashion and track medication use. Their principal advantage lies in permitting nurses to obtain medications for inpatients at the point of use. Most systems require user identifiers and passwords, and internal electronic devices track nurses accessing the system, track the patients for whom medications are administered, and provide usage data to the hospital's financial office for the patients' bills.

These automated dispensing systems can be stocked by centralized or decentralized pharmacies. Centralized pharmacies prepare and distribute medications from a central location within the hospital. Decentralized pharmacies reside on nursing units or wards, with a single decentralized pharmacy often serving several units or wards. These decentralized pharmacies usually receive their medication stock and supplies from the hospital's central pharmacy.

INTRAVENOUS THERAPY

Intravenous (IV) therapy may be used to provide fluids, medications, and nutrition directly into the patient's bloodstream through a vein. The difference between an IV route for a medication and IV therapy is the time of administration. With an IV route for medication, the medication is administered into an IV needle or catheter inserted into the vein and the order is completed. With IV therapy, the fluids, medication, or nutrition is continuously flowing into the IV catheter or needle. IV therapy orders refer to continuous IV solution infusions. The fact that it is continuous is what differentiates IV therapy orders from intermittent medications given via an IV route.

For IV therapy orders, a needle or catheter is inserted into the patient's vein. The IV access is commonly referred to as a line. A peripheral line is usually accessed in the hand or arm. The term *peripheral* means away from the center. A central line is accessed through the subclavian artery. Tubing is used to connect a plastic bag containing fluid, referred to as an IV bag, to the IV needle or catheter.

IV ORDER COMPONENTS

Just as there is a structure for medication orders, there is also a structure for IV therapy orders. IV therapy orders can be divided into four parts: amount, solution, rate, and additives.

IV Amount

The amount answers the question "How much fluid is in the IV bag," or "What is the size of the bag?" The amount of fluid is indicated in cubic centimeters (cc) or milliliters (ml). For adult patients, the most common size or amount is one liter. One liter is the same amount as 1000 cc or 1000 ml.

IV Solution

The solution answers the question "What kind or type of solution is in the IV bag?" Common IV solutions are saline or dextrose or a combination of both (Table 28-7). IV solutions are packaged in plastic bags or glass containers (Figure 28-8).

IV Rate

The rate answers the question "How fast should the IV fluid drip?" or "What is the length of time the IV should be infused?" The rate may be written in hours or milliliters per hour. The flow rate may be regulated mechanically with special tubing sets called volume-control sets or electronically through an infusion pump. The volume-control sets have roller clamps or dials that allow for the adjustment of the flow rate. An infusion pump is a machine for injecting a precise amount of fluid during a specific interval of time.

To determine the length of time an IV should run, one would divide the size of the bag (in milliliters) by the rate (in milliliters per hour). For example, if a 1000-ml bag is infusing at 125 ml/hour, divide 1000 by 125. The answer is 8, so a 1000-ml bag infusing at 125 ml/hour will last 8 hours.

TABLE 28-7   Common IV Solutions and Their Abbreviations

Solution	Abbreviation
Dextrose 5% water	D5W
Normal saline	NS or 0.9NaCl
Dextrose 5% water and one half normal saline	D5 ½ NS or D5.45NaCl
Dextrose 5% water and one-fourth normal saline	D5 ¼ NS or D5.25NaCl
Ringer's lactated or lactated Ringer's	RL or LR

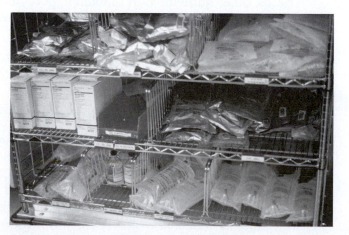

Figure 28-8 • *Prepackaged IV bags*

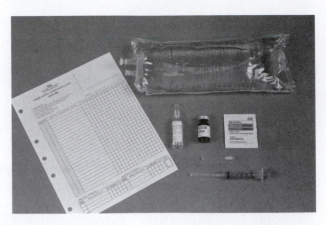

Figure 28-9 • *Medications may be added to IV solutions.*

To determine the drip or flow rate in milliliters per hour, divide the size of the bag (in milliliters) by the length of time (in hours). For example, if a 1000-ml bag is to infuse over 10 hours, divide 1000 by 10. The answer is 100, so a 1000-ml bag infusing over 10 hours should be regulated to flow of 100 ml/hour.

Additives

The additives answers the question, "What medications should be added to the continuous IV infusion?" An IV with a mixture of fluids and medications is called an IV admixture (Figure 28-9). Common additives include potassium chloride (KCl), vitamins, and heparin.

TOTAL PARENTERAL NUTRITION

Total parenteral nutrition (TPN), or hyperalimentation, is the practice of feeding a person by bypassing the gastrointestinal system and infusing the nutrients directly into the bloodstream. TPN is given to someone who cannot eat anything and must receive all nutrients through an intravenous line. A solution containing all the required nutrients including protein, fat, calories, vitamins, and minerals, is infused intravenously. TPN is given via a central, not a peripheral, intravenous line. A dextrose solution of greater than 10% concentration is usually the base for TPN. Depending on the patient's needs, other nutrients such as sodium, potassium, magnesium, calcium, insulin, multivitamins, and trace elements will be added. Most facilities have a special order form for TPN orders (Figure 28-10).

DRUG RESOURCES

There are many printed and online resources about pharmacology and medications. The health unit coordinator may use these resources to assist in the transcription of medication orders. The *United States Pharmacopeia* (USP) and *National Formulary* (NF) are books of drug standards for usage in the United States. The USP and NF are recognized by the U.S. Food and Drug Administration. Another commonly used drug reference is the *Physician's Desk Reference* (PDR). Information about drug names, doses, routes, and contraindications can be found in drug resources.

Aurora Health Care® *Milwaukee, Wisconsin*
- ☐ Aurora Medical Center, Hartford   ☐ St. Luke's South Shore
- ☐ Aurora Sinai Medical Center   ☐ West Allis Memorial Hospital
- ☐ St. Luke's Medical Center   ☐ Other: _____

PHYSICIAN'S ORDERS
24 Hour Adult Total Parenteral Nutrition Orders

PLEASE USE BALLPOINT PEN
Formulary approved equivalent will be dispensed unless the words "**NO SUBSTITUTES**" are written.

DATE/TIME OF ORDER	

CHECK ALLERGIES BEFORE WRITING MEDICATION ORDERS

Orders must be received in Pharmacy by 1600 hrs
Housewide Admixture Administration Time 2200 hrs
Dosing weight _____ (Kg)
Site of Administration: (check one)   ☐ Central   ☐ Peripheral

☐ **Standard Central**		☐ **Standard Peripheral**	
Non-prot. kcals:	25 kcals/kg/day (30% as Lipid)	Non-prot. calories:	1200 kcals (50% Dextrose/50% Lipid)
Protein:	1.5 gm/kg	Protein:	60 gm

These solutions are infused at **100 ml/hr** and contain standard electrolytes unless otherwise noted below

For additions/deletions or specialized solutions *(other than standard)*, complete appropriate information below
1. **Fluid Volume:** _____ ml/24 hrs or _____ ml/hr or Check ☐ for Minimum Volume
   or Cycle — on time: _____   off Time: _____
2. **Non-Protein Calories:** _____ K cal/24 hrs (average: 25–30 kcal/Kg/day)
3. **Lipid Requirements:** _____ % (as % of total non-protein calories: average 20–40%)
4. **Protein Requirements:** _____ Gm/24 hrs or _____ Gm/Kg/day
   (avg range 1–1.5 Gm/Kg/day)

5. **Additives are all per 24 hrs** *(check box and/or complete blanks)*

☐ STANDARD ELECTROLYTES	☐ Plus the following ADDITIONS (Please Complete Below)	☐ CUSTOMIZED (Please Complete Below)
Standard Electrolytes		
NaCl 18 mEq	_____ mEq	Sodium Chloride
Na Acetate 96 mEq	_____ mEq	Sodium Acetate
KCL 65 mEq	_____ mM	Sodium Phosphate
KP04 20 mM (30 mEq k+)	_____ mEq	Potassium Chloride
Mg++ 16 mEq	_____ mEq	Potassium Acetate
Ca++ 15 mEq	_____ mM	Potassium Phosphate
10 ml Multivitamin	_____ mEq	Magnesium Sulfate
3 ml Trace Elements	_____ mEq	Calcium Gluconate
	_____ mL	Multivitamins
	_____ mL	Trace Elements
	_____ units	Regular Human Insulin

Additions: _____

6. Check box below to order:
   ☐ Phytonadione (Vitamin K) 5 mg (SC) q Monday (HOLD if patient receiving warfarin)
   ☐ Vitamin B-12 1 mg (IM) today & q 30 days
7. **Monitoring Parameters: (except for 24 hr UUN, these are default values and should be considered orders)**

Comprehensive Metabolic Panel q Monday or _____	Fingerstick Blood Glucose: q 8 or _____ hours
Magnesium: q Monday or _____	I & O q 8 hours or _____
Basic Metabolic Panel: q Wednesday & Friday or _____	Weight: Daily or _____
Phosphate: q Monday & Friday or _____	
Other Labs: _____	
☐ Check for 24 Hour Urine Collection for Urca Nitrogen: q Monday or _____	

Physician Signature: _____   Date/Time _____

MD 342 PPO 00000836
PHYSICIAN'S ORDERS

Page 1 of 1
(Rev. 10/01)

Figure 28-10 • *Total parenteral nutrition order form (Reprinted with permission of Aurora Health Care, Milwaukee, WI)*

For example, a health unit coordinator is transcribing an order that is written as "Change Lanoxin to 0.25 mg po q am." The health unit coordinator accesses the patient's medication administration record (MAR) and Kardex or care plan to find where the medication Lanoxin was written so the dose can be changed. The health unit coordinator does not find the medication Lanoxin but sees where the medication digoxin is listed. The health unit coordinator looks up the drug Lanoxin to confirm that digoxin is the generic name for the drug Lanoxin. The health unit coordinator then proceeds with transcription and notes the dose change for the digoxin.

TRANSCRIBING MEDICATION AND IV ORDERS

As with all orders, extreme caution is necessary to prevent transcription errors. The health unit coordinator must be aware of the serious implications caused by medication errors.

The transcription of medication orders requires communication with the pharmacy and with the patient care staff. The pharmacy needs to know about the orders so they can dispense the medication, and the patient care staff need to know about the medication order so they can administer the medication.

The health unit coordinator may also need to order equipment such as IV tubing or infusion pumps for the patient care staff to complete the order. There may also be supplemental chart forms that are added to the patient care record, such as a TPN order form or a PCA order form.

MEDICATION ADMINISTRATION RECORD

The medication administration record (MAR) is a standard chart form (Figure 28-11). Usually, one form is used for each 24-hour period. In most health care facilities, the MAR is generated by the pharmacy's information system. Medication orders are entered into the pharmacy information system directly from the photocopy or NCR copy of the physician's orders. As new medication orders are written after the pharmacy has generated the MAR, they are hand-written onto the existing MAR. The MAR should include the patient's name, age, weight, allergies, diagnosis, and physician in addition to the medications ordered. The MAR is used by the patient care staff to document who administered the medications and when they were administered.

Table 28-8 lists transcription steps as they apply to medication and IV therapy orders.

PHARMACY MAR

START	STOP	MEDICATION	SCHEDULED TIMES	OK'D BY	0001 HRS. to 1200 HRS.	1201 HRS. to 2400 HRS.
08/31/xx 1800 SCH		PROCAN SR 500 MG TAB-SR 500 MG Q6H PO	0600 1200 1800 2400	JD	0600 GP 1200 GP	1800 MS 2400 JD
09/03/xx 0900 SCH		DIGOXIN (LANOXIN) 0.125 MG TAB 1 TAB QOD PO ODD DAYS-SEPT.	0900	JD	0900 GP	
09/03/xx 0900 SCH		FUROSEMIDE (LASIX) 40 MG TAB 1 TAB QD PO	0900	JD	0900 GP	
09/03/xx 0845 SCH		REGLAN 10 MG TAB 10 MG AC&HS PO GIVE ONE NOW!	0730 1130 1630 2100	JD	0730 GP 1130 GP	1630 MS 2100 MS
09/04/xx 0900 SCH		K-LYTE 25 MEQ EFFERVESCENT TAB 1 EFF. TAB BID PO DISSOLVE AS DIR. START 9-4	0900 1700	JD	0900 GP	1700 GP
09/03/xx 1507 PRN		NITROGLYCERIN 1/50 GR 0.4 MG TAB-SL 1 TABLET PRN* SL PRN CHEST PAIN		JD		
09/03/xx 1700 PRN		DARVOCET-N 100* 1 TAB Q4-6H PO PRN MILD-MODERATE PAIN		JD		
09/03/xx 2100 PRN		MEPERIDINE*(DEMEROL) INJ 50 MG Q4H IM PRN SEVERE PAIN W PHENERGAN		JD		2200 (H) MS
09/03/xx 2100 PRN		PROMETHAZINE (PHENERGAN) INJ 50 MG Q4H IM PRN SEVERE PAIN W DEMEROL		JD		2200 (H) MS

Gluteus	Thigh	Nurse's Signature	Initial	Allergies: NKA		Patient:	Patient, John D.
A. Right	H. Right					Patient #:	3-81512-3
B. Left	I. Left	7-3 G. Pickar, R.N.	GP				
Ventro Gluteal						Admitted:	08/31/xx
C. Right	J. Right	3-11 M. Smith, R.N.	MS	Diagnosis: CHF		Physician:	J. Physician, MD
D. Left	K. Left						
E. Abdomen	1 2 / 3 4	11-7 J. Doe, R.N.	JD			Room:	PCU-14 PCU

Figure 28-11 • *Medication administration record*

TABLE 28-8	Transcription Steps for Medication and IV Therapy Orders

Transcription Step	Key Points
1. Read the entire order set thoroughly.	Careful reading of the orders allows the health unit coordinator to review, prioritize, and check for incomplete or illegible orders.
2. Prioritize orders.	Determine the urgency of the orders in all the charts needing transcription. Decide what orders in the order set need to be transcribed first.

(continues)

TABLE 28-8 *(continued)*

Transcription Step	Key Points
3. If medications are included in the order set, send the order carbon or a copy to the pharmacy.	It is crucial that the pharmacy receive the physician's medication orders.
4. Communicate the order to the individual or department that will be performing the order.	The health unit coordinator will communicate medication orders to the pharmacy department and to the patient care staff responsible for the patient. The health unit coordinator may also need to contact central supply if IV tube supplies are needed. The health unit coordinator may need to add additional chart forms for PCA, TPN, or anticoagulant orders.
5. Record the orders on the patient Kardex or care plan.	Record the medication or IV order as written from the physician's order form to the patient Kardex or care plan.
6. Record medication orders on the medication administration record (MAR).	Record the medication or IV order as written from the physician's order form to the MAR.
7. Check off each order in the set as completed.	Placing a check mark by each order as it is transcribed can help the health unit coordinator track orders even when interrupted.
8. Re-read and check all work for accuracy.	Because of multiple requests received by the health unit coordinator, re-reading and checking work is a necessity.
9. Sign off the order with name, title, date, and time.	The health unit coordinator is accountable for the orders transcribed.

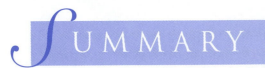

SUMMARY

Medications and intravenous therapy play a large part in the patient's plan of care. Medications and IVs may be ordered to cure or treat a disease or to alleviate symptoms. The health unit coordinator needs to be able to recognize orders that need to be communicated to the pharmacy department. Knowledge of the components of medication and intravenous therapy orders will make recognizing medication orders and communicating with the pharmacy department easier.

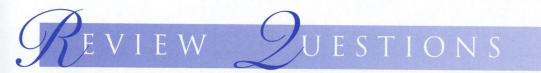

Write out the complete term represented by the following abbreviations.

1. ac

2. cap

3. cc

4. D5

5. gm

6. gr

7. gtt

8. ID

9. IM

10. INT

11. IVP

12. IVPB

13. L

14. LR

15. MAR

16. mcg

17. mEq

18. mg

19. ml

20. NaCl

21. PCA

22. subl

23. subq

24. List and describe the components of a medication order.

25. Convert the following times to military time: 9:30 A.M., 9:30 P.M., 2:30 A.M., 2:30 P.M., midnight.

26. List and describe the four components of an IV order.

TRANSCRIPTION PRACTICE

Go to the CD-ROM for transcription exercises that support the content in this chapter.

$\mathcal{N}$AHUC CERTIFICATION EXAM

CONTENT AREAS

I. A. 2   Interpret medical symbols, abbreviations, and terminology

I. A. 6   Enter orders on a Kardex

I. A. 11   Enter orders onto a medication administration record

I. A. 17   Process medication orders

I. A. 18   Process orders for parenteral fluids

I. B. 1   Notify staff of new orders

III. B. 4   Enter orders via computers

$\mathcal{T}$HROUGH THE EYES

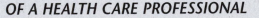

OF A HEALTH CARE PROFESSIONAL

A medication nurse shares her thoughts.

As a registered nurse, I am responsible for administering medications to the patient. I have to be sure the right patient is getting the right amount of the right medication at the right time via the right route. Fortunately, most health care facilities have a system of checks and balances to prevent medication errors. The health unit coordinator plays a crucial role in that system of checks and balances. The health unit coordinator must first recognize that there is a medication order that needs to be transcribed. Because the pharmacist must have an exact copy or replica of the medication order, the health unit coordinator must fax, tube, or deliver the medication order to the pharmacy. The health unit coordinator may also write the new medication on the MAR or care plan for the nurse. If there are stat medication orders, the health unit coordinator will bring it to the attention of the nurse. I know that the health unit coordinator is doing her best to communicate the medication orders to the pharmacy and the nursing staff.

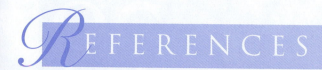

REFERENCES

Agency for Healthcare Research and Quality. Murray, M. D., & Shojania, K. G. Chapter 10 Unit-Dose Drug Distribution Systems. *http://www.ahcpr.gov/clinic/ptsafety/chap10.htm* Accessed January 2004.

Agency for Healthcare Research and Quality. Murray, M. D. Chapter 11 Automated Medication Dispensing Services. *http://www.ahcpr.gov/clinic/ptsafety/chap11.htm* Accessed January 2004.

U.S. Food and Drug Administration, Center for Drug Evaluation and Research. Drug Forms. *http://www.fda.gov/cder/dsm/DRG/drg00201.htm* Accessed January 2004.

U.S. Drug Enforcement Administration. Controlled Substances Act. *http://www.usdoj.gov/dea/agency/csa.htm* Accessed January 2004.

Altman, G. B. (2004). *Delmar's fundamental and advanced nursing skills* (2nd ed.). Clifton Park, NY: Thomson Delmar Learning.

DeLaune, S. C., & Ladner, P. K. (2002). *Fundamentals of nursing: Standards and practice* (2nd ed.). Clifton Park, NY: Thomson Delmar Learning.

Spratto, G. R., & Woods, A. L. (2004). *2004 edition PDR nurse's drug handbook.* Clifton Park, NY: Thomson Delmar Learning.

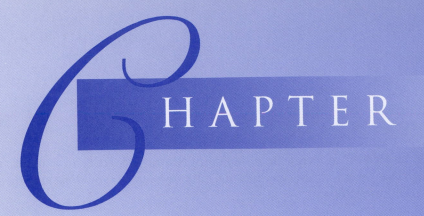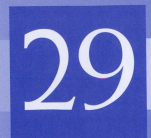

CHAPTER 29

Therapy Orders

Learning Objectives

Upon completion of this chapter and review questions, the learner should be able to:

1. Define vocabulary and abbreviations related to therapies.

2. List three types of treatments performed by the respiratory care department.

3. List three types of tests performed by the respiratory care department.

4. List the divisions within the physical medicine and rehabilitation department.

5. List two main types of dialysis.

6. Interpret and transcribe physicians' orders related to therapy.

Abbreviations

ABG Arterial Blood Gases

ADL Activities of Daily Living

AROM Active Range of Motion

AV Arteriovenous

BiPAP Bi-level Positive Airway Pressure

CPAP Continuous Positive Airway Pressure

CPM Continuous Passive Motion

CPT Chest Physical Therapy

EMG Electromyogram

EPC Electronic Pain Control

ET Endotracheal

FiO$_2$ Fraction of Inspired Oxygen

FWB Full Weight Bearing

HBO Hyperbaric Oxygen

IPPB Intermittent Positive Pressure Breathing

IS Incentive Spirometer

lpm Liters per Minute

MDI Metered-Dose Inhaler

nc Nasal Cannula

NCS Nerve Conduction Study

NWB Non-Weight Bearing

O$_2$ Oxygen

OT Occupational Therapy

Peep Positive End Expiratory Pressure

PFT Pulmonary Function Test

PM&R Physical Medicine and Rehabilitation

PROM Passive Range of Motion

PT Physical Therapy

Pulse ox Pulse Oximetry

PWB Partial Weight Bearing

RR Respiratory Rate

RT Recreational Therapy

SaO$_2$ Arterial Oxygen Saturation

ST Speech Therapy

TCDB Turn, Cough, Deep Breathe

TENS Transcutaneous Electrical Nerve Stimulation

TV Tidal Volume

vent Ventilator

vib & perc Vibration and Percussion

VT Tidal Volume

THERAPY

Many types of therapy and treatments are administered to patients to treat their illnesses and their symptoms. Specially trained personnel within each specialty department perform most therapies and treatments. The health unit coordinator transcribes orders that are performed by the staff within the specialty departments. In this chapter, the treatments provided by respiratory care, physical medicine and rehabilitation, dialysis, radiation therapy, and hyperbaric oxygen therapy and wound, ostomy, and continence care are discussed.

RESPIRATORY CARE

Respiratory care provides therapy, treatments, and tests related to breathing and lung function. Respiratory care may be its own department within a health care facility, or it may be its own stand-alone health care facility that provides care to outpatients. Other names given to respiratory care are respiratory therapy, inhalation therapy, and pulmonary function. In large facilities, breathing therapy and lung function tests may be divided into two departments or divisions, respiratory care and pulmonary function.

OXYGEN THERAPY

Body cells need oxygen (O_2). If a patient is not getting enough oxygen naturally through breathing or respiration, supplemental oxygen may be administered. A metal connector with a gauge or flow meter is inserted into an oxygen tank or a special wall outlet that provides oxygen (Figure 29-1). The flow meter consists of a cylinder marked at intervals with lines and numbers to measure the oxygen. A ball floats inside the cylinder when the valve is opened. The bottom of the gauge has a fitting for a water bottle or humidifier attachment. A tube leads from the humidifier to a device that fits on the patient.

There are different types of devices that fit on the patient to administer oxygen. Devices include a nasal cannula (nc), single face mask, open face tent, reservoir mask, and venturi mask (Figure 29-2).

Oxygen is measured by percentage (%) or liters per minute (lpm). The air one breathes naturally, referred to as room air, is approximately 23% oxygen.

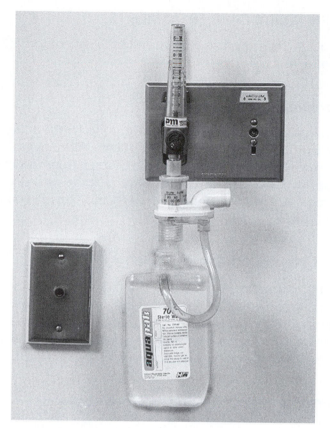

Figure 29-1 • *Oxygen flow meter*

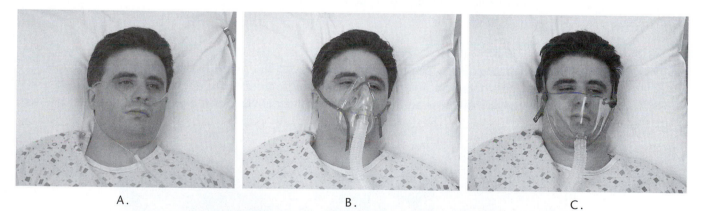

A.   B.   C.

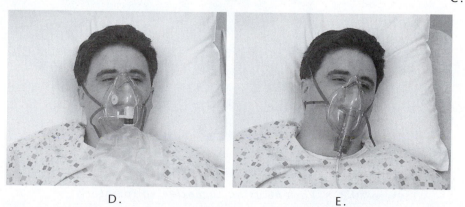

D.   E.

Figure 29-2 • *Devices used for oxygen administration: (A) nasal cannula, (B) single face mask, (C) open face tent, (D) reservoir mask, (E) Venturi mask*

RESPIRATORY CARE TREATMENTS

A variety of treatments can be given to the patient to facilitate adequate respiration and lung function.

Incentive Spirometer

An incentive spirometer (IS) is a device to teach the patient to breathe deeply. IS is often ordered for the postoperative patient to encourage deep breathing to open airways after receiving a general anesthetic. The respiratory therapist teaches the patient how to use the device and leaves the device with the patient to use as ordered (Figure 29-3). The respiratory therapist may also teach and assist the patient to turn, cough, and deep breathe (TCDB).

Chest Physical Therapy

Chest physical therapy (CPT) is a technique in which the patient is placed in various positions that aid in the removal of lung secretions. Positioning is combined with percussions to the chest wall. The percussions may be done manually or with a pneumatic percussor. Other terms used may be vibration and percussion (vib & perc), pummeling, cupping, and postural drainage.

Intermittent Positive Pressure Breathing

Intermittent positive pressure breathing (IPPB) is a device that forces air into the patient's lungs and allows the patient to breathe out. The device can also be used to administer medication in an aerosol form.

Nebulizer

A nebulizer is a type of inhaler that sprays a fine, liquid mist of medication. The device works by converting medication into a mist and delivering it through a mask worn over the nose and mouth. The mist is delivered using oxygen or air under pressure

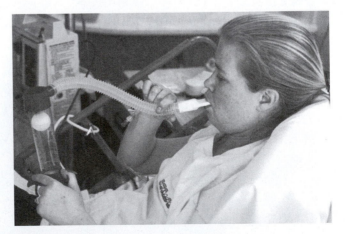

Figure 29-3 • *Patient using incentive spirometer*

or an ultrasonic machine. A mouthpiece is connected to a machine via plastic tubing to deliver the medication. This treatment may also be referred to as an updraft.

Metered-Dose Inhaler

A metered-dose inhaler (MDI) delivers a specific amount of medicine in aerosol form. Respiratory care may instruct the patient on the use of an MDI.

Continuous Positive Airway Pressure

Continuous positive airway pressure (CPAP) is administering positive pressure to airways by having the patient breathe through pressurized tubing (Figure 29-4). Bi-level positive airway pressure (BiPAP) is an alternative form of ventilation in which the ventilator reduces air pressure during exhalation.

Intubation

Intubation is the insertion of an endotracheal (ET) tube into the patient's windpipe to introduce air when the patient is unable to breathe on his or her own. This may also be referred to as an artificial airway. Intubation is required to place a patient on a breathing machine or ventilator (Figure 29-5).

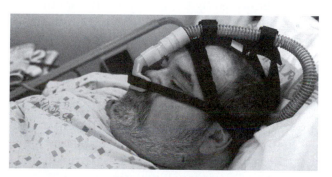

Figure 29-4 • *CPAP mask*

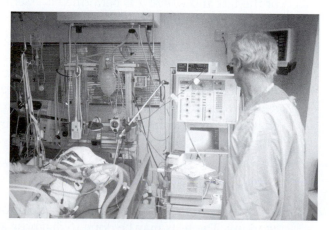

Figure 29-5 • *A patient connected to a mechanical ventilator*

Ventilator

A ventilator (vent) is a machine that assists or controls the patient's breathing. The health unit coordinator may transcribe orders for the regulation of ventilator settings and controls. Terms include:

- Tidal volume (TV or VT)
- Fraction of inspired oxygen (FiO_2)
- Respiratory rate (RR)
- Positive end expiratory pressure (Peep)
- Continuous positive airway pressure (CPAP)

RESPIRATORY AND PULMONARY TESTS

In addition to treatments, respiratory care may perform breathing and lung function tests.

Induced Sputum

Sputum is the required specimen for some laboratory tests. Although the actual test is performed by the laboratory, the sputum specimen may have to be obtained by respiratory care. When an induced sputum is needed, respiratory care assists the patient in producing the specimen. If the patient is not able to produce the specimen, respiratory care may suction the patient.

Blood Gases

Arterial blood gases (ABG) is a test that measures the concentration of oxygen and carbon dioxide in the blood, which shows how efficient the gas exchange is in the lungs. Again, the respiratory care department may collect the specimen, arterial blood, and the laboratory will perform the test.

It is the health unit coordinator who orders the tests from respiratory care. Knowledge of the test and where it is performed is essential to contacting the correct department for the test.

Pulse Oximetry

Pulse oximetry (pulse ox) is a noninvasive method of measuring arterial blood oxygen saturation (SaO_2). A device that is attached to the patient's finger has a photon sensor that measures the amount of light absorbed by oxygenated and unoxygenated hemoglobin (Figure 29-6).

Pulmonary Function Tests

Pulmonary function tests (PFTs) are a group of tests that measure how the lungs are working. The tests may be done to diagnose and confirm diseases or before surgery to make sure the patient's lungs will tolerate anesthesia and surgery. Tests may include spirometry, lung volume measurement, and diffusion capacity.

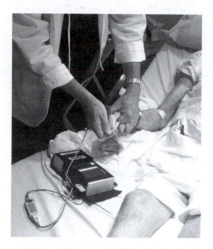

Figure 29-6 • *A pulse oximeter on a patient's finger*

Medline explains the tests as:

> Spirometry: a person performs the test by breathing into a mouthpiece that is connected to an instrument called a spirometer. The spirometer records the amount of air and the rate of air that is breathed in and out over a specified time. Some of the test measurements are obtained by normal, quiet breathing, and other tests require forced inhalation or exhalation after a deep breath.

> Lung volume measurement can be performed in two ways. The most accurate way is for a person to sit in a body plethysmograph, a sealed, transparent box that resembles a telephone booth, while breathing in and out of a mouthpiece. Changes in pressure inside the box allow determination of the lung volume. Lung volume can also be measured when a person breathes nitrogen or helium gas through a tube for a specified period of time. The concentration of the gas in a chamber attached to the tube is measured, allowing estimation of the lung volume.

> The diffusion capacity is measured when a person breathes carbon monoxide for a very short time (often one breath). The concentration of carbon monoxide in exhaled air is then measured. The difference in the amount of carbon monoxide inhaled and the amount exhaled allows estimation of how rapidly gas can travel from the lungs into the blood.

It is the health unit coordinator who will order these tests from respiratory care. Knowledge of the test and where it is performed is essential to contacting the correct department for the test.

PHYSICAL MEDICINE AND REHABILITATION SERVICES

The focus of physical medicine and rehabilitation (PM&R) is to restore function and improve the quality of life. Care is provided to patients who have had a stroke, amputation, paralysis, orthopedic injuries, and neurological injures, to name a few. PM&R may be provided by a division of a health care facility or as a stand-alone facility.

PM&R may consist of a variety of divisions, most commonly physical therapy (PT), occupational therapy (OT), speech therapy (ST), and recreational therapy (RT). PM&R may also include rehabilitation psychology services, chronic pain clinics, and electrodiagnostic studies. There are trained medical specialists in each division of PM&R. A rehabilitation physician is referred to as a physiatrist.

PHYSICAL THERAPY

Physical therapy uses natural forces such as water, heat, light, exercise, and electricity. PT is ordered for the patient to help restore motion and aid in recovery.

Water

Hydrotherapy is water therapy provided by PT. The physician may write orders for the whirlpool or Hubbard tank.

Heat and Light

PT may provide heat and light treatments to muscles and joints with heating pads, wax, ultrasound, or ultraviolet and infrared light.

Exercise

PT provides a wide variety of exercise. Exercise orders may indicate the range of motion the patient can tolerate. Abbreviations in these types of orders include:

◆ Active range of motion (AROM)

◆ Passive range of motion (PROM)

◆ Continuous passive motion (CPM)

The physical therapist may also provide ambulation and assistive device training for the use of parallel bars, crutches, canes, and walkers. Ambulation orders may indicate how much of his or her own weight the patient can bear. Abbreviations include:

◆ Non-weight bearing (NWB)

◆ Partial weight bearing (PWB)

◆ Full weight bearing (FWB)

Electricity

PT uses electricity for treatments and tests. Electrical nerve stimulation or electronic pain control (EPC) is also called transcutaneous electrical nerve stimulation (TENS). Healthatoz describes TENS:

TENS is a noninvasive, drug-free pain management technique. The TENS device is a small battery-powered stimulator that produces low-intensity electrical signals through electrodes on or near a painful area, producing a tingling sensation that reduces pain. There is no dosage limitation, and the patient controls the amount of pain relief. By sending electrical signals to underlying nerves, the battery-powered TENS device can relieve a wide range of chronic and acute pain. Some experts believe TENS works by blocking pain signals in the spinal cord, or by delivering electrical impulses to underlying nerve fibers that lessen the experience of pain. Others suspect that the electrical stimulation triggers the release of natural painkillers in the body.

An electromyogram (EMG) is an electrical recording of muscle activity. An EMG may be ordered to diagnose a neuromuscular disease. Healthatoz describes the EMG:

> During an EMG test, a fine needle is inserted into the muscle to be tested. Recordings are made while the muscle is at rest, and then during the contraction. A slightly different test, the nerve conduction velocity test or nerve conduction study [NCS], is often performed at the same time with the same equipment. In this test, stimulating and recording electrodes are used, and small electrical shocks are applied to measure the ability of the nerve to conduct electrical signals. This test may cause mild tingling and discomfort similar to a mild shock from static electricity.

OCCUPATIONAL THERAPY

Occupational therapy helps people regain and develop skills that are important for self-care and self-sufficiency. The most commonly ordered therapy from OT is activities of daily living (ADL). When ADL is ordered, the occupational therapist will assist the patient in learning self-care skills such as dressing, bathing, preparing meals, and driving (Figure 29-7).

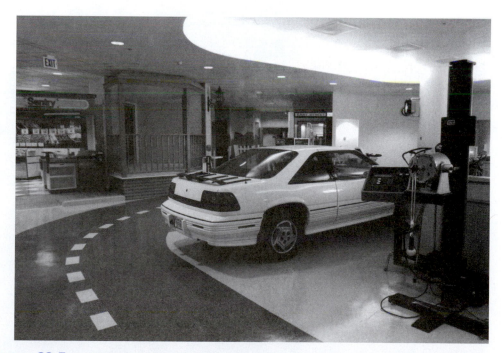

Figure 29-7 • *Props and equipment used to simulate activities of daily living (Courtesy of Aurora Health Care, Milwaukee, WI)*

SPEECH THERAPY

The speech therapy department provides services for patients with language and speech difficulties. They also provide services for patients with dysphagia, a swallowing disorder. A videofluorographic swallowing study may be ordered to evaluate the dysphagia.

RECREATIONAL THERAPY

Recreational therapy provides recreation and leisure services to patients with disabilities and illnesses. The recreational therapist may asses the patient's past leisure activities and create goals for new recreational activities that suit the patient's abilities and interests.

DIALYSIS

Dialysis is the treatment given to patients when their kidneys are unable to remove wastes or impurities from the blood (Figure 29-8). There are two types of dialysis: peritoneal dialysis and hemodialysis.

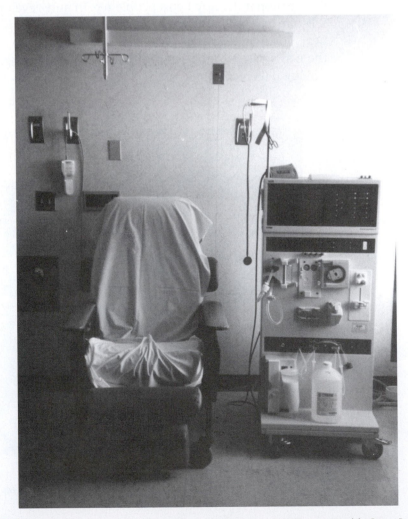

Figure 29-8 • *Hemodialysis equipment (Courtesy of All Saints Health Care, Racine, WI)*

PERITONEAL DIALYSIS

Medline explains peritoneal dialysis: "Peritoneal dialysis works by using the peritoneal membrane inside the abdomen as the semipermeable membrane. Special solutions that facilitate removal of toxins are infused in, remain in the abdomen for a time, and then are drained out. This form of dialysis can be performed at home, but must be done on a continuous everyday basis."

HEMODIALYSIS

Medline states:

> Hemodialysis works by circulating the blood through special filters. The blood flows across a semipermeable membrane (the dialyzer or filter), along with solutions that help facilitate removal of toxins. Before hemodialysis can be performed, there needs to be adequate access to the vascular system. A special type of arterial and venous access is therefore established.

> The access can be either external or internal. External access involves two catheters—one that is placed in an artery, and one in an adjacent vein, or two catheters positioned within different parts of a large vein. External access is typically only used in emergency situations.

> Internal access can be either an arteriovenous (AV) fistula or AV graft. An AV fistula involves the surgical joining of an artery and vein under the skin. The increased blood volume stretches the elastic vein to allow a larger volume of blood flow.

> After 4 to 6 weeks the fistula needs to heal, needles can be placed so that arterial blood can be pulled off for dialysis, and the cleansed blood returns through the dilated vein. Turbulent blood flow over the AV fistula is commonly felt and termed a thrill.

> An AV graft may be used for people whose veins are not suitable for an AV fistula. This procedure involves surgically grafting a donor vein from the patient's own saphenous vein (in the leg), a carotid artery from a cow, or a synthetic graft from an artery to a vein.

> After there is adequate access with two ports, a hemodialysis machine is connected. The port from the artery leads into the machine, and the port returning from the machine leads into the vein. Inside the machine, your blood is run through tubes with semipermeable membranes, and the tubes are bathed with solutions that help remove specific soluble materials from your blood.

RADIATION THERAPY

Radiation therapy is a treatment that uses radioactive substances to destroy cancer cells. Medline states: "Since radiation is most harmful to rapidly reproducing cells, radiation damages cancer cells more than the normal cells of the body. It prevents these cells from continuing to reproduce and thus prevents the tumor from growing further."

HYPERBARIC OXYGEN THERAPY

Hyperbaric oxygen therapy (HBO) uses a pressure chamber to enable a patient to breathe 100% oxygen (Figure 29-9). This type of therapy may be used for wound healing, tissue infections, smoke inhalation, and burns.

WOUND, OSTOMY, AND CONTINENCE CARE

Health care professionals with special training and skills in wound care are called wound, ostomy, and continence nurses or enterostomal therapists. An ostomy is a surgical opening created for the discharge of body wastes. Special care must be given to the skin around the ostomy to prevent irritation and infection. These professionals may also treat chronic wounds such as pressure ulcers. Pressure ulcers are open wounds that form whenever prolonged pressure is applied to skin. Pressure ulcers may be called bedsores or decubitus ulcers.

TRANSCRIPTION OF THERAPY ORDERS

Table 29-1 lists the transcription steps as they apply to therapy orders.

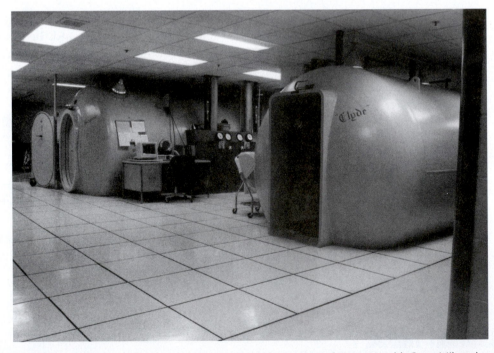

Figure 29-9 • *Hyperbaric oxygen chamber. (Courtesy of Aurora Health Care, Milwaukee, WI)*

TABLE 29-1 Transcription Steps for Therapy Orders

Transcription Step	Key Points
1. Read the entire order set thoroughly.	Careful reading of the orders allows the health unit coordinator to review, prioritize, and check for incomplete or illegible orders.
2. Prioritize orders.	Determine the urgency of the orders in all the charts needing transcription. Decide what orders in the order set need to be transcribed first.
3. If medications are included in the order set, send the order carbon or a copy to the pharmacy.	Medications may be included in IPPB and MDI orders.
4. Communicate the order to the individual or department that will be performing the order.	The health unit coordinator communicates therapy and treatment orders to the appropriate department and to the patient care staff responsible for the patient. This step is where the memorization of treatments and abbreviations will be useful.
5. Record the orders on the patient Kardex or care plan.	Record the therapy or treatment order as written from the physician's order form to the patient Kardex or care plan.
6. Record medication orders on the medication administration record (MAR).	This step may be omitted for treatment and therapy orders.
7. Check off each order in the set as completed.	Placing a check mark by each order as it is transcribed can help the health unit coordinator track orders even when interrupted.
8. Re-read and check all work for accuracy.	Because of multiple requests received by the health unit coordinator, re-reading and checking work is a necessity.
9. Sign off the order with name, title, date, and time.	The health unit coordinator is accountable for the orders transcribed.

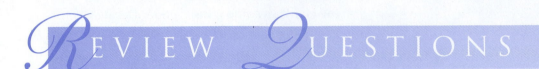

SUMMARY

Treatments and therapies are ordered for the patients to aid in their recovery. The treatments and therapies may help to heal the patients or may ease their symptoms or may assist them in living with their illness. The health unit coordinator must be aware of the many treatment and therapy departments and the services they provide.

REVIEW QUESTIONS

Write out the complete terms represented by the following abbreviations.

1. ABG

2. ADL

3. CPT

4. EMG

5. ET

6. IS

7. lpm

8. nc

9. NWB

10. O_2

11. PFT

12. PROM

13. SaO_2

14. TCDB

15. List three devices used to administer oxygen.

16. What is the name of the treatment in which the patient is placed in various positions that aid in the removal of lung secretions?

17. What is the name of the device used to teach the patient to breathe deeply?

18. What is the termed used for the insertion of an endotracheal (ET) tube into the patient's windpipe to introduce air when the patient is unable to breathe on his own?

19. What is the name of the noninvasive method of measuring arterial blood oxygen saturation?

20. List the divisions within the physical medicine and rehabilitation department and name one service that each provides.

21. What type of dialysis works by using the peritoneal membrane inside the abdomen as the semipermeable membrane?

22. What type of dialysis works by circulating the blood through special filters using a special type of arterial and venous access?

TRANSCRIPTION PRACTICE

Go to the CD-ROM for transcription exercises that support the content in this chapter.

*N*AHUC CERTIFICATION EXAM

CONTENT AREAS

I. A. 2   Interpret medical symbols, abbreviations, and terminology

I. A. 6   Enter orders on a kardex

I. A. 9   Schedule diagnostic tests and procedures

I. A. 10   Initiate and follow test preparation procedures

I. A. 13   Process orders for diagnostic and therapeutic tests and procedures

I. B. 1   Notify staff of new orders

III. B. 4   Enter orders via computers

THROUGH THE EYES

OF A HEALTH CARE PROFESSIONAL

A respiratory therapist shares his thoughts.

I work as a respiratory therapist in an intensive care unit where many of the patients are on a ventilator. On this type of unit, it is crucial that the respiratory therapist and the health unit coordinator have a good working relationship. At the beginning of each shift, I'll introduce myself to the health unit coordinator and give him my pager number. Throughout the shift, the health unit coordinator will bring new respiratory therapy orders to my attention either by pager or in person. The health unit coordinator may also assist me by letting me know what other tests and treatments a patient has scheduled so I can plan the respiratory treatments around other events in the patient's day. This exchange of information can prevent delays in treatments. If I need to talk to a specific physician, the health unit coordinator may assist me by notifying me when he is on the unit. When the health unit coordinator and I have good communication, it eases some of the stress in a very stress-filled environment.

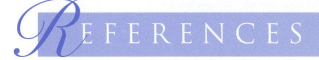

REFERENCES

Altman, G. B. (2004). *Delmar's fundamental and advanced nursing skills* (2nd ed.). Clifton Park, NY: Thomson Delmar Learning.

DeLaune, S. C., & Ladner, P. K. (2002). *Fundamentals of nursing: Standards and practice* (2nd ed.). Clifton Park, NY: Thomson Delmar Learning.

Health A to Z. *http://www.healthatoz.com* Accessed January 2004.

Medline Plus National Library of Medicine, National Institutes of Health. *http://www.nlm.nih.gov/medline* Accessed January 2004.

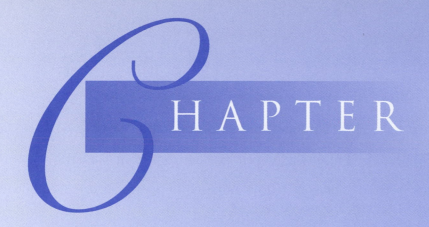

Surgery Orders

Learning Objectives

Upon completion of this chapter and review questions, the learner should be able to:

1 List four items that must be on a patient's chart before the patient can go to the operating room.

2. Describe preop orders.

3. Describe postop orders.

4. Discuss the role of the health unit coordinator in the preparation process for a patient to go to the operating room.

5. Explain the operation schedule and how the health unit coordinator uses the schedule.

Key Terms

elective surgery Surgery that is being done at the request of the patient but is done to correct a problem that is not life threatening at the moment.

emergency surgery Surgery that must be done right away to save the patient's life or limb.

holding area The room or area where a patient waits before going into the operating room; usually located next door to the operating room.

operating room The room or area where surgery is performed.

postoperative The period of time after the surgical procedure has been completed.

preoperative The time frame before a surgical procedure.

surgeon A physician who specializes in performing surgery.

surgical center A facility that operates solely to perform surgery.

surgical patient Someone who is admitted to the health care facility with the primary intent to have an operation.

Abbreviations

CRNA Certified Registered Nurse Anesthetist

ECG Electrocardiogram

EKG Electrocardiogram

ICU Intensive Care Unit

IV Intravenous

NPO Nothing by Mouth

OPS Outpatient Surgery

OR Operating Room

PACU Postanesthesia Care Unit

PAR Postanesthesia Room

PAT Preadmission Testing

Postop Postoperative

Preop Preoperative

Prep Preparation

RR Recovery Room

SDS Same Day Surgery

SDCS Same Day Cardiac Services

TF To Follow

SURGICAL PATIENTS

Persons admitted to the health care facility with the primary intent to have an operation are called **surgical patients**. These patients may be admitted as scheduled admissions or emergency admissions. They may be inpatients, outpatients, or same-day surgery (SDS)

TABLE 30-1 Surgeons and Their Specialty	
Surgeon	**Specialty**
Orthopedic surgeon	Bone surgeries, limb surgeries
Vascular surgeon	Vein and artery surgeries
Cardiovascular surgeon	Heart surgeries (cardiac), vascular surgeries
GYN surgeon	Surgeries involving women's reproductive organs

patients. A health care facility that operates solely for the purpose of performing surgical procedures is termed a **surgical center**. Surgical patients may also be admitted to a general hospital. Surgical centers often are connected to a general hospital, but they may also be stand-alone clinics privately owned and operated. All surgical centers must adhere to rules and regulations set forth by the federal and state governments.

A physician who specializes in performing surgery is called a **surgeon**. There are surgeons who specialize in particular types of surgery. Table 30-1 lists some of the more common types of surgeons.

ROUTINE SURGICAL PATIENT

A routine surgical patient is a person who has meet with the physician and decided to have a surgical procedure preformed. This procedure may be necessary for health reasons, or it may be cosmetic. **Elective surgery** is surgery that the patient chooses to have done to correct a condition that is not a life-or-death emergency.

SCHEDULING THE PATIENT

Routine surgical patients are scheduled by their surgeon's office for surgery before being admitted to the health care facility. The surgeon's office staff and the health care facility staff complete the surgical scheduling process. This process may include the surgeon's office and the facility's coordinating the date and time of the surgery according to the procedures at the facility. Most facilities have a certain day of the week that a surgeon is scheduled to perform elective surgeries. This type of scheduling allows the facility to schedule cases for all the surgeons on staff according to the number and types of operating suites available. It also allows for the best possible use of the operating area and staff. In small health care facilities, the operating room may be open for elective surgeries only Monday through Friday from 7 A.M. to 3 P.M., whereas in large facilities the operating room may be scheduled 24 hours a day 7 days a week. Often, the health care facility preadmission staff calls the patients a few days before they are to be admitted to collect personal information such as minor medical history and insurance information. They then start to process the paperwork required as well as provide the patient with instructions before surgery. The patient is notified of the time and day he or she should report to the health care facility. These instructions must be followed in order to have the surgery performed. If the surgery is to be performed before noon, the patient is usually asked to not eat or drink anything after midnight. "NPO after midnight" is how this request is often written.

The physician orders certain tests be to completed before surgery. These tests are called preoperative testing. Each facility has specific testing requirements before surgery. These requirements are stated in a health care system policy and procedures manual. Common preoperative tests are:

◆ Chest x-ray

◆ EKG, or ECG

◆ Laboratory tests

This testing must be completed and the results reported before the surgery time. If the results are found to be out of the normal limits, the surgeon may order certain medications or postpone the surgery. The testing may take place before the surgery in a department called preadmission testing (PAT). In this department, the nursing staff start completing the patient admission paperwork, perform the preoperative testing, and provide the patient and family with information and education related to the scheduled surgical procedure. Surgeries may be canceled if the preoperative testing is not within the normal limits required, if the patient has not followed the preoperative instructions correctly, or if the patient is not feeling well because of reasons not associated with the pending surgical procedure performed.

ADMITTING THE PATIENT

Often, patients are admitted to a holding area or outpatient surgery (OPS) department before surgery even if they will be staying overnight as an inpatient after the surgery has been performed. These departments are staffed to provide the care required by patients before going to the operating room. Other times the patients are admitted to the room in the department they will be returning to after the surgery and recovery process has been completed. All orders written before surgery are called **preoperative** (preop) orders. These orders must be completed before the patient can go to surgery. Preoperative orders will include:

◆ Nutrition orders

◆ Preparation (prep) orders

◆ Preoperative medication orders

◆ Activity orders

◆ Surgery to be performed

While the nurse is admitting the patient, the health unit coordinator prepares the chart that will accompany the patient to the operating room. This preparation consists of retrieving all the required paperwork, including test results from the various departments within the health care facility. To assist the health unit coordinator in double-checking that all the required paperwork is in order, the health care facility may have a preoperative checklist, which is used for every patient going to the operating room (OR). All requirements on this list must be completed before the patient can be sent to the operating room. A copy of a preop, or OR, checklist is shown in Figure 30-1.

The staff on the nursing unit are provided with a surgical schedule that lists key information about the number of surgical cases scheduled for surgery. The first copy of the

MARQUETTE GENERAL HEALTH SYSTEM

✓ **CHECKLIST** — ☐ SURGICAL   ☐ CARDIOVASCULAR

PATIENT LABEL

UNIT CLERK RESPONSIBILITIES:

1. ____ Surgical permit on chart. Limb disposal permits (2 copies) on chart.
2. ____ Anesthesia permit signed. (Not needed for Cardiac Cath Lab) ☐ Anes. to see   ☐ Parents to see Anes.   ☐ Local
3. ____ Pt. in isolation—OR notified: Date:_____ Time:_____   Type of isolation:_____.
4. ____ Latex allergy—OR notified: Date:_____ Time:_____.
5. ____ Labs within 60 days. ☐ Drawn on admission.
6. ____ EKG report on chart (within 24 hrs. for Cardiac Cath Lab).
7. ____ Chest x-ray report on chart. ☐ On admission.
8. ____ History and physical on chart.   ☐ MD notified   ☐ To see in pre-op   ☐ Other:_____.
9. ____ Old records on chart.   ☐ No old records   ☐ Microfilm/microfiche
10. ____ Type & screen ordered per transfusion service policy #100-028.
11. ____ Height and weight of patient entered into computer. IP.
12. ____ Height and weight of pediatric patient to pharmacy
13. ____ Pt. allergies or NKA entered into computer. IP.
14. ____ Two full pages of patient labels on inpatient chart.
15. ____ Urine or serum pregnancy test. ☐ To Lab at:_____.
16. ____ Physician Post Procedure Progress Notes placed in front of the progress notes.

CHART COMPLETED BY: _____ Date: _____ Time: _____

RN OR LPN RESPONSIBILITIES:

17. ____ Surgical permit signed. If not, please explain:_____
18. ____ Limb disposal permits signed (2 witnesses).
19. ____ ID band on non-operative side.
20. ____ Allergy band on.   ____ No allergy band needed.
      Patient has latex allergies ☐ YES   ☐ NO.   Latex Allergy Band on _____.
21. ____ Dentures removed. (Dentures, contact lenses, glasses and hearing aid should be left on patients for Cardiac Cath Lab).
22. ____ Contact lenses or glasses removed.
23. ____ Hearing aid removed.
24. ____ Jewelry removed (O.R. notified if unable to remove). Time:_____   Person Notified:_____.
25. ____ Make-up, nail polish, hair pins and hair pieces removed.
26. ____ Head cap and gown on. (No metal snaps for Cardiac Cath Lab patients).
27. ____ Prep completed.
28. ____ Catheter in place or voided.
29. ____ Lab values within normal limits (potassium must be 3.5 or above).
30. ____ TPR and B/P taken and charted.   B/P: _____   AP: _____   Temp: _____
      O_2 Sat_____   Resp._____.
31. ____ Pre-op medication given. (Administer preop sedation one hour prior to scheduled start of CABG surgery.)
32. ____ Antibiotic to be given in holding area taped to front of chart. If not why:_____.
33. ____ Chart with patient and patient ready for transport.
34. ____ Patient states hasn't had anything to eat or drink past midnight.
35. ____ Verify Surgical Site location.

Patient checked by **floor nurse:**_____ Date:_____ Time:_____

Holding Room RN verifies #32:_____ Date: _____ Time: _____

TIME OUT:

37. ____ Circulation has reviewed all information above & the surgical team agrees that they have:
      ☐ Correct Patient
      ☐ Correct Side: R_____ L_____
      ☐ Correct Site   ☐ Correct Procedure   ☐ Correct Position
      ☐ Correct implants/special equipment/other requirements
The permit/H&P agree with site, side & procedure to be completed.

Circulator:_____ Date:_____ Time:_____

Comments:_____
_____
_____
_____

D:\IC MGH\CheckList.pmd   1/89, Rev. 3/04 MRUR-subApprove: 8/5/03   Item# 760416

Figure 30-1 • *An OR checklist must be completed for each patient before the patient can be sent to the OR for surgery. (Courtesy of Marquette General Health System, Marquette, MI)*

CONFIDENTIAL OR Schedule

Second Copy

Estimated Time subject to change

OR #	Start Time	Patient Name	Sex	Age	Procedure	Surgeon	Anesthesia
1	07:30	Williams, Sally	F	41	TAH/BSO	Connors	White
	08:45	Brown, Lynn	F	35	Vag Hyster	Connors	White
2	07:30	Barry, Tim	M	57	CABG	Marren	Gross
	12:00	Winslow, Sally	F	65	CABG	Marren	Gross
	TF	Frommer, Ken	M	76	Exc. Anal Mass	Brown	Anderson
3	07:30	Krammer, Liz	F	34	IDET L-S1 C-Arm	Long	Thomas

Figure 30-2 • *The OR schedule is used by the health unit coordinator for needed information for patients going to the OR.*

schedule is usually distributed the night before surgery, and the second copy early on the morning of surgery (Figure 30-2).

This schedule lists the patient name, the surgery to be performed, the surgeon performing the surgery, and any other information that the health care facility requires. The first case of the day is denoted as such, with the next case listed with a specific time or listed as a "to follow (TF)" case. A TF case will be started after the first case has been completed. This information allows the health unit coordinator to know the approximate time that the patient should be transported to the OR. With this information, the health unit coordinator can plan when to have the chart ready as well as let the family know what time to arrive to see the patient before surgery. As can anything in a health care facility, times and events can change because of emergencies, so it is best to let the families know that this information is only an estimate. When the patient is ready and the operating room staff are ready for the patient, the patient will be transported to the area outside the operating room, where he or she is prepared for surgery. This area is called the **holding area**. In the holding area, the patient waits, the IV is started, medications may be given, and the anesthesia is started by the certified registered nurse anesthetist (CRNA) under the direction of the anesthesiologist.

The Patient Chart

The patient chart or charts must accompany the patient to the operating room. The chart is the device used to communicate with the health care team information regarding the patient when the patient is not able to communicate. The chart contains the following information in addition to the information found in a nonsurgical patient chart:

> *Surgical permit.* This permit, called informed consent, must be completed correctly (Figure 30-3). The name of the surgical procedure must be spelled out using no abbreviations. Before surgery, the patient must sign the permit indicating that the procedure has been explained along with all the information included in the permit.

MARQUETTE GENERAL HEALTH SYSTEM
Confirmation of Informed Consent

Patient Name: _____ Date of Birth: _____

The procedure, treatment or therapy is: _____

_____

_____

_____

_____

_____

My signature on this form confirms that the general purpose, potential benefits, possible risks, complications, and inconveniences of the procedure have been explained to my satisfaction by my physician or care provider, and the alternatives have been discussed. The possible outcomes of this procedure have been explained to me, and I understand there is no guarantee that any particular result will be obtained.

I voluntarily consent to the performance of the procedure named above by:

_____ (and his/her designated
Physician/Provider Name and Title
assistants) using whatever anesthetic, treatment, medical devices, equipment, medication, or transfusion necessary. *(See back for further information).* I further authorize my physician to do what is necessary in the event that unforseen conditions arise during the course of the procedure.

I also authorize the Hospital to dispose of body parts, tissue or fluids, if removed, and/or to preserve them for diagnostic, research of teaching purposes. I agree that any photographs or video recordings, if taken, may be used for medical, scientific or educational purposes with my identify protected.

Patient, physician, or staff may add comments or explanations. Each entry should be initials and dated.

_____

_____

_____

_____

_____

_____	_____
Signature of Patient Date	Signature of Witness Date
(Signature of Parent/Guardian if patient is a minor or incompetent. Signature of Patient's Advocate as appointed under Medical Durable Power of of Attorney	(Staff Member, physician/provider's office staff, patient's family member, or other person present when patient signed)

Confirmation of Informed Consent

Figure 30-3 • *The surgical permit must be filled out using no abbreviations. (Courtesy of Marquette General Health System, Marquette, MI) (continues)*

Description of Transfusion:

Blood is introduced into one of your veins using a sterile, disposable needle. The amount of blood transfused, and whether the transfusion will be of blood, or blood components such as plasma, is a judgment your physician will make based on your particular needs.

Risks of Transfusion:

Transfusions are a common procedure of relatively low risk. Some of the risks include:
- Bruising
- Hives or Rash
- Fever and Chills
- Shortness of Breath
- Immediate or delayed transfusion reaction, including shock, heart failure, and death
- Transmission of diseases, including but not limited to infections such as hepatitis or HIV

Alternatives:

If loss of blood poses serious threats in the course of your treatment, THERE MAY BE NO EFFECTIVE ALTERNATIVE TO BLOOD TRANSFUSION. However, if you have any further questions on this matter, your physician or his/her colleagues will fully explain the alternatives to you if it has not already been done.

Figure 30-3 • *continued*

Anesthesia permit. This permit is completed by the anesthesiologist and explained to the patient and the patient's family or guardian if the patient is not able to sign (Figure 30-4). A patient signature is required on this permit.

Required testing results for the surgical procedure.

Limb disposal permit. This permit needs to be filled out if the patient is having a limb removed so that the OR staff will know what to do with the removed limb (Figure 30-5). The patient may request that the health care facility dispose of the removed limb or that the limb be sent to a funeral home.

The health unit coordinator completes the permits for the patient and physician to sign. All information entered on permits must be spelled correctly, and the permit must contain no abbreviations. The patient's formal name must be used. The patient must sign the permits unless the patient is unable to sign. The following situations would require that the patient not sign the permits:

If the patient is under 18 years of age, and not an emancipated minor, the parent would sign.

If the patient has a guardian, the guardian would be required to sign.

If the patient is not able to sign, the next of kin would be required to sign.

If the patient has been given drugs that impair decision-making, the next of kin must sign the permit.

All of the appropriate signed permission forms must be within the patient's chart when he or she has a surgical procedure. The health unit coordinator is responsible for checking for these items and signing off that the chart contains the required items before the elective surgery patient can be sent to the operating room.

MARQUETTE GENERAL HEALTH SYSTEM   PRE-ANESTHESIA EVALUATION
PERMIT FOR ANESTHESIA

I do hereby consent to any anesthesia with the exception of: _____.
I fully understand that anesthesia is not an exact science. **Major complications include, but are not limited to:** death, stroke, heart attack, paralysis, liver and kidney failure, asthma, seizures, and brain damage. **Minor complications include, but are not limited to:** Phlebitis, nerve damage, rash and/or skin damage, broken dental work and/or damaged teeth, nausea, vomiting, sore throat, headaches, and infection. Potential adverse effects include recall of surgical events. Anesthesia at Marquette General is provided by both M.D. Anesthesiologists and Nurse Anesthetists under Anesthesiology supervision. I have received no commitment as to whom will administer my anesthetic. My signature on this form confirms that the general purpose, potential benefits, possible risks, complications, inconveniences and alternatives to care for the procedure have been explained to my satisfaction by my physician.

_____   _____   _____
Anesthesiologist/Witness   Patient or Legal Guardian   Date

NAME OF PATIENT _____

AGE _____   WEIGHT _____   HEIGHT _____

PROPOSED OPERATION _____

ALLERGIES _____

MEDICATIONS _____

ANESTHETIC HISTORY _____

_____

COULD YOU BE PREGNANT   ☐ YES   ☐ NO   ☐ NA

HISTORY OF JAUNDICE POSTSURGICAL   ☐ NO   ☐ YES _____

HISTORY OF LIVER DISEASE _____

FAMILY OR PERSONAL HISTORY OF ANESTHESIA COMPLICATIONS   ☐ NO   ☐ YES _____

H/O SMOKING   ☐ NO   ☐ YES _____   DENTAL PROBLEMS   ☐ NO   ☐ YES _____

RESPIRATORY	CARDIAC	DIABETES: ☐ NO ☐ YES
ASTHMA: ☐ NO ☐ YES	MI: ☐ NO ☐ YES	HYPERTENSION: ☐ NO ☐ YES
COPD: ☐ NO ☐ YES	ANGINA: ☐ NO ☐ YES	Kidney: _____
Auscultation _____	Auscultation _____	C.N.S. _____
HGB _____		
OTHER: _____		

ASA Classification   1   2   3   4   5   E   **ANESTHETIC PLAN**

Patient seen and evaluated by the undersigned who agrees that patient is an appropriate candidate for proposed anesthetic.

M.D. _____   Date _____

D:\IC MGH\PermitAnesth.pm6   4/97, Rev. 10/00, 4/01, 1/02   MRURsubApprove: 01/08/02   Item # 760233

Figure 30-4 • *The anesthesia permit must be signed by the anesthesiologist and patient or patient representative before the patient has surgery. (Courtesy of Marquette General Health System, Marquette, MI)*

MARQUETTE GENERAL HOSPITAL
CONSENT FOR DISPOSAL OF AMPUTATED MEMBER

Date _____

Hospital No. _____

This is to certify that I, _____, consent to the

disposal of my surgically removed _____
(fill in name of member)

by the following procedure:

1) I wish Marquette General Hospital to assume the responsibility for the disposal.

_____
Signature of Patient

Date: _____

Witnesses:

_____

_____

2) I wish Marquette General Hospital to release the amputated member to the

_____ **Funeral Home.**

_____
Signature of Patient

Date: _____

Witnesses:

_____

_____

C:PROJECTS/CONSENT/AMPUTATE.DOC   4/79, Rev. 2/96

Figure 30-5 • *The limb disposal permit must be completed if a limb is going to be removed during surgery. (Courtesy of Marquette General Health System, Marquette, MI)*

OPERATING ROOM

The **operating room** is the department where surgery is usually preformed in a hospital. This area is considered a nursing unit and is staffed with health care professionals. The staff includes:

Anesthesiologist. A physician who specializes in anesthesiology

Certified Registered Nurse Anesthetist (CRNA). The nurse who assists the anesthesiologist

Circulating nurse. The nurse who circulates in the operating room assisting with the different surgeries

Surgical technicians. Technicians who assist the surgeons

Scrub nurses. Nurses who scrub in and assist the surgeon

Health unit coordinator. Responsible for transcribing the orders on the patients while they are in the operating room and for preparing the correct paperwork and coordinating the flow of the operating room traffic

The operating room is protected from visitors. The patient's family is not permitted to go into the operating room with the patient. It is a sterile environment. After the surgery is completed, the patient goes either directly to the intensive care unit (ICU) or to the recovery room (RR). These areas may also be referred to as the postanesthesia room (PAR) or postanesthesia care unit (PACU). The health unit coordinator in the PACU will call to let the unit know the patient is in recovery. The health unit coordinator on the patient care unit has the responsibility to notify the nurse and the patient's family that the patient is on the unit. The health unit coordinator should not say anything to the family, other than that the surgery has been completed and the patient is now in the PAR. The decision as to which area the patient is sent to after surgery is based on the type of surgery performed and how the patient has responded to the anesthesia and surgical process.

POSTSURGICAL PATIENT

The patient is sent to the nursing unit after the surgery has been completed. This is called the **postoperative** (postop) period, the time after surgery has been completed. The chart accompanies the patient to the unit. The health unit coordinator should discontinue all physician and nursing orders written before the surgical procedure. The physician will have written a new set of orders. These orders are called postoperative orders, orders written after surgery (Figure 30-6). These orders contain activity orders, nutrition orders, medication orders, and other orders required for the postsurgical patient. The health unit coordinator transcribes these orders to the correct forms and requests services from the support service departments as ordered. After surgery, the forms used to document the patient's activities in the OR and recovery room are filed in the correct areas of the patient record so that the health care team can easily access the information. It is important that these forms be filed correctly.

PHYSICIAN'S ORDERS

MARQUETTE GENERAL HOSPITAL, INC.
MARQUETTE, MICHIGAN

Attending Physician	
J.R. LOVELL, M.D.	PATIENT LABEL

PROTOCOL FOR POST-OP ABDOMINAL SURGERY

DATE & HOUR	USE BALLPOINT PEN ONLY	PAGE 1 OF 1

1. NPO except for ice chips (clarify insulin orders if patient is diabetic). Clear liquid in a.m.

2. Strictly confined to bed. Up at bedside x 1 in p.m. Ambulate in a.m.

3. Cough and deep breathe every 2 hours for first 12 hours.

4. Routine post operative vital signs.

5. Hct and Hbg on 1st, 2nd and 4th post operative day.

6. I&O's.

7. Foley to dependent drainage. Remove in a.m. if urine clear. Obtain UA and culture on removal.

8. **Medications to be given together:** Demerol 100mg IM, every 3-4 hours. PRN for pain x 24 hours *and* Vistaril 50mg, IM, every 3-4 hours. PRN for pain x 24 hours.

9. Percodan, 1 or 2 PO, every 3 hours, PRN for pain for duration of stay.

10. Halcion, 0.25mg, PO, HS, PRN for insomnia, SOS x 1 for duration of stay.

11. Colace, 100mg, 1 BID, PO, until BM. Start in a.m.

12. Compazine, 10mg, IM, every 6 hours. PRN for nausea and vomiting.

_____, M.D.

Date/Time _____

C:\PhyOrd\Surgical\POAbdSrgyLov.pmd 4/01, Rev. 6/03

Figure 30-6 • *Postoperative orders are written by the surgeon after surgery has been completed. (Courtesy of Marquette General Health System, Marquette, MI)*

EMERGENCY SURGERY

A patient requiring emergency surgery may be admitted to the health care facility. **Emergency surgery** cannot wait to be scheduled but must be done as soon as possible to save the patient's life. This type of emergency may interrupt the OR schedule, causing the next scheduled patient to wait longer than planned. If the OR is closed, an emergency crew must be called in to perform the surgery. Most health care facilities have staff on call for these types of emergencies. On-call staff must be prepared to come to work if they are needed. A health unit coordinator may be on call for the operating room or recovery room. In emergencies, the patient requirements for surgery are waived, because there may not be time to get the preoperative tests completed. If the patient is unable to sign the OR and anesthesia permits, the next of kin may sign, or, if there is a guardian, he or she may sign. Emergency situations require the health care team to work together quickly and efficiently.

TRANSCRIPTION STEPS

Table 30-2 lists the steps that should be taken when transcribing postoperative orders.

TABLE 30-2   Transcription Steps for Postoperative Orders

Transcription Step	Key Points
1. Read the entire order set thoroughly.	Careful reading of the orders allows the health unit coordinator to review, prioritize, and check for incomplete or illegible orders.
2. Prioritize orders.	Determine the urgency of the orders in all the charts needing transcription. Decide what orders in the order set need to be transcribed first.
3. If medications are included in the order set, send the order carbon or a copy to the pharmacy.	The pharmacy requires a copy of a signed order. The pharmacy may supply the items used by completed the nursing orders. The pharmacy needs to know that the patient had a surgical procedure performed and must discontinue all previous medication orders.
4. Communicate the order to the individual or department that will be performing the order.	The health unit coordinator may schedule appointments, notify ancillary departments of needs, order equipment necessary to perform the order, and contact the nursing personnel responsible for the patient.

(continues)

TABLE 30-2 *(continued)*	
Transcription Step	**Key Points**
5. Record the orders on the patient Kardex or care plan.	Most health care facilities have a form used to keep track of current orders and the plan of care for a patient. It is important to document the type of surgery performed along with the date the surgery was performed.
6. Record medication orders on the medication administration record (MAR).	Most health care facilities automatically generate medication administration records every 24 hours based on orders entered into a computer. When a patient returns from the OR, a new set of MARs must be generated or written. All previous medications are discontinued, and only the postop orders are followed.
7. Check off each order in the set as completed.	Placing a check mark by each order as it is transcribed can help the health unit coordinator track orders even when interrupted. Discontinue all orders written before surgery.
8. Re-read and check all work for accuracy.	Because of multiple requests received by the health unit coordinator, re-reading and checking work is a necessity.
9. Sign off the order with name, title, date, and time.	The health unit coordinator is accountable for the orders transcribed.

SUMMARY

Patients who are admitted to the health care facility for elective or emergency surgery will have the surgery performed in the operating room. The operating room has specially trained staff and equipment needed to perform surgical procedures. The needs of the surgical patient vary depending on the surgery performed and the recovery of the patient. It is important to remember that after a surgical procedure has been performed, the physician must write postoperative orders; all orders written before surgery are discontinued.

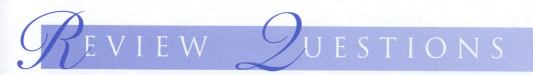

REVIEW QUESTIONS

Write out the terms for the following abbreviations.

1. Pre op

2. OR

3. CRNA

4. Post op

5. PACU

6. RR

7. List three items that would be included on the patient chart when the patient is going to the OR.

8. List three different health care professionals who work in the OR.

9. Describe what information is found on the operating schedule.

TRANSCRIPTION PRACTICE

Go to the CD-ROM for transcription exercises that support the content in this chapter.

NAHUC CERTIFICATION EXAM

CONTENT AREAS

I. A. 2   Interpret medical symbols, abbreviations, and terminology

I. A. 6   Enter orders on a Kardex

I. A. 15   Prepare surgical charts

I. A. 16   Process postoperative charts

I. B. 1   Notify staff of new orders

II. H. 4   Demonstrate knowledge of informed consent

III. B. 4   Enter orders via computers

THROUGH THE EYES

OF A HEALTH CARE PROFESSIONAL

The OR staff share their thoughts.

The health unit coordinators are an important link in readying the patient for surgery. They are the key personnel in preparing the chart by locating the required test results, completing the permits, filing the reports, and coordinating the transportation of the patient to the OR holding areas. The health unit coordinator communicates with the OR health unit coordinator solving any issues they can so as not to delay the surgical procedures. This allows for smooth patient flow and keeping the activity on schedule.

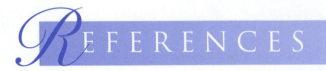

REFERENCES

Hegner, B. R. (2004). *Nursing assistant: A nursing process approach* (9th ed.). Clifton Park, NY: Thomson Delmar Learning.

Smith, S. F. (2004). *Clinical nursing skills* (6th ed.). Upper Saddle River, NJ: Prentice-Hall Health.

Support Services Orders

Learning Objectives

Upon completion of this chapter and review questions, the learner should be able to:

1. Demonstrate knowledge of information systems terminology.

2. List two reasons why health unit coordinators contact the hospital information management department.

3. Define which support service department should be contacted when a solicitor is noticed in the facility.

4. Explain the role of the health unit coordinator with managed care.

5. List the eight the rules of e-mail etiquette.

6. Identify the reasons why the health unit coordinator will need to contact social services.

7. List two ways to contact pastoral care.

8. Discuss some examples of when the health unit coordinator would need to call the maintenance department.

Key Terms

central processing unit   The central part of a computer system.

continuity of care Uninterrupted and consistent care of a patient.

downloading The copying of information from one computer to another.

hardware The visible parts of a computer system.

home page The first page you see when you start your browser.

HTML tags Special words that have different effects; a tag starts with the < symbol and ends with the > symbol.

hyperlink Refers to a link embedded in a document.

hypertext document (Web page). Contains hyperlinks to other documents stored locally or anywhere on the World Wide Web.

icon A picture used to represent an object.

incident report A form that is used to document accidents and thefts in a health care facility.

interface Refers to the connection between two computer components.

local area network (LAN) A data communications system often confined to a limited geographic area with moderate to high data rates.

mainframe A large-scale computer system that can house comprehensive software and several peripherals.

managed care A system of providing health care that controls costs through the cooperation of many programs in which physicians accept constraints on the amount charged for medical care and the patient is limited in the choice of a physician.

maximize To make a window take up the full screen.

menu The list of available functions for selection by the operator, usually displayed on the computer screen once a program has been entered.

minimize To shrink a program down so that it is displayed only on the task bar.

modem A device that allows your computer to communicate with another computer over phone lines.

old records Patient medical charts or records from a previous hospitalization.

port A place of access to a device or network, used for input and output of digital and analog signals.

Read Only Memory Computer memory in which data can be routinely read but written to only once using special means when the ROM is manufactured; used for storing data or programs (e.g., operating systems) permanently.

real time Data acted upon immediately instead of being accumulated and processed at a later time.

resolution The smallest significant number to which a measurement can be determined.

response time The elapsed time between the generation of the last character of a message at a terminal and the receipt of the first character of the reply.

server A computer running software that allows it to control the sharing of resources among many computers.

shutdown command A command issued before turning off the computer so that any data in memory can be saved to disk.

software The nonphysical parts of a computer system that include computer programs such as the operating system, high-level languages, and applications programs.

taskbar The portion of the screen including the Start button, the time display, and everything in between.

toolbar A collection of buttons, usually organized by category.

Webmaster One who develops and maintains a Web site.

Web page All the text, graphics, and sound visible with a single access to a Web site; what you see when you request a particular URL.

Web server The hardware and software required to make Web pages available for delivery to others on networks connected with yours.

Web site A collection of electronic "pages" of information on a Web server.

Abbreviations

CAD Coronary Artery Disease

CHF Congestive Heart Failure

CPU Central Processing Unit

ISP Internet Service Provider

NHP Nursing Home Placement

SS Social Services

LAN Local Area Network

PHI Personal Health Information

ROM Read Only Memory

URL Uniform Resource Locator or Universal Resource Locator

SUPPORT SERVICES

This chapter expands on the introductory information of support services in Chapter 7. The focus of this chapter is *communication* with support service personnel. Information needed to communicate and work with the other departments is important in providing accurate and timely patient care.

BUSINESS OFFICE

Medical bills do not often reach patients until they have been discharged. However, the patient or patient family may be concerned about a payment system. If the health unit coordinator receives questions about the facility's billing and payment plan, the health unit coordinator must refer the requester to the business office or patients' accounts department. It will be very helpful for the health unit coordinator to provide the telephone number as well as directions on how to find the business office when billing questions are asked.

THE LANGUAGE OF INFORMATION SERVICES

Computers are everywhere in health care. Throughout this textbook, there are many examples of computer usage. For instance, the admissions department has specific patient insurance information, and the laboratory may need to send personnel to collect blood work on a patient or have the results from tests done earlier in the day.

When the computer is not working properly, the computer services department needs to be notified. Because most computer services personnel do not have medical or health-related backgrounds and most health unit coordinators have not continued their studies in computers, it may be difficult for the two to communicate. Knowing the following terms will assist in this communication.

Central processing unit (CPU). The central part of a computer system that performs operations on data. In a personal computer, the CPU is typically a single microprocessor integrated circuit.

Downloading. The copying of information from one computer to another.

Hardware. The visible parts of a computer system, such as the circuitboards, chassis, enclosures, peripherals, and cables. It does not include data or computer programs.

Home page. The first page you see when you start your browser; often used (erroneously) to mean the first of a logical set of related Web pages or the welcome page or even the entire Web site.

HTML tags. Special words that have different effects; a tag starts with the < symbol and ends with the > symbol.

Hyperlink. This refers to a link embedded in a document. The link can point to a predefined position in the same document or another document or file stored locally or on a different server or computer.

Hypertext document (Web page). Contains hyperlinks to other documents stored locally or anywhere on the World Wide Web.

Icon. A picture used to represent an object. Each type of object has a different icon. That is, different types of files each have an icon representing the file type. Microsoft Word files have the MS Word icon; Microsoft Excel files have the MS Excel icon.

Interface. Refers to the connection between two computer components and/or a computer and its peripherals, printers, scanners, and so on.

ISP. Internet Service Provider.

Local area network (LAN). A data communications system confined to a limited geographic area with moderate to high data rates. The area served may consist of a single building, a cluster of buildings, or a campus-type arrangement. The network uses some type of switching technology and does not use common carrier circuits (i.e., telephone lines), although it may provide access to other public or private networks.

Mainframe. A large-scale computer system that can house comprehensive software and several peripherals.

Maximize. To make a window take up the full screen.

Menu. The list of available functions for selection by the operator, usually displayed on the computer screen once a program has been entered.

Minimize. To shrink a program down so that it is displayed only on the task bar.

Modem. A device that allows your computer to communicate with another computer over phone lines. Usually, the modem is inside the computer (internal), but there are external modems that plug into the back of a computer.

Port. A place of access to a device or network, used for input and output of digital and analog signals.

Real time. Data acted upon immediately instead of being accumulated and processed at a later time.

Resolution. The smallest significant number to which a measurement can be determined. For example, a converter with 12-bit resolution can resolve 1 part in 4096.

Response time. The elapsed time between the generation of the last character of a message at a terminal and the receipt of the first character of the reply. It includes terminal delay and network delay.

ROM, Read Only Memory. Computer memory in which data can be routinely read but written to only once using special means when the ROM is manufactured. ROM is used for storing data or programs (e.g., operating systems) permanently.

Server. A computer running software that allows it to control the sharing of resources among many computers.

Shutdown command. A command issued before turning off the computer, so that any data in memory can be saved to disk. To do this, click the Start button on your taskbar, then click "shutdown," then click "yes."

Software. The nonphysical parts of a computer system that include computer programs such as the operating system, high-level languages, and applications programs.

Taskbar. The portion of the screen including the Start button, the time display, and everything in between. The Start button gives access to the programs installed on the computer, the system settings, a shutdown command, and more. Immediately to the right of the Start button are buttons for each program currently running. There also will probably be little icons to the left of the time display for miscellaneous programs that make the computer work.

Toolbar. A collection of buttons, usually organized by category.

Webmaster. One who develops and maintains a Web site.

Web page. All the text, graphics, and sound visible with a single access to a Web site; what you see when you request a particular URL (Universal Resource Locator).

Web server. The hardware and software required to make Web pages available for delivery to others on networks connected with yours.

Web site. A collection of electronic "pages" of information on a Web server.

Electronic mail, or e-mail, is becoming more popular and is being increasingly used in health care. E-mail saves time by eliminating the need to make many phone calls throughout the day, for instance when the person on the other end is busy, so the caller has to hold, or if the receiver is not available and follow-up calls need be to made. E-mail has its own language and rules. E-mail should be used as a means to inform and persuade. Eight rules on e-mail etiquette are listed below.

1. Ensure that the subject line reflects the message.

2. Double-check the To: and CC: fields.

3. Keep messages short. If a lengthy message needs to be sent, a separate document should be made and sent as an attachment in the e-mail.

4. Be informal but not too casual.

5. Send a complete message. Do not expect people to read things into the message.

6. Proofread before sending. Go on to something else for a while, then come back and reread the message before sending it.

7. Do not use all capital letters; this can be construed to mean shouting.

8. Never swear or be abusive.

Contacting the computer services department just requires a telephone call. Once the call has been placed, explaining the situation will be easier and more effective by knowing the correct terminology.

EDUCATION DEPARTMENT

Health care facilities are designed so that patients with a certain diagnosis are cared for on a unit that specializes in that field of care. The advancement of health care research and technology has made for any one area of care to be divided into very separated and complex fields. For example, saying that a patient has heart disease can mean the person has congestive heart failure (CHF), coronary artery disease (CAD), long QT syndrome, or one or more of many other heart-related conditions. Keeping current with the ever-changing discoveries, treatments and technology is crucial in health care today. The nurse educator has multiple responsibilities, ranging from coordinating the orientation of new nursing staff to providing continuing education to the staff. The staff nurse, in turn, is responsible for educating the patient.

MANAGED CARE DEPARTMENT

Managed care is a system of providing health care that controls costs through the cooperation of many programs in which physicians accept constraints on the amount charged for medical care and the patient is limited in the choice of a physician. In promoting managed care, health care facilities have developed managed care initiatives. Managed care initiatives are multidisciplinary in that a team of clinical experts coordinate the approach to health care delivery. These team members develop tools to assist the health care providers in implementing specific strategies to improve patient outcomes. The tools may include treatment guidelines, standing order sets, teaching records, and provider and patient education materials. See Figure 31-1 and 31-2 for examples of managed care tools.

The role of the health unit coordinator is to know which specialists to contact, notifying the various team members of upcoming meetings, and ensuring that the workstation

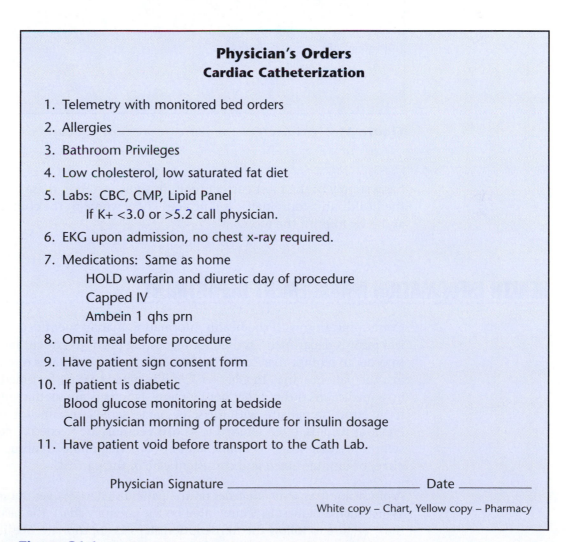

Physician's Orders
Cardiac Catheterization

1. Telemetry with monitored bed orders
2. Allergies _____
3. Bathroom Privileges
4. Low cholesterol, low saturated fat diet
5. Labs: CBC, CMP, Lipid Panel
     If K+ <3.0 or >5.2 call physician.
6. EKG upon admission, no chest x-ray required.
7. Medications: Same as home
     HOLD warfarin and diuretic day of procedure
     Capped IV
     Ambein 1 qhs prn
8. Omit meal before procedure
9. Have patient sign consent form
10. If patient is diabetic
     Blood glucose monitoring at bedside
     Call physician morning of procedure for insulin dosage
11. Have patient void before transport to the Cath Lab.

Physician Signature _____ Date _____

White copy – Chart, Yellow copy – Pharmacy

Figure 31-1 • *Sample managed care standing orders*

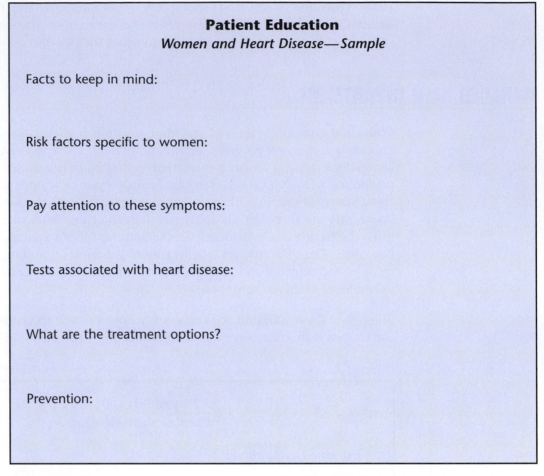

Patient Education
Women and Heart Disease—Sample

Facts to keep in mind:

Risk factors specific to women:

Pay attention to these symptoms:

Tests associated with heart disease:

What are the treatment options?

Prevention:

Figure 31-2 • *Sample managed care patient education materials*

has a supply of the most current tools. In some facilities, these tools are kept online so the health unit coordinator will need to know where in the computer to locate them and how to print the tools.

HEALTH INFORMATION MANAGEMENT DEPARTMENT

Communication with the health information management department, or the medical records department, is used for requesting previous patient records and charts. In order to request these records, the health unit coordinator often needs more than just the patient name. In Chapter 7, it was stated that patient medical records are filed by a medical record number not by name. Numbers are used in an effort to reduce filing errors on patients with the same name, same last name, or even a similar name. Previous records, often referred to as **old records** are needed to compare previous symptoms, diagnoses, recommendations, and treatments to ensure **continuity of care**, or uninterrupted and consistent care of the patient.

A physician may write an order on the patient's chart to "get old records on the unit." When such a request is documented on the patient's chart, the health unit coordinator must be sure to follow the transcription steps as appropriate. See Table 31-1 and note that, in this case, steps 3 and 6 may be eliminated.

Some facilities require just a phone call to the department to request the records; others require that the request be made via the computer. When old records are requested immediately, even if the facility requires a computer conversation for requests, a telephone call should be placed to express the urgent need. Using the list of support services telephone extensions, as shown in Figure 31-3, will help expedite the call. Table 31-1 lists the transcription steps for requests to the medical records department.

In some health care facilities, it is the medical records department's responsibility to photocopy records when necessary. When a patient is going to be transferred to another facility, such as a nursing home, the receiving facility will require various records documenting that the patient is ready to be transferred and to ensure continuity of care. In order to ensure confidentiality of PHI, or personal health information, a consent form to release medical records has to be completed and signed by the patient. This form limits the number of forms to be copied. A sample release is shown in Figure 31-4.

TheBestHospital
Quick List Phone Numbers
5th Floor

		UNIT PHONE #S		
Admitting Dept.	2234		**Room**	**Phone**
Business Office	2237		101	555
Cardiology	2221		**102**	**556**
Central Services	2243		103	557
Computer Services	2238		**104**	**558**
Diagnostic Xray	2227		105	559
Dietary	2228		**106**	**560**
Employee Health	2239		107	561
Environmental Services	2244		**108**	**562**
GI Lab	2222		109	563
Human Services	2240		**110**	**564**
Maintenance	2241		111	565
Medical Records	2242		**112**	**566**
Occupational Therapy	2232		113	567
Pastoral Care	2236		**114**	**568**
Path Lab	2223		115	569
Pharmacy	2229		**116**	**570**
Pharmacy	2230		117	571
Physical Therapy	2231		**118**	**572**
Pulmonary Dx	2224		119	573
Pulmonary Rehab	2225		**120**	**574**
Respiratory Therapy	2226		121	575
Security	**2235**			
Speech Therapy	2233			

Figure 31-3 • *Quicklist of support services telephone extensions*

TABLE 31-1 Transcription Steps for Requests to Medical Records

Transcription Step	Key Points
1. Read the entire order set thoroughly.	Careful reading of the orders allows the health unit coordinator to review, prioritize, and check for incomplete or illegible orders.
2. Prioritize orders.	Determine the urgency of the orders in all the charts needing transcription. Decide what orders in the order set need to be transcribed first.
3. If medications are included in the order set, send the order carbon or a copy to the pharmacy. (This step may be eliminated if no medication orders are included in the order set.)	It is crucial that the pharmacy receive the physician's medication orders.
4. Communicate the order to the individual or department that will be performing the order.	The health unit coordinator will request the old records via the telephone or the order will be entered into the computer to notify the department of the order.
5. Record the orders on the patient Kardex or care plan.	Most health care facilities have a form used to keep track of current orders and the plan of care for a patient. Documentation on the Kardex is usually done in pencil and updated as orders are changed, discontinued, and added.
6. Record medication orders on the medication administration record (MAR). (This step may be eliminated if no medication orders are included in the order set.)	If the order contains preprocedure medications, the health unit coordinator may be responsible for writing the medication on the MAR. Check your facility's policies and procedures.
7. Check off each order in the set as completed.	Placing a check mark by each order as it is transcribed can help the health unit coordinator track orders even when interrupted.
8. Re-read and check all work for accuracy.	Because of multiple requests received by the health unit coordinator, re-reading and checking work is a necessity.
9. Sign off the order with name, title, date, and time.	The health unit coordinator is accountable for the orders transcribed.

TheBestHospital
RELEASE OF MEDICAL INFORMATION FORM

1. **Patient Full Name** _____

2. **Date of Birth** _____ / _____ / _____

   Address _____

   City/State _____

3. **Health Information to Be Disclosed:**

   Laboratory Reports—specify report and date _____

   Radiology Reports—specify report and date _____

   Billing Records _____

   Other _____

4. **Purpose of Disclosure** _____

5. **Persons/Organizations Authorized to Release Information:**

   Name of Health Care Provider _____

   Address _____

   City _____ State _____ Zip Code _____

6. **Persons/Organizations Authorized to Receive Information:**

   Self _____

   Name of Health Care Provider _____

   Address _____

   City _____ State _____ Zip Code _____

7. **Signature of Patient/Legal Representative**

   _____ Date _____

8. **Witness** (when applicable) _____

You are not obliated to authorize a disclosure of your health information. You may limit the amount of information as you wish.

You have the right to inspect or copy the health information to be released for this authorization.

You have the right to receive a copy of this consent form.

You have the right to refuse to sign this authorization.

You have the right to revoke this authorization.

Figure 31-4 • *Release of medical information form*

SECURITY DEPARTMENT

One of the responsibilities of the security department is to make rounds of the entire health care facility inside and out. Security personnel patrol all of the workstations, so the health unit coordinator sees and greets them on a daily basis. The security officer is responsible for providing protection from assault, robbery, and solicitation. Solicitation of personnel and especially of patients and patients' families and friends is never allowed on the health care facility's property. At times, solicitors do get into the building without being noticed. A health unit coordinator who notices a solicitor should call the security department immediately and report the person. At times, theft of personal or facility property occurs. At such times, it is the health unit coordinator who calls the security department to report the theft. In addition to calling the security department, the health unit coordinator needs to file a report. This report is known as an **incident report**. The health unit coordinator knows where the incident reports are kept and should retrieve and start completing the report before the arrival of security. This incident report will also be completed if an employee or visitor falls on the grounds and injures himself or herself. Figure 31-5 shows an incident report.

Requesting services from the security department always requires just a phone. The health unit coordinator should memorize the security department's phone number.

SOCIAL SERVICES

A common order seen by a health unit coordinator is "SS for NHP." This means the social services (SS) department should see the patient and assist the patient and family in choosing a nursing home (NHP, nursing home placement). Once the nursing home has been selected, the social worker will assist the health unit coordinator by listing all the forms the facility of choice requires when receiving the transferred patient. The social worker will assist in arranging the transportation for these transfers as well.

Social workers also may be requested to help the patient find help from the community, such as drug and alcohol abuse support groups.

Communication with social services is really a two-way process. Once again, it is the health unit coordinator who initiates the communication by contacting social services first. The social services department will be contacted according to the employer's policy. Many facilities require only a phone call to the department; other facilities requires that this notification be made via the computer. No matter how the request is made, the complete request needs to be shared when initially contacting social services. This may be done by repeating the order verbatim. When the order to contact social services is a written order on the physician's order sheet, the steps of transcription must be followed, as shown in Table 31-2.

CHAPLAIN SERVICES DEPARTMENT

The original request for chaplain services may come from the patient's nurse. The patient herself or the patient's family member or friend may call or stop at the workstation and talk to the health unit coordinator to see if such services are available. Requests such as this need to be handled empathetically and professionally.

TheBestMedicalCenter
INCIDENT REPORT

If patient, addressograph

Last Name	First Name
Address	
City	State Zip

DESCRIPTION OF INCIDENT:

INCIDENT LOCATION

INCIDENT DATE & TIME

WITNESS(ES)

PROPERTY LOSS OR DAMAGE

Person Completing the Report

NOT A PERMANENT PART OF THE CHART, FORWARD TO SECURITY.

Figure 31-5 • *Incident report*

TABLE 31-2 Transcription Steps for Social Services Orders

Transcription Step	Key Points
1. Read the entire order set thoroughly.	Careful reading of the orders allows the health unit coordinator to review, prioritize, and check for incomplete or illegible orders.
2. Prioritize orders.	Determine the urgency of the orders in all the charts needing transcription. Decide what orders in the order set need to be transcribed first.
3. If medications are included in the order set, send the order carbon or a copy to the pharmacy.	It is crucial that the pharmacy receive the physician's medication orders.
4. Communicate the order to the individual or department that will be performing the order.	The health unit coordinator will request the social services via the telephone, or the order will be entered into the computer to notify the department of the order.
5. Record the orders on the patient Kardex or care plan.	Most health care facilities have a form used to keep track of current orders and the plan of care for a patient. Documentation on the Kardex is usually done in pencil and updated as orders are changed, discontinued, and added.
6. Record medication orders on the medication administration record (MAR).	If the order contains preprocedure medications, the health unit coordinator may be responsible for writing the medications on the MAR. Check your facility's policies and procedures.
7. Check off each order in the set as completed.	Placing a check mark by each order as it is transcribed can help the health unit coordinator track orders even when interrupted.
8. Re-read and check all work for accuracy.	Because of multiple requests received by the health unit coordinator, re-reading and checking work is a necessity.
9. Sign off the order with name, title, date, and time.	The health unit coordinator is accountable for the orders transcribed.

The health unit coordinator may contact the chaplain services department when emergencies or expirations occur. The health unit coordinator develops various skills, one of which is to be alert and aware of all the activity going about on the unit. This awareness may alert the health unit coordinator to a need for action even before a request is made. Chaplains have been trained to handle situations in which they go to consult a patient or family and find their services are not wanted.

MAINTENANCE DEPARTMENT

Knowing how to prioritize communications with the maintenance department is beneficial to the nursing unit, to the maintenance department, and to the health unit coordinator. For example, the nursing assistant comes to the workstation and tells the health unit coordinator that the light bulb at the end of the B wing is burnt out and needs replacement. This request should be communicated the same day, but it is not something that should interrupt the transcription of orders or the organizing of nursing home papers that the health unit coordinator may be in the middle of completing. On the other hand, a statement to the health unit coordinator that the elevator is stuck between the third and fourth floor must be relayed to the maintenance department immediately.

There are various commercial computer programs that a health care facility may purchase to be used for sending and receiving maintenance requests. Some facilities may have their own computer conversation to use or use just a phone call to the department to contact the maintenance department. If the service is needed immediately, both a written request via the computer and a phone call will be necessary. When contacting the maintenance department, it is important for the health unit coordinator to remain calm and give as much detail about the situation as possible. Whether or not the health care facility has a computer conversation for the maintenance department, the phone number for this department should be kept near the telephone. Refer to Figure 31-3.

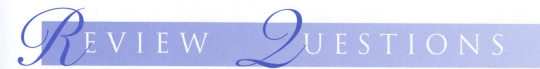

SUMMARY

There are many departments that are responsible for keeping a health care facility operating smoothly and safely. It takes a lot of teamwork to organize a safe recovery and discharge of the patient. It is the health unit coordinator who is at the hub of all the communication involved in organizing this teamwork. Each patient has personal needs. In order for the health unit coordinators to share these needs with the appropriate departments, they must learn the means of communication with all departments.

REVIEW QUESTIONS

1. List two reasons why health unit coordinators contact the hospital information management department.

2. Define which support service department should be contacted when a solicitor is noted in the facility.

3. Define managed care.

4. List the eight the rules of e-mail etiquette.

5. Identify the reasons why the health unit coordinator needs to contact social services.

6. List two ways to contact pastoral care.

TRANSCRIPTION PRACTICE

Go to the CD-ROM for transcription exercises that support the content in this chapter.

NAHUC CERTIFICATION EXAM

CONTENT AREAS

I. A. 2   Interpret medical symbols, abbreviations, and terminology

I. A. 6   Enter orders on a Kardex

I. A. 8   Initiate pathway protocols

I. B. 1   Notify staff of new orders

II. D. 9   Arrange for maintenance and repair of equipment

III. B. 1   Maintain computer census (i.e., ADT functions)

III. B. 4   Enter orders via computers

III. B. 6   Prepare documents using computer software

III. B. 7   Generate reports using computers

III. B. 8   Operate computers safely and correctly

III. B. 9   Troubleshoot problems with computers

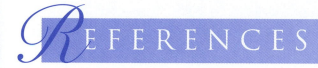

THROUGH THE EYES

OF A HEALTH CARE PROFESSIONAL

Health unit coordinators are vital in implementing managed care initiative orders. Managed care initiatives must be implemented as soon as possible. It is the alert health unit coordinator who identifies the need to pull the appropriate managed care initiative and place it on the patient's chart so the physician and nurse have it readily available. Health unit coordinators are instrumental in ensuring completeness by reading through the initiatives and carefully noting standards which may be embedded such as patient-controlled analgesic orders included in postoperative pathways.

REFERENCES

http://www.dell.com/glossary Accessed November 11, 2003.

http://www.helpwithpcs.com/jargonmenu.htm/ Accessed November 11, 2003.

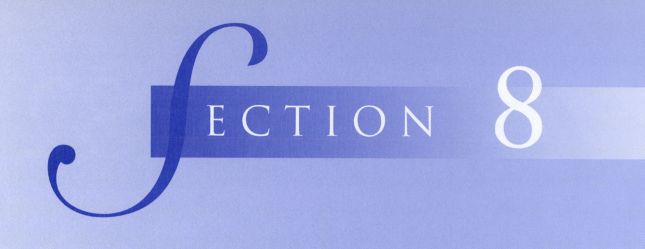

SECTION 8

Professional Development

Professional Development

Learning Objectives

Upon completion of this chapter and review questions, the learner should be able to:

1. List five potential employers of health unit coordinators.

2. List three guidelines for completing employment applications.

3. List and describe five sections of a résumé.

4. List five questions that may be asked in a job interview.

5. Explain how to become nationally certified as a health unit coordinator.

6. Explain how to maintain current certification status.

7. List two professional development activities.

Key Term

transferable skills Tasks that one may have learned in one job or setting that can be used within another setting.

PROFESSIONAL DEVELOPMENT

For most students, the final goal at the completion of an education program is to find employment within that field. Many of the students who complete this book will enter into a job search. Once employed, they may look for ways to continue their professional growth. This chapter addresses career and continuing education opportunities and strategies for a life-long process of professional development.

FINDING EMPLOYMENT

IDENTIFYING CAREER OPPORTUNITIES

One of the first steps in the job search process is to locate and research potential employers. There are many resources available to job seekers. A popular resource is the Career Resource Library at America's Career Infonet (*www.acinet.org/acinet/library*). This Web site offers tips and suggestions for all phases of the job search process including résumé writing, interviewing, and negotiating.

The more employers identified, the better one's chances in the job search. Do not limit the job search to inpatient acute care facilities only or to searching for a job under only one title. Identify employers that need employees with health unit coordinating skills. In the early chapters of this textbook, a coordinator was defined as one who facilitates the activities of people engaged in a common action to work together smoothly and harmoniously. A health unit coordinator is one who does this facilitating in the health care setting. Thinking of the employer as one who needs those types of skills opens the door to employment possibilities in almost any setting that provides health care services.

Clark and Mazza (1999) explain the role of the health unit coordinator in hospital departments such as a birth center, burn unit, dialysis, emergency department, geriatrics, pediatrics, oncology, mental health, neurology, rehabilitation, orthopedics, surgery, postanesthesia, and special intensive care units, to name a few. Clark and Mazza (1999) also write about health unit coordinators in settings other than acute care facilities such as agency staffing services, community mental health services, community and vocational colleges, criminal justice facilities, hospice, extended-care facilities, medical offices, home care, rehabilitation facilities, and research institutions.

To find names and addresses of health care facilities, access a local phone book or Web directory. Read through newspapers and health care publications. Look beyond the classified ads for news about expansions and new developments. That type of news may provide information about hiring. Networking is an important part of the job search. Telling people about the training one has completed and that one is in the market for a job will help in the job search.

APPLICATION PROCESS

Depending on the health care facility, one may be required to complete the application in person or electronically. It is important to prepare whether submitting the application in person or online. Gather the information for applications before completing one. Be sure to have complete names, addresses, and phone numbers of previous employers, schools, and references. One suggestion is to complete a sample application with all the information and bring the application when applying for jobs (Figure 32-1). The application may be the first impression the employer has of you. Make sure it is a positive first impression. Some application tips follow.

◆ Be prepared to complete the application on-site or online.

◆ Bring a pen.

◆ Bring a pocket dictionary to make sure there are no spelling errors on the application.

◆ Read the application carefully and follow the directions exactly. If there are spaces that require a check, mark a ✓; if there are spaces that require an _x_, mark an _x_. Be sure to list items in the order requested. For example, does the application indicate to list the most recent job first or to list previous jobs in chronological order? Be careful not to write in any space that states "for office use only."

◆ Complete applications in ink, being careful not to make errors.

◆ Fill in all the blank spaces or draw a line through or write "not applicable" to questions that do not apply. For example, if the application has a question about military service and you have none, do not just leave the space blank; write "not applicable."

◆ Before submitting the application, read through it carefully, checking for errors. If there are errors, it is better to ask for another application form than to submit an application with mistakes. If submitting an electronic application, proofread carefully before sending.

◆ Ask to attach a résumé, diplomas, and letters of recommendation with the application.

RÉSUMÉS

Health care facilities may vary in their requirement for a résumé. However, it is best to be prepared and have a résumé for the job search process (Figure 32-2). A neat and simple style of résumé is recommended, especially if submitting electronically. Most résumés are one page long and are divided into sections:

◆ Name and contact information

◆ Objective

◆ Education

◆ Employment

◆ Personal Interests and Activities

Name and Contact Information

Use your full name as listed on the job application. Include your address, phone number with area code, and e-mail address. If using a private phone number with an answering

Personal Information

First Name: _____

Middle Name: _____

Last Name: _____

Social Security Number: _____

Street Address: _____

City: _____ State: _____ Zip: _____ County: _____

Home Phone: _____

Business Phone: _____

Have you ever applied for employment with us?

Yes: _____ No: _____ If yes, when? _____

Position Desired

Title: _____

Desired Salary: $_____

Work Eligibility

Are you eligible to work in the United States?   Yes: _____ No: _____

Are you available to work holidays?   Yes: _____ No: _____

When will you be available to begin work?   _____ /_____ (Month/Year)

Availability

Days Available

Sun. _____ Mon. _____ Tues. _____ Wed. _____ Th. _____ Fri. _____ Sat. _____

Total Hours Available: _____ Hours Available: from _____ to _____

Have you been convicted of or pleaded no contest to a felony within the last five years?

Yes: _____ No: _____

If yes, please explain: _____

_____

Have you been convicted of, pleaded guilty to, or pleaded no contest to, an act of dishonesty, or breach of trust or mural turpitude, such as misdemeanor petty theft, burglary, fraud, writing bad checks, and other related crimes within the last five (5) years?   Yes: _____ No: _____

If yes, please explain: _____

_____

Do you have other special training or skills (additional spoken or written languages, computer software knowledge, machine operation experience, etc.)?

_____

_____

Education

High School: _____ City: _____ State: _____

College: _____ City: _____ State: _____

Course of Study _____ No. of Years Completed: _____

Did You Graduate? Yes: _____ No: _____ Degree: _____

Figure 32-1 • *Sample job application (continues)*

Employment History

Please give accurate and complete full-time employment record. Start with present or most recent employer. Include military experience if applicable.

Position 1

Company Name: _____ City: _____ State: _____

Company Phone Number: _____

Job Title: _____

Name of Supervisor: _____

Employed (Month and Year) From: _____ To: _____

Weekly Pay: _____

Describe your work: _____

_____

May we contact this employer? Yes: _____ No: _____

If not, why not? _____

Reason for leaving: _____

Position 2

Company Name: _____ City: _____ State: _____

Company Phone Number: _____

Job Title: _____

Name of Supervisor: _____

Employed (Month and Year) From: _____ To: _____

Weekly Pay: _____

Describe your work: _____

_____

May we contact this employer? Yes: _____ No: _____

If not, why not? _____

Reason for leaving: _____

Agreement of the Transfer of Information

I declare the information provided by me in this application is true, correct, and complete to the best of my knowledge. I understand that if employed, any falsification, misstatement, or omission of fact in connection with my application, whether on this document or not, may result in immediate termination of employment. I authorize you to verify any and all information provided above.

I acknowledge that employment may be conditional upon successful completion of a substance abuse screening test as part of the company's pre-employment policy. I acknowledge that if I become employed, I will be free to terminate my employment at any time for any reason, and that the company retains the same rights. No company representative has the authority to make any contrary agreement.

I understand it is unlawful to require or administer a lie detector test as a condition of employment or continued employment. Any employer who violates this law shall be subject to criminal and/or civil liabilities.

Signature: _____ Date: _____

Printed Name: _____

Figure 32-1 • *(continued)*

CATHERINE L. THOMAS
123 Main Street
Anytown, TX 12345
(555) 222-3333
cthomas@yippie.com

Objective

Looking to apply health unit coordinator training and skills within a health care setting.

Education and Certifications

Health Unit Coordinator Program Certificate 2004	Fine Community College, Anytown, TX
High School Diploma 2002	Scholar High School, Anytown, TX
NAHUC Certification	June 2004 through May 31, 2007

Employment Experience

Scheduler (2002–2004)   Allgood Staffing Services, Anytown, TX

Performed scheduling and staffing activities. Recorded requests for staffing. Operated multi-line phone, facsimile, and personal computer. Proficient with word processing and spreadsheet software. Assisted with payroll.

Retail Clerk (2001–2002)   The Department Store, Anytown, TX

Assisted customers with purchases. Operated cash register. Assisted with inventory control.

Personal Interests Activities

Hospital Auxiliary Volunteer (2001–2003)	Memorial Hospital, Anytown, TX
Young Leaders of Tomorrow (2000–2002)	Scholar High School, Anytown, TX

References Available Upon Request

Figure 32-2 • *Sample résumé*

machine, be sure to have a short, professional outgoing message and to answer the phone professionally during the job search. If using a shared phone number, make sure all parties using the number are aware of the job search process and that it is important to take thorough messages.

Objective

An objective is a brief sentence about what one wants to do. Again, do not limit the options by using a specific title in the objective. Rather than stating "Looking for a health unit coordinator position in a hospital," one could state "Looking to apply health unit coordinator training and skills within a health care setting."

Education

Normally, education is listed with the most recent education first. Therefore, if one has just completed health unit coordinator training, that would be listed first. For most jobs, it is not necessary to go back any further than high school. Be sure to include any seminars or certificate programs that are applicable to the desired job. For example, a seminar on Spanish in the Workplace would be appropriate for a résumé, but a seminar on Spanish Music would not need to be included unless there were skills learned that were applicable to the desired job. If one is nationally certified as a health unit coordinator, include that information in the education section of the résumé.

Employment

When writing about previous employment, list the title of the position; the employer's name, city, and state; and the dates of employment. When describing previous work responsibilities, list the most important and relevant duties, using action words. Examples of action words include:

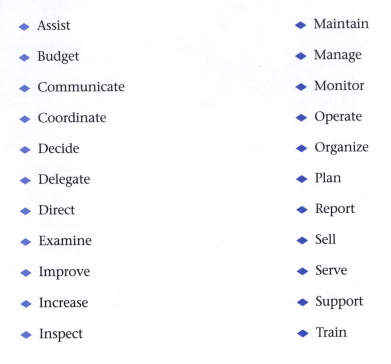

- ◆ Assist
- ◆ Budget
- ◆ Communicate
- ◆ Coordinate
- ◆ Decide
- ◆ Delegate
- ◆ Direct
- ◆ Examine
- ◆ Improve
- ◆ Increase
- ◆ Inspect
- ◆ Maintain
- ◆ Manage
- ◆ Monitor
- ◆ Operate
- ◆ Organize
- ◆ Plan
- ◆ Report
- ◆ Sell
- ◆ Serve
- ◆ Support
- ◆ Train

Transferrble Skills

When listing skills, think about **transferable skills**. Transferable skills are tasks that one may have learned in one job or setting that can be used within another setting. For example, if you learned word-processing skills in an educational environment, you could transfer those word-processing skills to a health care environment. If you trained new employees in a food service environment, you could transfer the training skills to the health care environment. If you learned customer service skills in a retail setting, you could transfer those skills to the health care environment.

Personal Interests and Activities

The personal interests and activities section can be used for information that does not fit into the other sections. This section can be what sets one apart from other applicants.

Although the title of this category is personal interests, the interests listed should be related to the job search and described as transferable skills. It is appropriate to list achievements and skills learned in volunteer, church, and community work and in sports and hobbies. For example, it is relevant to list involvement in a community walk-a-thon but maybe not relevant to list that one's hobby is playing cards.

INTERVIEWS

Be prepared for the interview. Know that appearance and attitude are just as important as experience and your responses to the interviewer's questions.

- Know something about the employer.
- Practice answering questions out loud.
- Dress conservatively.
- Project a positive, interested attitude.
- Ask questions.

An interviewer may ask open-ended questions to learn more about the applicant and to find out about the applicant's work ethic. Open-ended questions cannot be answered with a simple yes or no. They force the applicant to think and talk. Preparing for these types of questions can reduce anxiety during interviews. Typical open-ended interview questions are:

1. Tell me about yourself.

2. Why do you want to work as a health unit coordinator?

3. Why do you think you are the best candidate for the job?

4. What would you bring to this organization?

5. How do you know you will be at work every scheduled day? What are your attendance records at school and work?

6. Why did you leave your previous employer?

7. What would someone who knows you well identify as your strengths and your weaknesses?

8. Where do you want to be in five years and how do you plan to get there?

You may be asked to answer at least one question for which you have not prepared. If necessary, ask for a minute to think about the answer or ask to come back to that question. It is important to think before speaking.

Asking the interviewer questions shows interest in the job. Have a few questions prepared to ask. Avoid questions about salary and benefits until after a position has been offered. You may want to bring paper and pen to record the answers. This can assist in the next step, follow-up. Questions you may want to ask the interviewer are:

1. In what type of department will I be working?

2. How many patients receive services in an average day?

3. What type of computer system does the department have?

4. How is the department organized or managed?

FOLLOW-UP

Within 2 days of the interview, send a thank you letter to the employer. A short note thanking them for their time and reinforcing your interest in the position is appropriate. Be sure to spell the name of the interviewer correctly. If you have interview notes, refer to something specific you were told and liked about the employer.

JOB OFFER

The time to discuss salary and benefits is after the job offer has been made. If possible, get the job offering in writing, with the specific job description and hours. Getting as much information as possible can aid in making an informed decision. A preemployment physical and orientation may be scheduled once the job offer has been accepted.

PROFESSIONAL DEVELOPMENT WITHIN THE PROFESSION

The first step in one's professional development is becoming proficient in the job for which one was hired. It may be 6 to 12 months before a health unit coordinator feels fully confident in the new role. Once he or she has attained that comfort level, the health unit coordinator may be ready to expand or enhance the role. There are a number of ways to enhance one's job, both within and outside of the profession. Ways to enhance one's profession within the profession include certification, continuing education, committee work, precepting, training, taking on additional responsibilities, and "climbing" the career ladder.

CERTIFICATION

The national certification exam for health unit coordinators was discussed in Chapter 2. There has been national certification for health unit coordinators since 1983. The exam is based upon a national job task analysis completed by health unit coordinators. The certification exam content outline is based upon the results of the national job task analysis (Figure 32-3).

Frequently asked questions about certification and recertification are answered in the National Association of Health Care Coordinators' (NAHUC) Certification/Recertification Fact Sheet (Figure 32-4).

RECERTIFICATION

The recertification process is essentially that of maintaining certification or demonstrating continued competency to practice. The recertification program strives to serve the profession, the health care industry, and consumers fairly and observe all relevant

National Association of Health Unit Coordinators Certification Exam Content Outline

I. Transcription of Orders (35%)
 A. Processing
  1. Check charts for orders that need to be transcribed
  2. Interpret medical symbols, abbreviations, and terminology
  3. Clarify questionable orders
  4. Prioritize orders and tasks
  5. Process orders according to priority
  6. Enter orders on a Kardex
  7. Enter orders on patient treatment plan
  8. Initiate pathway protocols
  9. Schedule diagnostic tests and procedures
  10. Initiate and follow test preparation procedures
  11. Enter orders onto a medication administration record
  12. Enter patient charges
  13. Process orders for diagnostic and therapeutic tests and procedures
  14. Process nursing treatment orders
  15. Prepare surgical charts
  16. Process postoperative charts
  17. Process medication orders
  18. Process orders for parenteral fluids
  19. Recognize order categories (i.e., standing, one-time, prn, and stat)
 B. Notification
  1. Notify staff of new orders
  2. Notify and document consulting physicians of consult requests
  3. Indicate on the order sheet that each order has been processed
  4. Sign off orders (e.g., signature, title, date, and time)
  5. Flag charts for co-signature
 C. Requests
  1. Request services from ancillary departments
  2. Request services from support departments
  3. Request supplies and equipment
  4. Request patient information from external facilities

II. Coordination of Health Unit (47%)
 A. Admissions
  1. Label and assemble patient charts upon admission
  2. Obtain patient information prior to admission
  3. Assign beds to patients coming into the unit
  4. Inform nursing staff of patient admissions, transfers, discharges, and returning surgical patients
  5. Process patient registration
 B. Patient results processing
  1. Receive diagnostic test results
  2. Notify physicians of diagnostic test results
  3. Report diagnostic test results to nursing staff
 C. Discharges/Transfers
  1. Assemble necessary forms and perform clerical tasks for patients being transferred to an external facility
  2. Prepare patient charts and perform clerical tasks for discharge or transfer to other units within the health facility
  3. Notify appropriate departments and individuals when patients are discharged (i.e., home, expired, AMA, transferred, etc.)
  4. Disassemble patient charts, put in appropriate order, and send to medical records office upon expiration or discharge
  5. Schedule follow-up appointments
  6. Schedule appointments for diagnostic work at other facilities
  7. Follow organ procurement procedures
  8. Schedule ground transportation for patients
 D. Unit Responsibilities/Clerical
  1. Maintain a supply of chart forms
  2. Maintain stock of patient care supplies and equipment
  3. Maintain stock of clerical and desk supplies
  4. Maintain patient charts by thinning and adding forms as needed
  5. File forms and reports
  6. Maintain unit bulletin board
  7. Maintain policy and procedures manuals
  8. Monitor patients' off-unit locations
  9. Arrange for maintenance and repair of equipment
 E. Reports and Record Keeping
  1. Report unit activities to on-coming shift
  2. Maintain patient census logs
  3. Record patient acuity
  4. Record unit/department statistics
  5. Graph and chart information onto appropriate forms
  6. Maintain patient census boards
  7. Maintain on-call schedules
  8. Maintain patient assignment board

Figure 32-3 • *Certification exam content outline* (Reprinted with permission from the National Association of Health Unit Coordinators) *(continues)*

9. Perform quality assurance on charts (i.e., verify that chart forms are filed and labeled correctly, all orders have been transcribed, allergies are noted in appropriate places, prepare incident reports, etc.)
10. Reconcile patient charges/credits
11. Retrieve test results
12. Recopy medication administration records
13. Recopy Kardex/patient treatment plan
14. Inventory unit equipment

F. Personnel management
1. Orient new staff members to the unit
2. Precept new or student unit coordinators
3. Communicate facility policies to visitors, patients, and staff (i.e., visiting hours, no smoking, etc.)
4. Maintain staff assignment logs
5. Assist with unit staffing
6. Greet patients, physicians, visitors, and facility staff who arrive on the unit
7. Respond to patient, physician, visitor, and facility staff requests and complaints

G. Safety and Security
1. Maintain a hazard-free work environment
2. Maintain unit security
3. Participate in emergency and disaster plans
4. Respond to cardiac or respiratory arrests
5. Initiate call to cardiac or respiratory arrests
6. Comply with regulatory agency guidelines/rules

H. Confidentiality and Patient Rights
1. Screen telephone calls and visitor requests for patient information to protect patient confidentiality
2. Restrict access to patient information (i.e., charts, computer)
3. Assist with Advance Directives documentation
4. Demonstrate knowledge of informed consent

III. Equipment/Technical Procedures (15%)
A. Communication
1. Communicate with patients and staff via intercom
2. Send and receive documents via fax machine
3. Contact personnel via telecommunications systems (e.g., pagers, cell phones)
4. Answer and process unit telephone calls

B. Computers
1. Maintain computer census (i.e., ADT functions)
2. Retrieve diagnostic result from computers
3. Follow established computer down-time procedures
4. Enter orders via computers
5. Schedule appointments via computers
6. Prepare documents using computer software
7. Generate reports using computers
8. Operate computers safely and correctly
9. Troubleshoot problems with computers

C. Monitoring Systems
1. Register patient into monitor system
2. Print and mount strips

D. Miscellaneous Equipment
1. Duplicate documents using a copy machine
2. Transport patient specimens, supplies, and medication using pneumatic tubes

IV. Professional Development (3%)
A. Training
1. Attend in-service training sessions
2. Attend department, staff, or health unit coordinator meetings

B. Individual development
1. Review job-related publications (e.g., NAHUC Standards of Practice, journals)
2. Review facility-specific publications, memos, policies
3. Pursue and maintain certification

Figure 32-3 • *(continued)*

laws. There are two options for recertification: continuing education and retesting. The recertification process is described in NAHUC's recertification manual as,

Contact Hours Option—Meet eligibility requirements for CHUC recertification and acquire 36 NAHUC contact hours over a three-year period. Submit recertification application and fee. Recertification requires 36 NAHUC contact hours earned during a three-year recertification cycle. It is the certified health unit coordinator's responsibility to collect, save, and submit all documentation of recertification activities.

Certification Exam Option—Meet eligibility requirements for NAHUC recertification and successfully complete the NAHUC Certification Examination.

What is the purpose of certification?

Certification as a health unit coordinator by the NAHUC Certification Board provides proof to your employer, other health care professionals, the public, and your peers that you have demonstrated the basic knowledge and skills in areas of health unit coordinating. Certification can be a source of recognition nationwide, an aid for career advancement, and a condition of employment.

What are the eligibility requirements?

Anyone who is currently a health unit coordinator or has completed training to become a health unit coordinator or anyone who is involved with unit coordinator activities may test for certification. A high school diploma or GED is required.

Candidates for certification need not be members of NAHUC, but we strongly encourage all health unit coordinators to join NAHUC so that they may participate and receive the benefits of their professional association. You may request a membership application from the NAHUC office.

How do I register for the national certification exam?

The first step is to obtain a candidate handbook by visiting the Web site at www.nahuc.org or contacting the NAHUC national office toll free at 888-22-NAHUC. The candidate handbook contains vital information and should be kept for reference until after you receive your certification.

How is the examination developed?

The examination is prepared, administered, and graded by a testing agency, Promissor. Health unit coordinator practitioners, supervisors, and educators write the exam questions. The Examination Review Committee of the NAHUC Certification Board (a representative group of practitioners, an educator, and a supervisor) reviews all test questions before they are used on examinations. This committee helps to provide the job related perspective that underlies valid examinations.

How do I prepare for the certification exam?

An outline of the material to be tested, a list of study materials, and sample test questions are included in the candidate handbook. The exam questions are based on the certification exam content outline created from the national job task analysis. The content outline is also posted on the Web site, www.nahuc.org.

When and where is the examination held?

Promissor offers year-round electronic testing in most states. Check the list of exam sites for the location most convenient for you. The blue card lists them or you can call Promissor at 800-274-8719 or www.promissor.com for locations.

How is the exam scored?

All tests are reported as "scaled scores" to insure that all candidates have the same advantage regardless of which test they take. The questions are multiple choice and are adjusted for minor differences in difficulty. Exam results are reported on a scale of 300–600 points (the minimum score is 450).

How soon will I get the results of the exam?

One of the advantages of electronic testing is that candidates receive their scores immediately at the test site.

When will I receive my certificate?

You will receive your certificate 4–6 weeks after you have passed the exam.

How may I obtain the certification pin and/or patch?

Send your name, address, certification number, and year certified with the fee indicated on the order form to NAHUC.

How do I obtain the handbook?

A certification exam handbook is posted on the web site, www.nahuc.org.

Figure 32-4 • *Certification/Recertification Fact Sheet (Reprinted with permission from the National Association of Health Unit Coordinators)*

CONTINUING EDUCATION

It is the responsibility of the health unit coordinator to remain current in the field. Because of the many continuing education opportunities for health unit coordinators, remaining current is relatively easy to do. Many health care facilities are teaching facilities and have many in-services and workshops on a wide variety of health care topics. Education that is offered and targeted to other health care professionals such as physicians and nurses can be beneficial to health unit coordinators as well.

NAHUC currently offers continuing education through its member newsletter, the Web site questionnaires, the NAHUC Lending Library, and various workshops. Information about the Lending Library, Web questionnaires, and the workshop calendar can be found on the NAHUC Web site.

COMMITTEE WORK

Another way to enhance one's job is to become an active participant in the employer's goals. Once can participate by serving on committees. Some committees may have a community focus. For example, there may be committees for the work and activities the facility participates in throughout the community, such as blood pressure clinics or well-baby outreach. Other committees may have a problem-solving or quality improvement focus. There may be committees that address medication errors or patient falls. Chances are there is a committee that would welcome the perspective of a health unit coordinator.

PRECEPTING AND TRAINING

Teaching is another way to enhance one's job. One's first experience in teaching may be to orient a new employee to one's own job. If one enjoys precepting, one may want to look for other training opportunities. Often, health unit coordinators are asked to provide computer training to the other staff within the facility. There may also be opportunities to present information at health unit coordinator staff meetings. Volunteer to explain a new policy or procedure at a staff meeting. One could also contact the staff education or human resource development department and ask for opportunities to plan and present training.

ADDITIONAL RESPONSIBILITIES

A valuable employee seeks out new responsibilities. Perhaps the health unit coordinator could relieve the department manager of some of the administrative duties. In some facilities, the health unit coordinator may perform staffing and scheduling duties and assist with budgeting and payroll functions. The health unit coordinator might also assist the department manager by managing the calendar and performing some secretarial duties.

CAREER LADDERS

In Chapter 2, a career ladder was defined as grade levels of increasing complexity and responsibility within a job description. In some facilities, the health unit coordinator job description may be written as two or three levels. Often, the job-enhancing suggestions above are included in the more advanced level of the health unit coordinator job description.

PROFESSIONAL DEVELOPMENT OUTSIDE OF THE PROFESSION

As a health unit coordinator, one is in the unique position of communicating with almost every department within the facility. This position affords the health unit coordinator with an advantageous networking pool. Networking is about maintaining effective relationships with others. Within those relationships, there is a give and take of information and support. As a health unit coordinator, one has the opportunity to learn about a wide variety of jobs within the health care field. There is a wealth of career information at the fingertips of a health unit coordinator who is interested in changing jobs.

SUMMARY

Health unit coordinating is a fascinating job that provides opportunities for professional growth. Whether one plans on working as a health unit coordinator for a short time or for many years, the job is as interesting and challenging as one makes it. An experienced health unit coordinator can enhance the job through continuing education, committee work, teaching, and being willing to take on different responsibilities. For someone who is planning on changing careers in the future, the knowledge gained in the health unit coordinator position is transferable to many other roles within health care. The authors' wish for the reader of this textbook is to rise to the challenge of professional growth.

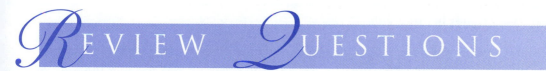

REVIEW QUESTIONS

1. List three types of employers, other than hospitals, that hire health unit coordinators.

2. "The job application should be completed in ink." Is this statement true or false?

3. "It is okay to leave sections of the application blank." Is this statement true or false?

4. List and describe the five sections of a résumé.

5. "The only way to become certified is to successfully pass the national certification exam." Is this statement true or false?

6. What is the continuing education requirement for recertification as a health unit coordinator?

7. List and describe four methods of professional development.

NAHUC CERTIFICATION EXAM

CONTENT AREAS

II. E. 7   Maintain on-call schedules

II. F. 4   Maintain staff assignment logs

II. F. 5   Assist with unit staffing

IV. A. 2   Attend department, staff, or health unit coordinator meetings

IV. B. 1   Review job-related publications (e.g., NAHUC Standards of Practice, journals)

IV. B. 2   Review facility-specific publications, memos, policies

IV. B. 3   Pursue and maintain certification

THROUGH THE EYES

OF A HEALTH CARE PROFESSIONAL

A job seeker shares her thoughts.

The time between finishing school and receiving a job offer can be a very stressful time. It helped me to start preparing for the job search while I was still in school. Early in the process, I addressed what I thought was the most crucial component of the job search—networking. I took time to become acquainted with the instructors, the staff, and the other students. We had the opportunity to learn about each other's interests and goals. If I learned that someone had the same interest as someone else I knew, I would introduce the two to each other. Building this matrix of relationships was invaluable to me when I was exploring potential employers. It was amazing to me to learn how many people knew someone who was working in health care and how willing they were to share that information with me once we got to know each other. Now that I am employed, I still maintain my earlier networking relationships and look forward to new relationships. Networking opened many doors for me. In turn, I hope that I am able to open doors for others.

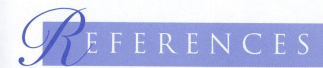

REFERENCES

America's Career Internet. Career Resource Library. *http://www.acinet.org/acinet/library* Accessed January 2004.

National Association of Health Unit Coordinators (NAHUC). Certification Exam Outline. *http://www.nahuc.org/certification/NAHUC%20* Accessed January 2004.

National Association of Health Unit Coordinators (NAHUC). Recertification Manual. *http://www.nahuc.org/certification/cb_recer.htm* Accessed January 2004.

National Association of Health Unit Coordinators (NAHUC). Recertification Manual. *http://www.nahuc.org/certification/cb_recer.htm* Accessed January 2004.

Clark, M. A., & Mazza, V. S. (1999). *Health unit coordinating: Expanding the scope of practice.* Philadelphia: W. B. Saunders.

APPENDIX A

NAHUC Certification Exam Content Outline Areas		Health Unit Coordinator: 21st Century Professional Textbook Chapter
IV. B. 1	Review job-related publications (e.g., NAHUC Standards of Practice, journals)	Chapter 2
IV. B. 3	Pursue and maintain certification	
I. A. 4	Prioritize orders and tasks	
I. C. 1	Request services from ancillary departments	Chapter 4
I. C. 2	Request services from support departments	Chapter 5
I. C. 3	Request supplies and equipment	
II. D. 1	Maintain a supply of chart forms	
II. D. 2	Maintain stock of patient care supplies and equipment	
II. D. 3	Maintain stock of clerical and desk supplies	
II. D. 6	Maintain unit bulletin board	
II. D. 7	Maintain policy and procedures manuals	
II. D. 8	Monitor patients' off-unit locations	
II. D. 9	Arrange for maintenance and repair of equipment	
II. E. 1	Report unit activities to on-coming shift	
II. E. 2	Maintain patient census logs	
II. E. 3	Record patient acuity	
II. E. 4	Record unit/department statistics	
II. E. 6	Maintain patient census boards	
II. E. 8	Maintain patient assignment board	
II. E. 14	Inventory unit equipment	
II. F. 7	Respond to patient, physician, visitor, and facility staff requests and complaints	

(continues)

NAHUC Certification Exam Content Outline Areas		*Health Unit Coordinator: 21st Century Professional Textbook Chapter*
(continued)		
I. C. 1	Request services from ancillary departments	Chapter 6
I. C. 2	Request services from support departments	Chapter 7
I. A. 12	Enter patient charges	Chapter 9
I. C. 3	Request supplies and equipment	
II. D. 1	Maintain a supply of chart forms	
II. D. 2	Maintain stock of patient care supplies and equipment	
II. D. 3	Maintain stock of clerical and desk supplies	
II. D. 9	Arrange for maintenance and repair of equipment	
II. E. 10	Reconcile patient charges/credits	
II. E. 14	Inventory unit equipment	
II. F. 3	Communicate facility policies to visitors, patients, and staff (i.e., visiting hours, no smoking, etc.)	Chapter 10
II. G. 1	Maintain a hazard-free work environment	
II. G. 2	Maintain unit security	
II. G. 3	Participate in emergency and disaster plans	
II. G. 4	Respond to cardiac or respiratory arrests	
II. G. 5	Initiate call to cardiac or respiratory arrests	
II. G. 6	Comply with regulatory agency guidelines/rules	
III. D. 2	Transport patient specimens, supplies, and medication using pneumatic tubes	
IV. A. 1	Attend in-service training sessions	
I. C. 4	Request patient information from external facilities	Chapter 11
II. H. 1	Screen telephone calls and visitor requests for patient information to protect patient confidentiality	
II. H. 2	Restrict access to patient information (i.e., charts, computer)	
IV. B. 1	Review job-related publications (e.g., NAHUC Standards of Practice, journals)	
IV. B. 2	Review facility-specific publications, memos, policies	

(continues)

(continued)

NAHUC Certification Exam Content Outline Areas		*Health Unit Coordinator: 21st Century Professional* Textbook Chapter
II. H. 3	Assist with Advance Directives documentation	Chapter 12
II. D. 4	Maintain patient charts by thinning and adding forms as needed	Chapter 13
II. D. 5	File forms and reports	
II. E. 5	Graph and chart information onto appropriate forms	
II. E. 9	Perform quality assurance on charts (i.e., verify that chart forms are filed and labeled correctly, all orders have been transcribed, allergies are noted in appropriate places, prepare incident reports, etc.)	
I. C. 4	Request patient information from external facilities	Chapter 14
II. A. 1	Label and assemble patient charts upon admission	
II. A. 2	Obtain patient information prior to admission	
II. A. 3	Assign beds to patients coming into the unit	
II. A. 4	Inform nursing staff of patient admissions, transfers, discharges, and returning surgical patients	
II. A. 5	Process patient registration	
II. C. 1.	Assemble necessary forms and perform clerical tasks for patients being transferred to an external facility	
II. C. 2	Prepare patient charts and perform clerical tasks for discharge or transfer to other units within the health facility	
II. C. 3	Notify appropriate departments and individuals when patients are discharged (i.e., home, expired, AMA, transferred, etc.)	
II. C. 4	Disassemble patient charts, put in appropriate order, and send to medical records office upon expiration or discharge.	
II. C. 5	Schedule follow-up appointments	
II. C. 6	Schedule appointments for diagnostic work at other facilities	
II. C. 7	Follow organ procurement procedures	
II. C. 8	Schedule ground transportation for patients	

(continues)

(continued)

NAHUC Certification Exam Content Outline Areas		*Health Unit Coordinator: 21st Century Professional Textbook Chapter*
II. B. 1	Receive diagnostic test results	Chapter 15
II. B. 3	Report diagnostic test results to nursing staff	
II. F. 6	Greet patients, physicians, visitors, and facility staff who arrive on the unit	
II. F. 7	Respond to patient, physician, visitor, and facility staff requests and complaints	
III. A. 4	Answer and process unit telephone calls	
II. B. 1	Receive diagnostic test results	Chapter 16
II. B. 3	Report diagnostic test results to nursing staff	
II. D. 6	Maintain unit bulletin board	
II. E. 6	Maintain patient census boards	
II. E. 8	Maintain patient assignment board	
II. F. 7	Respond to patient, physician, visitor, and facility staff requests and complaints	
III. A. 1	Communicate with patients and staff via intercom	
III. A. 2	Send and receive documents via fax machine	
III. A. 3	Contact personnel via telecommunications systems (e.g., pagers, cell phones)	
III. A. 4	Answer and process unit telephone calls	
III. B. 1	Maintain computer census (i.e., ADT functions)	
III. B. 4	Enter orders via computers	
III. B. 5	Schedule appointments via computers	
III. B. 6	Prepare documents using computer software	
III. B. 7	Generate reports using computers	
III. B. 8	Operate computers safely and correctly	
III. B. 9	Troubleshoot problems with computers	
III. D. 1	Duplicate documents using a copy machine	
III. D. 2	Transport patient specimens, supplies, and medication using pneumatic tubes	
II. F. 1	Orient new staff members to the unit	Chapter 17
II. F. 2	Precept new or student unit coordinators	

(continues)

(continued)

NAHUC Certification Exam Content Outline Areas	Health Unit Coordinator: 21st Century Professional Textbook Chapter
I. A. 2 Interpret medical symbols, abbreviations, and terminology	Chapter 20
I. A. 2 Interpret medical symbols, abbreviations, and terminology	Chapter 21
I. A. 2 Interpret medical symbols, abbreviations, and terminology	Chapter 22
I. A. 1 Check charts for orders that need to be transcribed I. A. 2 Interpret medical symbols, abbreviations, and terminology I. A. 3 Clarify questionable orders I. A. 4 Prioritize orders and tasks I. A. 5 Process orders according to priority I. A. 6 Enter orders on a Kardex I. A. 19 Recognize order categories (i.e., standing, one-time, prn, and stat) I. B. 1 Notify staff of new orders I. B. 3 Indicate on the order sheet that each order has been processed I. B. 4 Sign off orders (e.g. signature, title, date, and time) I. B. 5 Flag charts for co-signature II. E. 9 Perform quality assurance on charts (i.e., verify that chart forms are filed and labeled correctly, all orders have been transcribed, allergies are noted in appropriate places, prepare incident reports, etc.) III. B. 4 Enter orders via computers	Chapter 23
I. A. 2 Interpret medical symbols, abbreviations, and terminology I. A. 6 Enter orders on a Kardex I. A. 9 Schedule diagnostic tests and procedures I. A. 10 Initiate and follow test preparation procedures I. A. 13 Process orders for diagnostic and therapeutic tests and procedures I. B. 1 Notify staff of new orders	Chapter 24

(continues)

(continued)

NAHUC Certification Exam Content Outline Areas	*Health Unit Coordinator: 21st Century Professional Textbook Chapter*
II. B. 2 Notify physicians of diagnostic test results	Chapter 24
II. E. 11 Retrieve test results	
III. B. 2 Retrieve diagnostic result from computers	
III. B. 4 Enter orders via computers	
I. A. 2 Interpret medical symbols, abbreviations, and terminology	Chapter 25
I. A. 6 Enter orders on a Kardex	
I. A. 9 Schedule diagnostic tests and procedures	
I. A. 10 Initiate and follow test preparation procedures	
I. A. 13 Process orders for diagnostic and therapeutic tests and procedures	
I. B. 1 Notify staff of new orders	
II. H. 4 Demonstrate knowledge of informed consent	
III. B. 4 Enter orders via computers	
I. A. 2 Interpret medical symbols, abbreviations, and terminology	Chapter 26
I. A. 6 Enter orders on a Kardex	
I. B. 1 Notify staff of new orders	
III. B. 4 Enter orders via computers	
I. A. 2 Interpret medical symbols, abbreviations, and terminology	Chapter 27
I. A. 6 Enter orders on a Kardex	
I. A. 14 Process nursing treatment orders	
I. B. 1 Notify staff of new orders	
III. B. 4 Enter orders via computers	
I. A. 2 Interpret medical symbols, abbreviations, and terminology	Chapter 28
I. A. 6 Enter orders on a Kardex	
I. A. 11 Enter orders onto a medication administration record	
I. A. 17 Process medication orders	
I. A. 18 Process orders for parenteral fluids	
I. B. 1 Notify staff of new orders	
III. B. 4 Enter orders via computers	

(continues)

NAHUC Certification Exam Content Outline Areas		Health Unit Coordinator: *21st Century Professional* Textbook Chapter
I. A. 2	Interpret medical symbols, abbreviations, and terminology	Chapter 29
I. A. 6	Enter orders on a Kardex	
I. A. 9	Schedule diagnostic tests and procedures	
I. A. 10	Initiate and follow test preparation procedures	
I. A. 13	Process orders for diagnostic and therapeutic tests and procedures	
I. B. 1	Notify staff of new orders	
III. B. 4	Enter orders via computers	
I. A. 2	Interpret medical symbols, abbreviations, and terminology	Chapter 30
I. A. 6	Enter orders on a Kardex	
I. A. 15	Prepare surgical charts	
I. A. 16	Process postoperative charts	
I. B. 1	Notify staff of new orders	
II. H. 4	Demonstrate knowledge of informed consent	
III. B. 4	Enter orders via computers	
I. A. 2	Interpret medical symbols, abbreviations, and terminology	Chapter 31
I. A. 6	Enter orders on a Kardex	
I. A. 8	Initiate pathway protocols	
I. B. 1	Notify staff of new orders	
II. D. 9	Arrange for maintenance and repair of equipment	
III. B. 1	Maintain computer census (i.e., ADT functions)	
III. B. 4	Enter orders via computers	
III. B. 6	Prepare document using computer software	
III. B. 7	Generate reports using computers	
III. B. 8	Operate computers safely and correctly	
III. B. 9	Troubleshoot problems with computers	
II. E. 7	Maintain on-call schedules	Chapter 32
II. F. 4	Maintain staff assignment logs	
II. F. 5	Assist with unit staffing	
IV. A. 2	Attend department, staff or health unit coordinator meetings	

(continues)

(continued)

NAHUC Certification Exam Content Outline Areas	*Health Unit Coordinator: 21st Century Professional Textbook Chapter*
IV. B. 1 Review job related publications (e.g., NAHUC Standards of Practice, journals)	Chapter 32
IV. B. 2 Review facility specific publications, memos, policies	
IV. B. 3 Pursue and maintain certification	

(NAHUC Certification Exam Content Outline Areas reprinted with permission of the National Association of Health Unit Coordinators)

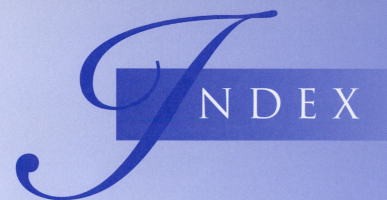

INDEX

Note: Page numbers in *italic* type reference non-text material, such as tables and illustrations.

License Agreement for Thomson Delmar Learning

IMPORTANT! READ CAREFULLY: This End User License Agreement ("Agreement") sets forth the conditions by which Thomson Delmar Learning, a division of Thomson Learning Inc. ("Thomson") will make electronic access to the Thomson Delmar Learning-owned licensed content and associated media, software, documentation, printed materials, and electronic documentation contained in this package and/or made available to you via this product (the "Licensed Content"), available to you (the "End User"). BY CLICKING THE "I ACCEPT" BUTTON AND/OR OPENING THIS PACKAGE, YOU ACKNOWLEDGE THAT YOU HAVE READ ALL OF THE TERMS AND CONDITIONS, AND THAT YOU AGREE TO BE BOUND BY ITS TERMS, CONDITIONS, AND ALL APPLICABLE LAWS AND REGULATIONS GOVERNING THE USE OF THE LICENSED CONTENT.

1.0 SCOPE OF LICENSE

1.1 *Licensed Content.* The Licensed Content may contain portions of modifiable content ("Modifiable Content") and content which may not be modified or otherwise altered by the End User ("Non-Modifiable Content"). For purposes of this Agreement, Modifiable Content and Non-Modifiable Content may be collectively referred to herein as the "Licensed Content." All Licensed Content shall be considered Non-Modifiable Content, unless such Licensed Content is presented to the End User in a modifiable format and it is clearly indicated that modification of the Licensed Content is permitted.

1.2 Subject to the End User's compliance with the terms and conditions of this Agreement, Thomson Delmar Learning hereby grants the End User, a nontransferable, non-exclusive, limited right to access and view a single copy of the Licensed Content on a single personal computer system for noncommercial, internal, personal use only. The End User shall not (i) reproduce, copy, modify (except in the case of Modifiable Content), distribute, display, transfer, sublicense, prepare derivative work(s) based on, sell, exchange, barter or transfer, rent, lease, loan, resell, or in any other manner exploit the Licensed Content; (ii) remove, obscure, or alter any notice of Thomson Delmar Learning's intellectual property rights present on or in the Licensed Content, including, but not limited to, copyright, trademark, and/or patent notices; or (iii) disassemble, decompile, translate, reverse engineer, or otherwise reduce the Licensed Content.

2.0 TERMINATION

2.1 Thomson Delmar Learning may at any time (without prejudice to its other rights or remedies) immediately terminate this Agreement and/or suspend access to some or all of the Licensed Content, in the event that the End User does not comply with any of the terms and conditions of this Agreement. In the event of such termination by Thomson Delmar Learning, the End User shall immediately return any and all copies of the Licensed Content to Thomson Delmar Learning.

3.0 PROPRIETARY RIGHTS

3.1 The End User acknowledges that Thomson Delmar Learning owns all rights, title and interest, including, but not limited to all copyright rights therein, in and to the Licensed Content, and that the End User shall not take any action inconsistent with such ownership. The Licensed Content is protected by U.S., Canadian and other applicable copyright laws and by international treaties, including the Berne Convention and the Universal Copyright Convention. Nothing contained in this Agreement shall be construed as granting the End User any ownership rights in or to the Licensed Content.

3.2 Thomson Delmar Learning reserves the right at any time to withdraw from the Licensed Content any item or part of an item for which it no longer retains the right to publish, or which it has reasonable grounds to believe infringes copyright or is defamatory, unlawful, or otherwise objectionable.

4.0 PROTECTION AND SECURITY

4.1 The End User shall use its best efforts and take all reasonable steps to safeguard its copy of the Licensed Content to ensure that no unauthorized reproduction, publication, disclosure, modification, or distribution of the Licensed Content, in whole or in part, is made. To the extent that the End User becomes aware of any such unauthorized use of the Licensed Content, the End User shall immediately notify Thomson Delmar Learning. Notification of such violations may be made by sending an e-mail to delmarhelp@thomson.com.

5.0 MISUSE OF THE LICENSED PRODUCT

5.1 In the event that the End User uses the Licensed Content in violation of this Agreement, Thomson Delmar Learning shall have the option of electing liquidated damages, which shall include all profits generated by the End User's use of the Licensed Content plus interest computed at the maximum rate permitted by law and all legal fees and other expenses incurred by Thomson Delmar Learning in enforcing its rights, plus penalties.

6.0 FEDERAL GOVERNMENT CLIENTS

6.1 Except as expressly authorized by Thomson Delmar Learning, Federal Government clients obtain only the rights specified in this Agreement and no other rights. The Government acknowledges that (i) all software and related documentation incorporated in the Licensed Content is existing commercial computer software within the meaning of FAR 27.405(b)(2); and (2) all other data delivered in whatever form, is limited rights data within the meaning of FAR 27.401. The restrictions in this section are acceptable as consistent with the Government's need for software and other data under this Agreement.

7.0 DISCLAIMER OF WARRANTIES AND LIABILITIES

7.1 Although Thomson Delmar Learning believes the Licensed Content to be reliable, Thomson Delmar Learning does not guarantee or warrant (i) any information or materials contained in or produced by the Licensed Content, (ii) the accuracy, completeness or reliability of the Licensed Content, or (iii) that the Licensed Content is free from errors or other material defects. THE LICENSED PRODUCT IS PROVIDED "AS IS," WITHOUT ANY WARRANTY OF ANY KIND AND THOMSON DELMAR LEARNING DISCLAIMS ANY AND ALL WARRANTIES, EXPRESSED OR IMPLIED, INCLUDING, WITHOUT LIMITATION, WARRANTIES OF MERCHANTABILITY OR FITNESS OR A PARTICULAR PURPOSE. IN NO EVENT SHALL THOMSON DELMAR LEARNING BE LIABLE FOR: INDIRECT, SPECIAL, PUNITIVE OR CONSEQUENTIAL DAMAGES INCLUDING FOR LOST PROFITS, LOST DATA, OR OTHERWISE. IN NO EVENT SHALL THOMSON DELMAR LEARNING'S AGGREGATE LIABILITY HEREUNDER, WHETHER ARISING IN CONTRACT, TORT, STRICT LIABILITY OR OTHERWISE, EXCEED THE AMOUNT OF FEES PAID BY THE END USER HEREUNDER FOR THE LICENSE OF THE LICENSED CONTENT.

8.0 GENERAL

8.1 *Entire Agreement.* This Agreement shall constitute the entire Agreement between the Parties and supercedes all prior Agreements and understandings oral or written relating to the subject matter hereof.

8.2 *Enhancements/Modifications of Licensed Content.* From time to time, and in Thomson Delmar Learning's sole discretion, Thomson Delmar Learning may advise the End User of updates, upgrades, enhancements and/or improvements to the Licensed Content, and may permit the End User to access and use, subject to the terms and conditions of this Agreement, such modifications, upon payment of prices as may be established by Thomson Delmar Learning.

8.3 *No Export.* The End User shall use the Licensed Content solely in the United States and shall not transfer or export, directly or indirectly, the Licensed Content outside the United States.

8.4 *Severability.* If any provision of this Agreement is invalid, illegal, or unenforceable under any applicable statute or rule of law, the provision shall be deemed omitted to the extent that it is invalid, illegal, or unenforceable. In such a case, the remainder of the Agreement shall be construed in a manner as to give greatest effect to the original intention of the parties hereto.

8.5 *Waiver.* The waiver of any right or failure of either party to exercise in any respect any right provided in this Agreement in any instance shall not be deemed to be a waiver of such right in the future or a waiver of any other right under this Agreement.

8.6 *Choice of Law/Venue.* This Agreement shall be interpreted, construed, and governed by and in accordance with the laws of the State of New York, applicable to contracts executed and to be wholly preformed therein, without regard to its principles governing conflicts of law. Each party agrees that any proceeding arising out of or relating to this Agreement or the breach or threatened breach of this Agreement may be commenced and prosecuted in a court in the State and County of New York. Each party consents and submits to the non-exclusive personal jurisdiction of any court in the State and County of New York in respect of any such proceeding.

8.7 *Acknowledgment.* By opening this package and/or by accessing the Licensed Content on this Web site, THE END USER ACKNOWLEDGES THAT IT HAS READ THIS AGREEMENT, UNDERSTANDS IT, AND AGREES TO BE BOUND BY ITS TERMS AND CONDITIONS. IF YOU DO NOT ACCEPT THESE TERMS AND CONDITIONS, YOU MUST NOT ACCESS THE LICENSED CONTENT AND RETURN THE LICENSED PRODUCT TO DELMAR LEARNING (WITHIN 30 CALENDAR DAYS OF THE END USER'S PURCHASE) WITH PROOF OF PAYMENT ACCEPTABLE TO THOMSON DELMAR LEARNING, FOR A CREDIT OR A REFUND. Should the End User have any questions/comments regarding this Agreement, please contact Thomson Delmar Learning at delmarhelp@thomson.com.